THE CONCEPT OF
HEALTH

Third Edition

THE CONCEPT OF HEALTH

Donald A. Read

Worcester State College

with the assistance of
JUDITH SUTTON

WALTER STOLL, JR., M.D.
medical advisor

Holbrook Press, Inc., Boston

WILLIAM MADISON RANDALL LIBRARY UNC AT WILMINGTON

CREDITS

Photographs on pages 3, 8, 45, 53, 73, 81, 121, 189, 201, 220, 252, 329, and 351 by Pat Torelli.

Figures on pages 144, 145, 148, 154, 162, 163, 165, 172, 175, 181, 187, 188, 192, 193, 195, 197, 206, and 241 by Charles H. Boyter; figures on pages 211, 221, 266, and 320 by D. Patrick Russell; and figures on pages 267, 280, 289, 313, and 335 by D. Patrick Russell and Marcia Williams, all of the Educational Media Support Center at the Boston University School of Medicine.

Cartoons on pages 51, 55, 63, and 64 by Bryan Hendrix.

Figures on pages 10, 12, 17, 37, 49, 50, 55, 61, 77, 85, 190, 204, 207, 208, 209, 210, 213, 223, 224, 226, 238-9, 263, 264, 294, 304, 314, 316, and 323 by Phil Carver & Friends.

Cover illustration by Bill Ogden of Phil Carver & Friends.
Cover design by Sally Bindari of Designworks.

© Copyright 1978 by Holbrook Press, Inc.

© Copyright 1973 by Holbrook Press, Inc.

© Copyright 1969 by Holbrook Press, Inc., 470 Atlantic Avenue, Boston. All rights reserved. Printed in the United States of America. No part of the material protected by this copyright notice may be reproduced or utilized in any form or by any means, electronic or mechanical, including photocopying, recording, or by any informational storage and retrieval system, without written permission from the copyright owner.

Library of Congress Cataloging in Publication Data

Read, Donald A
　　The concept of health.

　　Bibliography: p.
　　Includes index.
　　1. Health.　I. Title.　[DNLM:　1. Hygiene.　QT180 R282c]
RA776.R34　　1978　　613　　77–10323
ISBN　0–205–05686–5

RA776
.R34
1978

TO MY MOTHER, FLORENCE,
AND
MY BROTHER, HUGH

165061

Contents

56158, 262

PEOPLE AND DRUGS   200

5

Preface

Although most of us want to live long and joyful lives that are free of pain, few of us actually do what we know we should to maintain a high level of health. We give good health very little thought—until we are sick.

The Concept of Health is directed toward changing this. This text focuses on the idea that each individual is responsible for his own well-being, and he alone controls the direction of his growth—toward good health or ill health. Every individual must assume responsibility for avoiding the negative excesses that may lessen the pleasures of living.

The primary assumption of *The Concept of Health* is that strong feelings of self-worth—a positive self-image—may be the single most important factor in striving to maintain good health. A great deal of time is devoted to heightening the reader's awareness of his own values, in the hope that he may gain insight into the purposes and directions of his life. Good health can only serve to enhance an otherwise productive existence.

It seems that books are no longer simply written; they are produced by many people. I would like to take this opportunity to thank some of them: John DeRemigis, Manager of Holbrook Press, Inc., for his continued support of this project. Thanks and love to Walter Stoll, M.D., for his very close and critical reading and suggestions on the technical aspects of this text. And a very special thanks to Ann Butterfield Pettine and Judith Sutton, who spent so much time rewriting from my original draft.

Donald A. Read

1

HEALTH:
AN INTRODUCTION

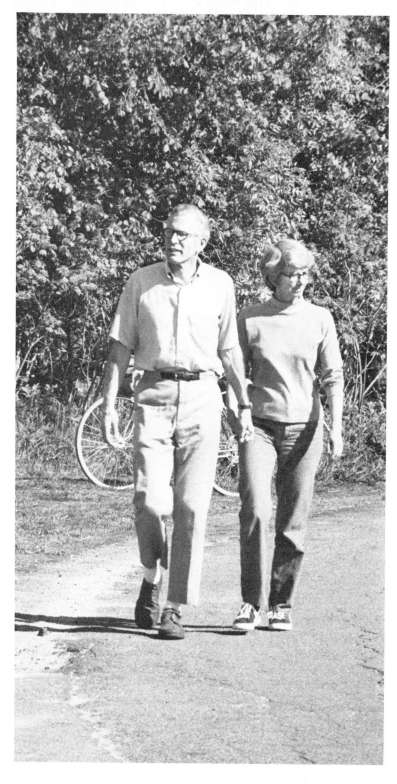

. . . The accidents of health had more to do with the march of great events than was ordinarily suspected.

Herbert A. L. Fisher
The Atlantic Monthly

Chapter 1

Health:
What Does
It Mean?

What does the word "health" mean to you? If you were asked this question, you would probably respond with a negative definition, seeing health as the *absence* of sickness. Until recent times, anyone free from disability or disease was considered to be a healthy person. In the past, ill health has always connoted disease. Today good health means more. The World Health Organization offers this definition: "Health is a state of complete physical, mental, and social well-being and not merely the absence of disease or infirmity."[1]

PREVENTIVE MEDICINE

This enlarged definition means that good health does not depend solely on the individual's doctor, who may cure him of disease; it is in great part the responsibility of the individual himself.

The focus now is on prevention rather than cure, on education for health rather than sickness. Health professionals feel that treatment and care for a specific illness contribute little to any improvement in general health of the individual. Basic changes towards better health come from the individual's own increased self-understanding, knowledge, and concern. Programs aimed at the promotion of optimal health for all people can help with this learning process.

The problem with defining "optimal health for all people" is that each person and the conditions under which he lives and survives are

[1] "Constitution of the World Health Organization," *Chronicle of the World Health Organization,* 1947, p. 3.

5

Life Expectancy

Perhaps because our memories are short, most of us are unaware of the remarkable contribution that public health measures and medicine have made to human longevity in the United States since 1900. A male born in Massachusetts in 1850 had a life expectancy of 38.3 years, a female, of 40.5 years. As the decades passed, life expectancy at birth inched upward—by 1880 a male could expect to live 41.7 and a female 43.5 years, by 1890 life expectancy was 42.5 and 44.5, respectively, and in the next decade for males it rose to 46 years and for females to nearly 50, at 49.4 years.

Comparable data for other states apparently do not exist for the years prior to 1900, when 10 states joined in a "birth and death registration area" to collect vital statistics with reasonable national validity. Inasmuch as Massachusetts data for 1900 correlate closely with those of states from the registration area for 1900, however, we may assume that the Massachusetts statistics provide a reliable picture of gains in longevity for the nation from 1850 to 1900. During that half century, life expectancy for U.S. citizens rose about 9 years.

In the next half century, by contrast, life expectancy for U.S. citizens rose 22 years. By 1973, average longevity for whites was 72 years, up from 48 in 1900; for nonwhites, average longevity stood at 66 years, doubling from only 33 years at the turn of the century.

The principal factor in this increased longevity was a sharp reduction in infant mortality, brought about by improved sanitation, health care, and the development of antibiotics. Between 1935 and 1972, the death rate for white infants dropped 68.6 percent, from 51.9 deaths per 1,000 to 16.3. Deaths among nonwhite infants showed a similar decline, 65.1 percent, from 83.7 per 1,000 live births in 1935 to 29 in 1972. The resulting increase in life expectancy for individuals who survived early infancy is illustrated in Table 1.1.

It is important to note that most of these improvements in life expectancy occurred early in the century. By the early 1950's the decline in the infant death rate had slowed and the average length of life had leveled off. Except for the influenza year of 1918, mortality rates (adjusted for the general aging of the population) declined steadily from 1900 to 1954; they have since stabilized.

Infant death rates continued to improve between the mid-1950's and the 1960's, but less rapidly than before. In fact, of the 10 largest metropolitan areas, only Los Angeles's and Houston's were lower in 1961 than in 1950, and in six of these areas infant death rates actually increased.

often very different. For example, what guides can be used to measure complete fitness of body, complete physical well-being, or soundness of mind for all mankind? How is one to measure social well-being when we consider the extremes of living conditions on this earth?

"Health" is a "polar word"—its meaning is relative to some standard or scale previously set up. Fraser Brockington suggested the polar view when he stated:

Table 1.1 *Life Expectancy, by Race and Sex*

Age, color, and sex	Average number of years of life remaining								
	1973	1972	1959–61	1949–51	1939–41	1929–31	1919–21	1909–11	1902–09
White, male									
0	68.4	68.3	67.55	66.31	62.81	59.12	56.34	50.23	48.23
15	55.1	55.0	54.93	54.18	52.33	50.39	49.74	46.91	46.25
30	41.4	41.3	40.97	40.29	38.80	37.54	37.65	34.87	34.88
45	27.8	27.6	27.34	26.87	25.87	25.28	26.00	23.86	24.21
60	16.2	16.1	16.01	15.76	15.05	14.72	15.25	13.98	14.35
75	8.1	8.1	7.92	7.77	7.17	7.02	7.30	6.75	6.34
All other, male									
0	61.9	61.5	61.48	58.91	52.33	47.55	47.14	34.05	32.54
15	49.5	49.1	50.39	48.23	43.95	39.83	41.75	36.77	38.26
30	36.7	36.4	37.05	35.31	32.25	29.45	32.51	27.33	29.25
45	24.9	24.8	24.89	23.59	22.02	20.59	23.55	18.85	20.09
60	15.6	15.6	15.29	14.91	14.38	13.15	14.74	11.67	12.62
75	9.2	9.3	8.93	8.83	8.09	6.99	7.61	6.58	6.60
White, female									
0	76.1	75.9	74.19	72.03	67.29	62.67	58.53	53.62	51.08
15	62.5	62.3	61.15	59.39	56.07	53.00	50.67	49.12	47.79
30	48.0	47.9	46.63	45.00	42.21	39.99	38.72	36.96	36.42
45	33.9	33.8	32.53	31.12	28.90	27.39	26.98	25.45	25.51
60	21.1	21.0	19.69	18.64	17.00	16.05	15.93	14.92	15.23
75	10.4	10.4	9.28	8.87	7.92	7.56	7.62	7.20	7.33
All other, female									
0	70.1	69.9	66.47	62.70	55.51	49.51	46.92	37.67	35.04
15	57.4	57.3	54.85	51.36	46.22	40.87	40.36	39.18	39.79
30	43.3	43.3	40.83	38.02	34.52	30.67	31.48	29.61	30.70
45	30.3	30.3	28.14	26.07	24.00	21.39	22.61	20.43	21.36
60	19.3	19.4	17.83	16.95	16.14	14.22	14.69	12.78	13.60
75	11.3	11.5	10.10	10.15	9.80	8.62	8.37	7.55	7.90

Source: U.S. Center for Health Statistics, *Vital Statistics of the United States, 1973*, Vol. II, Sec. 5, "Life Tables," DHEW Pub. No. (HRA) 75–1104 (Washington, D.C.: Government Printing Office, 1975), Table 5–5.

Health and disease must be intimately related, for if disease did not exist it would be nonsense to talk of health. . . . The difficulty is to determine, as with light and darkness, at what point health and disease meet and whether they are mutually exclusive. If the most perfect functioning of the body is the light of the sun's zenith, and death the "darkest hour," the point of distinction between health and disease can be anywhere in between. Health may be reckoned between a light and a dark, or anything less than the zenith may be counted as disease.[2]

[2] Fraser Brockington, *World Health*, Baltimore, Md.: Penguin Books, Inc., 1958, p. 15.

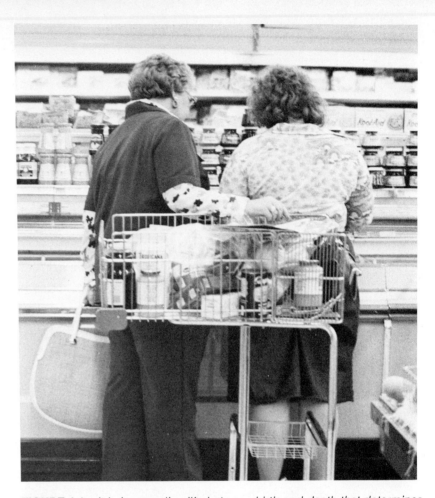

FIGURE 1.1 *It is how we live life between birth and death that determines to a great extent the quality of our health. As Sidney Jourard states in* The Transparent Self, *". . . illnesses arise for one reason, and one reason only: the people who live the ways of life typical to their social position become ill because they behave in ways exquisitely calculated to produce just those outcomes. They sicken because they behave in sickening ways."*

Many people would disagree with Brockington's suggestion that at one end of the health continuum is death and at the other is the most perfect functioning of the human body; they may feel that no upper limit can be fixed for the potentialities of human functioning. What is being suggested then is that it is really not possible to give a concise definition of health. How one chooses to live his life must ultimately be decided on the basis of his individual value system.

Table 1.2 *Leading Causes of Death, 1900, 1960, and 1970*

Rank	Causes of death	Deaths per 100,000 population	Percent of all deaths
	1900		
	(All causes)	(1,719)	(100)
1	Pneumonia and influenza	202.2	11.8
2	Tuberculosis (all forms)	194.4	11.3
3	Gastritis, etc.	142.7	8.3
4	Diseases of the heart	137.4	8.0
5	Vascular lesions affecting the central nervous system	106.9	6.2
6	Chronic nephritis	81.0	4.7
7	All accidents[1]	72.3	4.2
8	Malignant neoplasms (cancer)	64.0	3.7
9	Certain diseases of early infancy	62.5	3.6
10	Diphtheria	40.3	2.3
	Total		64
	1960		
	(All causes)	(955)	(100)
1	Diseases of the heart	366.4	38.7
2	Malignant neoplasms (cancer)	147.4	15.6
3	Vascular lesions affecting the central nervous system	107.3	11.3
4	All accidents[2]	51.9	5.5
5	Certain diseases of early infancy	37.0	3.9
6	Pneumonia and influenza	36.0	3.5
7	General arteriosclerosis	20.3	2.1
8	Diabetes mellitus	17.1	1.8
9	Congenital malformations	12.0	1.3
10	Cirrhosis of the liver	11.2	1.2
	Total		85
	1970		
	(All causes)	(945.3)	(100)
1	Diseases of the heart	362.0	38.3
2	Malignant neoplasms (cancer)	162.8	17.2
3	Cerebrovascular diseases	101.9	10.8
4	Accidents	56.4	6.0
5	Influenza and pneumonia	30.9	3.3
6	Certain causes of mortality in early infancy[3]	21.3	2.2
7	Diabetes mellitus	18.9	2.0
8	Arteriosclerosis	15.6	1.6
9	Cirrhosis of the liver	15.5	1.6
10	Bronchitis, emphysema, and asthma	15.2	1.6
	Total		85

[1] Violence would add 1.4 percent; horse, vehicle, and railroad accidents provide 0.8 percent.
[2] Violence would add 1.5 percent; motor vehicle accidents provide 2.3 percent; railroad accidents provide less than 0.1 percent.
[3] Birth injuries, asphyxia, infections of newborn, ill-defined diseases, immaturity, etc.

Source: President's Science Advisory Committee Panel on Chemicals, *Chemicals and Health* (Washington, D.C.: Government Printing Office, 1973), p. 152; U.S. Department of Health, Education, and Welfare, Public Health Service, *Facts of Life and Death,* DHEW Pub. No. (HRA) 74–1222 (Washington, D.C.; Government Printing Office, 1974), p. 31.

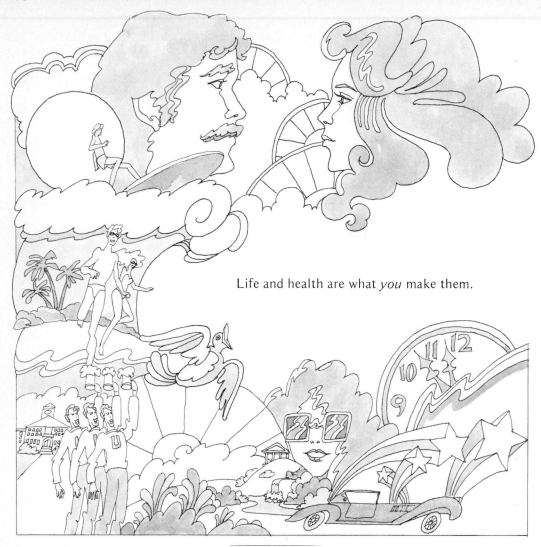

Life and health are what *you* make them.

FIGURE 1.2

HEALTH AND HUMAN VALUES: AN IMPORTANT RELATIONSHIP

Each of us faces confusion and conflict at some point in deciding how to live our lives. Values are guides to our behavior. They give direction to our decision making and can help provide some feeling of security and consistency in a changing world.

The problem with values or valuations in regard to health is that some values are fairly common to all people (e.g., the desire not to

---

Our Values are the Key to Our Well-Being

The value that one places on one's own health

affects

The level of health of others with whom one interacts

affects

The level of health of all living things

affects

The level of health of the individual

---

suffer, not to live without meaning or joy, and not to die needlessly) while others are not. This is not suggesting that people who have values in conflict with certain norms are bad or wrong. But what about those people who value things that may be in direct conflict with what is considered beneficial to good health or certain other of their values?

For example, consider the individual who places a high value on maintaining good health but continues to smoke cigarettes. He may try to offset the ill effects of smoking by concentrating on getting enough exercise or eating a good diet, but he is still indulging in a practice that will be harmful to his health.

In any discussion of health, therefore, it is important to take into consideration your own value system. If you value your health highly, you will work to maintain it. If health is of low priority, you will do little if anything to maintain and protect it. Modern medicine can do little to protect the health of those who devalue their own health and well-being. The greater tragedy is that those who devalue their own health often devalue the health of others as well and may harm others through their own careless actions (e.g., drunken drivers are a menace to others on the highway; smokers endanger the health of non-smokers around them).

The question of values and valuing in relation to health and well-being, then, is a key theme—perhaps the most important one—throughout this book. While reading this text, you should ask yourself, "What do I value?" "What are my values in relation to health?" "Do the values of my peers and friends affect my level of health?" "How do my values influence and affect my level of health?"

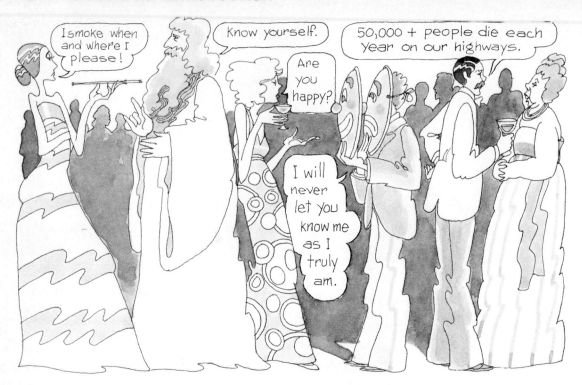

FIGURE 1.3 *Values in conflict? Do you call attention to people who smoke in No Smoking areas? What have you done to help cut down the number of accidents on our nation's highways? Do you present yourself to others as you truly are? Do you know yourself? Are you happy?*

FURTHER READINGS

Dubos, René. *Mirage of Health.* Garden City, N.Y.: Doubleday & Company, Inc. 1961.

Although more than ten years old, this book remains one of the most readable and comprehensive presentations of the meaning of health as it is related to man's general life and existence.

————. *Man Adapting.* New Haven, Conn.: Yale University Press, 1965.

The dominant theme of this book, according to the author "is that the states of health or disease are the expression of the success or failure experienced by the organism in its efforts to respond adaptively to environmental challenges."

Maslow, Abraham H. *Toward a Psychology of Being.* New York: D. Van Nostrand Company, Inc. 1962.

The author uses studies of psychologically healthy people and of the healthiest experiences and moments in the lives of average people to demonstrate that human beings can be loving, noble, and creative—that they are capable of pursuing the highest values and aspirations.

Selye, Hans. *The Stress of Life.* New York: McGraw-Hill Book Company. 1956.

This book incorporates the author's well supported theory on stress as a general factor in the etiology of disease and, in addition, includes his fascinating and logically presented philosophy of life as it relates to health and disease.

Chapter 2

Making Wise Health Decisions

WHEN TO SEEK MEDICAL ADVICE

Most people in the United States must seek medical advice at various times in their lives. Members of the health industry do not all agree on when or how often one should see a physician or other health professional. Some physicians recommend having a complete physical examination at least once every two years, while others feel that such an exam only every five years (or even less often[1]) is practical. However, it is usually the individual who decides when to see a doctor —and his decision is not always wise. Some people may visit the doctor more than necessary, for simple or imaginary ills. Others may make appointments very infrequently—even ignoring symptoms until the last possible minute—and thus may experience grave illness or problems that could have been avoided with earlier treatment or care. There are no hard-and-fast guidelines of when to see a doctor, but two general rules may prove helpful:

1. See a doctor or other health professional whenever you feel disturbed by any health problem.
2. See a physician whenever you notice changes in your health or the functioning of your body that may indicate illness.

[1] See Richard Spark, M.D., "The Case against Regular Physicals," *The New York Times* Magazine (July 25, 1976), pp. 10–11, ff.

15

Warning Signs   There are some specific signs that may indicate the need to seek professional help. Among these are:

1. Fever of undetermined origin lasting more than one day
2. Any symptoms you cannot deal with yourself (this is not advocating self-treatment, but you should practice discrimination—it is usually not necessary to see a doctor for a cold, for example)
3. Any recurring symptoms of unknown causes
4. Any problems with the urinary tract
5. Any swelling without a specific self-limiting cause
6. Any unexplained change in bodily functions, such as blurring of vision, vertigo, cramps, heartburn, diarrhea or constipation, rash, etc.
7. Foreign body lodged anywhere that cannot be removed
8. Absorption or ingestion of a toxic substance
9. A problem in daily living that affects sleep, concentration, etc.
10. Any injury that is painful longer than several days
11. Any of the seven danger signals of cancer
    · change in bowel or bladder habits
    · a sore that does not heal
    · unusual bleeding or discharge
    · thickening or lump, in the breast or elsewhere
    · indigestion or difficulty in swallowing
    · obvious change in a wart or mole
12. Chest pain caused by exertion
13. Exposure to a contagious disease

CHOOSING A DOCTOR

How do you go about choosing a doctor when you have moved or need a new physician for some other reason? Most people who have moved to a new city, for example, wait until an emergency arises to search for a doctor. However, it makes much more sense to seek out a doctor before the emergency, so that he knows you and your medical history, and so that you will feel comfortable and confident with him.

Types of Doctors   What kind of doctor should you select as your personal or family physician? There are basically three choices: the internist, the general practitioner, and the family specialist.

The *internist* is a specialist; he is an M.D. who has acquired advanced training in the diagnosis and treatment of the internal organs. The broad scope of this specialty enables an internist to treat the whole patient. Many people therefore choose an internist for their physician.

Several years ago, the family or personal physician was usually a *general practitioner*. The "G.P." is an M.D. who has chosen not to undergo additional years of specialized training in any one area. The G.P. is in most cases well qualified to handle routine medical needs. However, in recent years the G.P. has lost prestige for various reasons and far more medical students choose to specialize. One reason for this trend toward specialization is the ever-increasing amount of knowledge any doctor must acquire. It is more possible to keep up with new developments in a specialized area than in the entire field of medicine. However, most patients do not need the knowledge of a specialist, the G.P. serves an important function by answering their needs. The competent G.P. will know when to recommend that a patient see a specialist and when he can handle the case himself.

In an effort to maintain the necessary supply of general practitioners, a new specialty was created in 1969—the *family practitioner*. Physicians interested in general practice are thus able to acquire the additional training (and prestige) of the specialist. Perhaps because of the broad area covered by this specialty, the American Board of Family Practice (the particular medical board involved) requires these physicians to be re-examined every five to seven years to ensure that they have kept up with medical advances and are otherwise still fully qualified.

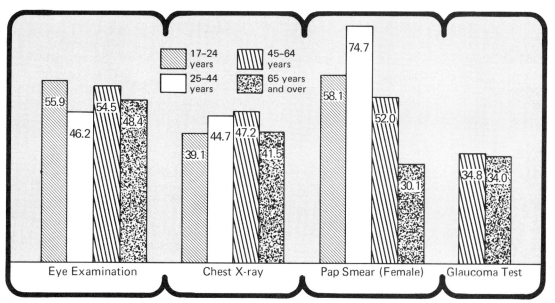

FIGURE 2.1 *Percent of population with selected preventive care examinations within past 2 years, 1973. Source: National Center for Health Statistics, Health Interview Survey.*

Specialists   At some point you may need to consult a specialist (other than the internist or family practitioner) for a certain disorder. A board certified specialist is probably the best choice. A general practitioner may become a self-styled specialist by limiting his practice to certain areas of medicine, or a physician may be a part time specialist, meaning he has had one or two years of residency training in a certain specialty. However, a board certified specialist must have fulfilled much more rigorous requirements. He must complete a full residency of from three to five (or even more) years and two years of satisfactory full time specialty practice. He must also pass oral and written exams in his specialty and fulfill several other requirements. He then becomes a board certified specialist (a diplomate). A board eligible physician is one who has fulfilled all the requirements except the passing of the oral exam; he may only be board eligible for three years before he must retake the exam.[2]

Among the major specialty areas are the following physicians:

- *allergist* treats conditions of allergic origin, such as hay fever or asthma
- *anesthesiologist* specializes in the administration of anesthesia during operations or diagnoses
- *cardiologist* treats cardiovascular diseases
- *dermatologist* treats diseases of the skin
- *endocrinologist* specializes in the diagnosis and treatment of diseases caused by disturbances in the functions of the endocrine glands (pituitary, thyroid, etc.)
- *gastroenterologist* specializes in diseases of the digestive system
- *geriatrician or gerontologist* specializes in diseases of older people
- *gynecologist* specializes in diseases of the female reproductive system
- *neurologist* specializes in the diagnosis and treatment of diseases of the nervous system
- *obstetrician* treats pregnant women
- *ophthalmologist* specializes in diseases of the eye and vision defects
- *orthopedist* specializes in diseases of the bones, joints, muscles, tendons, etc.
- *otolaryngologist* treats diseases of the ear and larynx
- *otologist* treats diseases of the ear
- *otorhinolaryngologist* specializes in diseases of the ear, nose, and larynx
- *pathologist* specializes in the identification of diseases through analysis of changes in body organs, tissues, and cells, and alterations of body chemistry.
- *pediatrician* specializes in the care of infants and children
- *proctologist* specializes in disorders of the colon, anus, and rectum
- *psychiatrist* specializes in the interpretation and treatment of mental and personality disorders

[2] Aubrey C. McTaggart and Lorna M. McTaggart, *The Health Care Dilemma,* 2d edition (Boston: Holbrook Press, 1976), pp. 16–17.

- *radiologist* specializes in the diagnostic and therapeutic uses of radiant energy, including x-rays, radium, and cobalt 60
- *rhinologist* treats disorders of the nose
- *surgeon* treats disease, injury, or deformity through operative measures. There are various specialties within surgery, and many specialists are also licensed to practice surgery within their specialties
- *urologist* diagnoses and treats diseases and abnormalities of the genitourinary tract

The Selection Process

Once you have determined the type of physician you would like, possible ways of finding a doctor include getting recommendations from friends or co-workers, calling the county medical society, or using the phone book. Recommendations from friends may sometimes provide good choices, but do not always work out. People are not always aware of the qualifications or quality of their physician.

The county medical society will provide a list of physicians but will not make specific recommendations. Furthermore, its listing does not include all the doctors in the area; only members of the American Medical Association (AMA) and the local medical society who desire to be included are on the list. Thus, some doctors of high quality may not be on the list.

Just as the county medical listing does not guarantee competency, neither does any listing in the Yellow Pages. Again, the list in the phone book includes only those who want to be listed. Using the phone book, then, is rarely a reliable method.[3]

There are certain guidelines that should prove helpful in locating a competent physician. One possibility for those who are moving is to secure recommendations from their present doctor. He will often know the reputations of doctors in other areas and may provide several names. If you trust your present doctor's judgment, you may find a good doctor through him.

If you live in an area with a medical school, you may be able to find a physician on the faculty there. Some members of the faculty have their own practices as well. They usually must demonstrate a fairly high level of capability to be included on the faculty. In addition, a physician who is teaching is expected to be aware of recent developments in the field of medicine.

Calling a hospital affiliated with a medical school (a teaching hospital) or any respected hospital should provide you with a list of competent physicians. Finding a doctor through a good hospital also means that he has staff privileges at a hospital you respect.

Finding a physician who is in group practice often will mean that he is a reputable practitioner. Physicians in a group usually are concerned that each member is competent. The physicians may

[3] Ibid., pp. 25–26.

refer patients to each other, and they want to be assured that "their" patients will receive good care from any of their associates. Good doctors like to work with other good doctors.

As you receive recommendations from various sources, you may be able to find out all you need to know about each physician's qualifications and educational background. If you decide upon a specialist, you should inquire about board certification. However, some hospitals or agencies may be reluctant to provide in-depth information about the names they list. The AMA publishes the *American Medical Directory* (found in most libraries), which provides biographical and educational information on all physicians who are members of the AMA, as well as some who are not.[4] The *Directory of Medical Specialists,* also available in most libraries, lists all board certified specialists in the United States and Canada, with biographical and training information.[5]

The Doctor-Patient Relationship

Once you acquire a list of possible physicians, there are several steps to take before establishing one as your own. Some questions you should be concerned with can be answered by the receptionist or nurse, and others must be answered by the doctor himself. First of course you must find out whether or not the doctor is accepting any new patients. Some good doctors may already have too many patients.

You should also determine the doctor's fee schedule and decide whether the prices are reasonable and comparable to those of other doctors in the area. A new patient should discuss other questions such as when the doctor would be willing to make house calls, what his procedure is during an emergency, and who will answer his calls when he is on vacation or otherwise unavailable.

The physician should stress preventive medicine. A competent doctor would rather prevent his patients from becoming ill at all. He will want to cure them of any disorders as soon as possible instead of treating them again and again for recurrent problems.

What To Expect on the First Visit

When you finally choose a doctor you feel you can depend on, you should make an appointment with him so that he can learn your medical history and give you a complete physical examination. There are three ways this is usually done—through a screening examination, a general examination, or a comprehensive examination.

The *screening exam* involves taking a relatively simple history and performing a complete physical exam. A urinalysis is also re-

[4] Ibid., p. 38.
[5] Ibid., p. 20.

CHOOSING A SURGEON

Last year some 12 million Americans underwent surgery. Of that number, experts estimate that in 2 million cases the surgery done was either questionable or totally unwarranted. Furthermore, up to 50 percent of all operations in this country are performed by doctors who are either untrained or unqualified to do them.

In view of these problems, some good advice to follow when considering surgery includes:

· Never seek the services of a surgeon directly; wait to be referred through your family physician
· Make certain, by checking the *Directory of Medical Specialists,* that the surgeon is certified by either the American Specialty Boards or the American Osteopathic Board of Surgery. The most competent surgeons are designated Fellows of the American College of Surgeons (F.A.C.S.) or the American College of Osteopathic Surgeons
· Try to find a surgeon affiliated with a teaching hospital
· Check to be sure the hospital with which the surgeon is affiliated is accredited. (See discussion on accreditation in text)

---

quired, and some other special studies are occasionally included. The *general exam* includes a complete history and a complete physical, involving checks of vision and hearing, a pelvic exam for women, and a rectal proctoscopy. A urinalysis, certain blood studies, a chest x-ray, and an electrocardiogram are also part of this evaluation. The *comprehensive exam* includes essentially a history and the extensive physical examination of the general examination. In addition, numerous laboratory procedures are called for: studies of the stomach and of the colon, x-rays of the gall bladder and perhaps of the back, and other studies as indicated.

The Medical History

Collecting a complete medical history on a new patient should usually take about half an hour. The physician or his nurse or physician's assistant may perform this task. The medical history is a way of recording a patient's previous health problems and any current problems.

The questions asked should cover:

· present illness or complaint (if any)
· personal health history

· review of the physiological systems
· family health history
· social/occupational history

The Physical Examination

There are a number of procedures used by the doctor in performing a physical exam, including observation, touching or feeling (palpation), and percussion (or thumping) and listening (auscultation), usually with a stethoscope. A complete physical examination should include the following:

· *head:* observation and palpation all over
· *eyes:* use of ophthalmoscope to look at retina for inflammation and discharge; checking pupillary reaction and visual acuity
· *ears:* palpation; observation of ear drum; checking of functioning
· *nose:* observation with nosescope; palpation; transillumination of sinuses
· *mouth:* observation of all areas with light and tongue depressor; palpation of all surfaces inside mouth (with gloved finger)
· *neck:* observation; palpation, auscultation of carotid arteries
· *breasts:* palpation
· *chest:* observation, front and back; palpation while breathing, especially over the heart; percussion over lungs—front, back, and sides; auscultation over both lungs (in at least six places); auscultation over heart (in at least four places), using both parts of the stethoscope, while sitting up and lying down
· *arms:* palpation; checking of joints and the range of motion; comparison of bilateral strength
· *abdomen:* (in this order) observation; auscultation; percussion; palpation
· *pelvis: male*—hernia check, observation and palpation of genitalia, rectal examination, prostate examination; *female*—vaginal examination, rectal examination
· *legs: standing up*—check for circulation and varicose veins, check for balance and pelvic support by shifting weight; *lying down*—check for range of motion
· *spine:* check flexibility and posture; palpation, percussion, and observation
· *feet:* check between toes; check circulation and structural integrity
· *neurological:* check for equal sensation, strength, and reflexes on both sides of the body

OTHER HEALTH PRACTITIONERS

There are several other types of health practitioners to whom people may turn. Among these are the osteopath, the chiropractor, and the acupuncturist.

The Osteopath   Osteopathy is a field of medicine that was founded in the late 1800s by Andrew T. Still. His philosophy was that disease is caused by disturbed nerve functions, so he practiced various forms of manipulative therapy. Today the philosophies and practices of osteopathy are much closer to those of traditional medicine. The osteopath (D.O.) now receives training that is generally comparable to that of the M.D.

Osteopaths are now licensed to practice medicine and surgery in every state. In fact, the AMA is interested in a merger with the American Osteopathic Association (AOA), recognizing the quality of osteopathic training and practice. The AOA opposes this merger, however, fearing that osteopaths would lose their distinction. Also, the medical philosophies of the AMA and the AOA are not entirely similar. For example, osteopathy stresses general medicine rather than any specialization, and the vast majority of D.O.'s are general practitioners (in contrast to the predominance of specialists among M.D.'s).[6]

California passed legislation in the 1960s enabling all D.O.'s to become M.D.'s and most osteopaths took advantage of this ruling. Osteopaths are also now accepted for residency training by many specialty boards and any osteopath can join the AMA. However, most of the approximately 15,000 osteopathic physicians choose to treat their patients in the more than 300 osteopathic hospitals in the United States, and to maintain an indepedent position relative to this alternative system of medicine and surgery.

The Chiropractor   Chiropractic is a system of therapeutics based upon the claim that disease is caused by abnormal function of the nerve system. A chiropractor believes that he can restore normal function of the nerve system (and consequently restore health) by manipulation and treatment of parts of the body, especially the spine. This emphasis on the nervous system may sound similar to some aspects of osteopathy, but the two fields are widely separated. A chiropractor does not have the medical training and experience of the osteopath or other physicians. Chiropractic training usually consists of only four additional years of education after high school.

Because of their lack of extensive medical training, chiropractors work within a very limited sphere. They are not trained to diagnose or treat serious illness, or even many common disorders. Furthermore, they are not licensed either to prescribe drugs or to perform surgery. Chiropractors are not granted hospital privileges, so they cannot treat any patients requiring hospitalization.

[6] Ibid., p. 85.

Some chiropractors are more reliable than others. In trying to establish the legitimacy of their field, chiropractic officials themselves have offered several warnings to any prospective chiropractic patient. One warning is to avoid anyone advertising free x-rays. Chiropractors make use of extensive x-rays in their treatments, but these should not be used as an advertising lure. The patient should ask the chiropractor if he refers patients to other health professionals. If the answer is no or the chiropractor disparages other professions and traditional medical treatment, he is not to be trusted. As mentioned above, chiropractors do not have hospital privileges and they have to refer patients who need hospital care to physicians. Any prospective patient should also beware of scare tactics, such as threats of "irreversible damage" if treatment is not begun immediately. The individual should also inquire about fee schedules. Most chiropractors have a flat office fee (and do not offer "discounts" for prepayment). There should not be any extra charges for "units of treatment," such as heat therapy and other chiropractic practices.[7] Before going to a chiropractor, it would probably be profitable to consult a licensed physician.

The Acupuncturist

Although acupuncture has been practiced in China for centuries, it is relatively new to the United States. It is a method of relieving pain through the use of hair-thin needles. There are many theories currently offered to explain this form of treatment. The most popular theory, the "two-gate theory of pain control," postulates that the acupuncture needles block pain impulses to the brain, where pain is actually felt.

Treatments consist of inserting six to eight stainless steel needles into strategic points (described on traditional ancient eastern charts) on the body. There have been some amazing results achieved through the use of acupuncture. Because of the recent controversy over complications (including infection and punctured lungs), one should seek this type of treatment only through a licensed physician.

CHOOSING A HOSPITAL

When a patient requires hospitalization, he usually goes to the hospital with which his physician is affiliated. However, the doctor often has privileges at more than one hospital so he will offer his patient a choice. How can the individual make an intelligent decision? There are several questions to consider.

[7] "Chiropractors: Healers or Quacks?" *Consumer Reports* (October 1975), p. 610.

Is the Hospital Accredited?   A hospital must meet certain standards of the Joint Commission on Accreditation of Hospitals (JCAH) to receive accreditation. A hospital must apply to be evaluated by the JCAH, so it is a voluntary process, and some good hospitals may not be accredited. Furthermore, these are only minimum standards; however, it is wiser to find a hospital that is accredited and has passed the evaluation. The evaluation process must be repeated every three years. A hospital given full accreditation usually displays its certificate prominently. A check with the state's regulatory agency will also assure you of a hospital's evaluation.

What Type of Hospital Is It?   Hospitals are usually classified according to three categories: type of ownership or control; type of patient treated; and type of care offered, either short- or long-term.

A hospital may be either government, voluntary nonprofit, or private. The federal government has set up hospitals to provide care for military personnel and their families, veterans, and other groups; it also maintains hospitals to deal with certain diseases, such as leprosy and drug addiction. State hospitals may offer either general care or treatment for specific disorders. City and county hospitals are usually general care facilities responsible for treating patients who cannot afford to pay for their hospitalization. They may also be concerned with controlling communicable diseases. The quality of treatment in government hospitals is usually high.

Government-financed hospitals are able to support long-term patient care that other hospitals are less likely to offer. Short-term hospitals are responsible for over 90 percent of all admissions in the United States. Short-term care is defined as thirty days or less of treatment. Chronic conditions or mental and neurological disorders usually require longer periods of hospitalization (in a long-term facility).[8]

The majority of hospitals in this country are voluntary nonprofit organizations. These are public institutions and may be run by religious or charitable organizations, other philanthropic organizations or individuals, or the community. They may receive some funding from local groups or the government. These hospitals usually provide general care on a short-term basis.

Private hospitals are owned and run by individuals or corporations on a profit-making basis. The standards of private hospitals, especially the smaller ones, may not be as high as those of government or voluntary hospitals. Some large private hospitals are highly regarded, but it is difficult for the patient to evaluate such a hospital.

[8] McTaggart and McTaggart, *Health Care Dilemma,* p. 164.

They may not have the facilities or high-caliber physicians and staff of the other types of hospitals. In fact, only about one-third of these private hospitals are accredited. Because of the profit motive, private hospitals are more interested in treating illness or disorders that require only short-term care and those that are unlikely to involve complications. Private hospitals rarely accept patients who are unable to pay.

Is the Hospital a Teaching Hospital?

The affiliations of a hospital are important. The quality of a hospital can sometimes be judged by whether it is associated with a medical and/or nursing school and whether it has been approved for training interns and residents. Such affiliations usually guarantee that the medical procedures and facilities of the hospital are up to date. However, there are only 114 medical schools in the United States, so the number of teaching hospitals is limited.

Some patients do not want to be involved in the research and training of medical students and personnel. These individuals may consider the affiliations of a hospital to be a drawback.

How Large Is the Hospital?

A hospital must have over twenty-five beds before it can even apply for accreditation; a larger hospital can usually afford a greater range of facilities and more modern equipment than a smaller one. A larger hospital is also more likely to have a wide range of specialists available. Good doctors and specialists are attracted to hospitals involved in research (a teaching hospital or a large institution) and to hospitals with a number of other specialists, i.e., a large staff.

CHOOSING A DENTIST

Finding a good dentist or other dental specialist can also be a problem. Again, there are certain guidelines in this process that should enable the individual to make a satisfactory choice.

Dentists and Specialists

To become a dentist requires two to four years of predental college study and four years of dental training. The dental student must acquire a base of knowledge about the physical and biological sciences, as well as clinical training so that he can deal with problems of disease. He must also be able to prescribe drugs and perform oral surgery. The dentist receives one of two types of degrees: a Doctor of Dental Surgery (D.D.S.) or a Doctor of Medical Dentistry (D.M.D.).

A dentist may become a specialist in several ways; although many practice as specialists, only 15 percent of all dentists are board certified in a specialty. There are eight dental specialty areas recognized by the American Dental Association:

- *endodontist:* specializes in diseases of the pulp or nerves of the tooth
- *oral pathologist:* diagnoses diseases, tumors, and injuries of the mouth
- *oral surgeon:* specializes in surgery for oral tumors, diseases, injuries, tooth extractions, and defects of the jaw
- *orthodontist:* specializes in straightening teeth and correcting improper bite
- *pedodontist:* specializes in dental treatment of children
- *periodontist:* specializes in treating the supporting tissues of the teeth
- *prosthodontist:* specializes in preparing crowns, dentures, and bridges
- *public health dentist:* is concerned with the prevention and control of dental diseases and the promotion of general dental health at the community level

Methods of Choice

Some of the possible options for finding a good dentist are similar to those used in choosing a doctor. The local dental society will provide a list of any dentists in your area who are society members, but it will not make recommendations on competency.

Contacting the faculty of a school of dentistry is a recommended method. The faculty members are highly qualified, and if they are too busy, they can usually make referrals to other capable dentists.

If you are seeking a specialist, you can usually secure recommendations from your regular dentist. The *Directory of Dental Specialists* lists all dentists who are certified diplomates, recognized by the American Dental Association (or you may write the ADA at 211 East Chicago Avenue, Chicago, Illinois to find a specialist in your area).

The First Visit

Once you have chosen a dentist, there are certain things you can watch for that should indicate whether he is capable and reputable. Discuss the dentist's fees with him; if you need extensive dental work be sure to get an estimate in advance. You may want to compare fees with those of other dentists in your area. You should find out how (or if) the dentist treats emergencies.

A good dentist will find out your dental history and background before treating you. He should also explain any procedures in detail and should allow you to evaluate alternatives. When taking x-rays, he should provide a lead apron (to protect the reproductive organs of both the male and female).

If the dentist will discuss these problems or questions with you freely and carefully, and to your satisfaction, you may be assured of the merit of your choice.

QUACKERY

The first part of this chapter has been concerned with enabling you to make good choices about health professionals and facilities. Another concern of the individual who is determined to make wise health decisions is the avoidance of quackery in all its forms.

Why do people believe any of the quacks? The quack's major resources are people's gullibility and fear. Most people are afraid of disease, but many people are also afraid of doctors.

Another explanation for the success of quack cures is the *placebo effect.* A placebo is a substance containing harmless and ineffective ingredients (e.g. the "sugar pill"). The placebo effect can be defined as improvement in a patient's condition during treatment of some sort, but not resulting from that treatment. It is one of the quack's most effective weapons. Placebos have been shown to relieve anxiety and tension, alleviate pain, and to bring about other "miraculous" reactions. These effects may occur because the patient expects the "medicine" to work or when an illness is of psychosomatic origin (tension headaches, for example). Whatever the explanation, the quack can often use the placebo effect as a demonstration of his efficiency.

Forms of Quackery

People suffering from chronic or incurable disease are among those most likely to respond to a quack's claim. Individuals suffering from cancer or arthritis then are among the many people victimized each year by quackery.

Cancer Cures

There are four categories of people susceptible to the quack who offers a "cure" for cancer. The first category includes the hypochondriacs who are afraid they have cancer. Every time one of these people seeks the cancer therapy a quack prescribes, the quack's cure rate will soar (since there was no cancer to cure in the first place).

The second type are those people who have been diagnosed incorrectly as having cancer. When they seek treatment from a quack, they are "miraculously" cured—of a nonexistent disease—and the quack's "success" may be favorably publicized.

The third group are those who have a treatable form of cancer, but because of poor advice, religious beliefs, or other reasons discontinue the scientifically advocated treatment in favor of a "quick cure" offered by a quack. These people are sometimes well on their way to being cured when they give up in favor of the quack's false hope for a quick cure.

The final group is made up of those people suffering from terminal cancer, with no cure in sight. These people are especially vulnerable because they may be constantly hoping for a miracle cure and are "grasping at straws."

Arthritis Cures

An estimated 17 million Americans suffer from some form of arthritis. Because of the constant pain these people suffer and their desperate need for relief, they are easy targets for the quack. It is estimated that quacks sell approximately $250 million worth of arthritis cures a year, even though the most serious type of arthritis, rheumatoid arthritis, has no cure. Because the person who suffers from rheumatoid arthritis has periods of improvement and relief from pain (remissions), he may feel that he has been cured.

Other Types of Quackery

There are many other claims made by these disreputable practitioners. Some of the more important areas the quack "specializes" in are nutrition, hair products (especially for growing hair), relief of pain, mental health, and weight reduction.

Avoiding the Quack Trap   How can the individual avoid quack cures and treatments? Here are some questions you should ask yourself before investing in any health care products or processes of treatment:

1. Does the advertisement cover specific problems recognized by the medical profession? Or, instead, does the product claim to cure a number of ailments, like the old "medicine man's" panacea?
2. Does the claim make good common sense? Is it within the range of technical knowledge? Claims such as a "cure" for the common cold are obviously false.
3. Does the claim use an overabundance of unsupported facts and figures ("most dentists recommend . . ." or "of all brands tested . . .")?

4. Does the product seem reliable merely because it is endorsed by celebrities? Remember that these people are being paid and even if they do use the product, it does not mean that it is either good or safe for every individual.

5. Is a time limit or supply shortage mentioned in the advertisement? This particular ploy is one of the most commonly used to stimulate buying.

6. Are there testimonial letters included in the advertising? There is a brisk market for the sale of testimonials and lists of people who will write and sell them. (A government study found that one man had over two hundred testimonials out on various products.)

7. Does the ad use such terms as "world famous research institute" and "tests conducted under a doctor's observation" or "use of a secret formula"? These claims are suspect unless they are supported by specifics.

8. Does the ad offer to diagnose by mail? This is impossible and no reputable firm would ever make such a statement.

9. Is there a request for payment in advance? In these cases, the consumer usually receives much less than he expected, both in quality and usefulness of the product.

10. Does the advertisement guarantee results? Reputable cures are not guaranteed; they may work for almost everyone, but some people may react differently.[9]

11. Does the practitioner offering treatment ask you to sign a contract for services? A written agreement for treatment is not customary practice.[10]

12. If you are seeking a remedy for a certain disorder, have you seen a qualified physician? If not, why not?

CONSUMER PROTECTION

The consumer in the health marketplace must educate himself to avoid incompetent health practitioners and unreliable health care products. There are a number of private and governmental organizations that have been established to protect and educate the consumer.

The American Medical Association is one such private organization. It works to prevent fraudulent and improper advertising of medical products and conducts research aimed at better products. The American College of Radiology and the National Health Council also are involved in finding and stopping fraudulent medical practices and products. The American Cancer Society and the Arthritis Foundation investigate fraud connected with those specific diseases. The Better Business Bureau investigates and acts upon complaints of unethical business practices. Other private organizations include testing and rating agencies such as the Consumers Research Institute, which conducts independent research on consumer products.

[9] "Chiropractors," loc. cit.
[10] Ibid.

The Food and Drug Administration (FDA) of the U.S. Government protects the consumer by insuring that (1) foods are safe, pure and wholesome; (2) drugs and therapeutic devices are safe and effective; (3) cosmetics are safe; (4) all foods, drugs, and cosmetics are honestly and informatively labeled and packaged; and (5) certain hazardous household cleaning aids and other poisons have adequate warning labels.

The Federal Trade Commission (FTC) is authorized to regulate unfair (to competitors) trade practices and to assure the truthfulness and fairness of advertising. Nevertheless, the legal tools in the hands of this agency are inadequate. The maximum fine for false or unfair advertising is only $5,000—a trivial sum for advertisers with nationwide sales. The FTC's main weapon against false advertising has been the "cease and desist" order, under which the advertiser is told only not to use exactly the same words in exactly the same advertisement again. In recent years, there have been some attempts to force the FTC to become more aggressive in its consumer protection activities. More and better enforcement methods, such as requiring false advertisers to run correctional ads in the same media in which the offending material appeared, are needed.

The U.S. Postal Service is authorized to prevent the sale of fraudulent products through the mail. The Consumer Products Safety Commission devises standards for product safety, sets up restrictions on the sale of flammable products, regulates laboratories engaged in interstate commerce, etc. The Department of Health, Education, and Welfare recently set up a Bureau of Health Education to provide leadership regarding that agency's health education responsibilities.

People Power

There are also a number of agencies set up by consumers themselves. Ralph Nader, one of the nation's leading consumer advocates, has been responsible in great part for a new era of consumer consciousness concerning the quality and safety of certain products being sold today.

One area that has received particular attention is advertising. A number of consumer advocates are zeroing in on products dangerous to children. They are asking for more extensive warnings on these products, many of which are promoted on TV during afternoon and early evening hours when children do 90 percent of their television watching. Certain consumer organizations are demanding that ads for these potentially dangerous products be aired only after 9 p.m., when far fewer children are watching television. At the least, these organizations want the Federal Communications Commission to require that the dangers as well as the benefits of such products be included in the advertising.

Patient's Bill of Rights

The American Hospital Association first issued a bill of rights for patients in November of 1972 and again in January of 1973 to its 7,000 member hospitals. Formulated by a committee appointed by the trustees of the American Hospital Association, discussed by its regional advisory boards and consumer representatives, the bill's twelve-point protocol is:

1. The patient has the right to considerate and respectful care.

2. The patient has the right to obtain from his physician complete current information concerning his diagnosis, treatment and prognosis in terms the patient can reasonably be expected to understand.

3. The patient has the right to receive from his physician information necessary to give informed consent prior to the start of any procedure and/or treatment.

4. The patient has the right to refuse treatment to the extent permitted by law, and to be informed of the medical consequences of his action.

5. The patient has the right to every consideration of his privacy concerning his own medical care program.

6. The patient has the right to expect that all communications and records pertaining to his care should be treated as confidential.

7. The patient has the right to expect that within its capacity a hospital must make reasonable response to the request of a patient for services.

8. The patient has the right to obtain information as to any relationship of his hospital to other health care and educational institutions insofar as his care is concerned.

9. The patient has the right to be advised if the hospital purposes to engage in or perform human experimentation affecting his care or treatment.

10. The patient has the right to expect reasonable continuity of care.

11. The patient has the right to examine and receive an explanation of his bill regardless of source of payment.

12. The patient has the right to know what hospital rules and regulations apply to his conduct as a patient.

FURTHER READINGS

Acupuncture and Moxibustion. New York: Schocken Books, 1976.

A "cookbook" for medical practice in the Chinese mode.

Belsky, Marvin. *How To Choose and Use Your Doctor.* Greenwich, Conn.: Fawcett Crest Book, 1975.

A "how to" book on being an assertive patient.

Cox, Edward et al. *The Nader Report on the Federal Trade Commission.* New York: Grove Press, 1969.

This book shows how credit frauds have bilked Americans of millions of dollars—and gone unpunished by a "sleepy FTC."

Crichton, Michael. *Five Patients.* New York: Alfred A. Knopf, Inc., 1970.

This popular book, written by a noted author (*The Andromeda Strain*) and medical school graduate, provides an intimate view of the problems faced by modern hospital patients and those who care for them.

Frank, Jerome. *Persuasion and Healing.* New York: Schocken Books, 1974.

Topics covered include nonmedical healing, religious healing, religious revivalism, and thought reform.

Hechtlinger, Adelaide. *The Great Patent Medicine Era.* New York: Madison Square Press, 1970.

A rather entertaining presentation of the story of American folk medicine—the nostrums, super-situations, and medicines of another era.

Jarvis, David C. *Folk Medicine.* Greenwich, Conn.: Fawcett Publications Inc., 1958.

A famous doctor's guide to folk medicine practices of Vermont.

Meyer, Clarence. *American Folk Medicine.* New York: Plume Books, 1973.

A complete collection of time-tested home remedies made from everything from herbs, garden vegetables, and fruits.

Nolen, William. *Healing: A Doctor in Search of a Miracle.* Greenwich, Conn.: Fawcett Publications Inc., 1974.

From hope to heartbreak to an authentic miracle, *Healing* is a doctor's compassionate, witty, and richly entertaining account of that search.

Organizing for Health Care. Boston: Beacon Press, 1974.

Information on resources and organizations in the area of health care.

Rothenberg, Robert. *The Complete Surgical Guide.* New York: A Signet Book, 1974.

The most comprehensive one-volume encyclopedia of surgical preparation, practice, and techniques.

Samuels, Mike and Bennett, Hal. *The Well Book.* New York: Random House, 1973.

This is the new home medical handbook covering physical exams, diagnosis of common diseases, etc.

The American Health Empire. New York: Vintage Books, 1971.

A report from the Health Policy Advisory Center on power, profits, and politics of the health care system.

Vickery, Donald and Fries, James. *Take Care of Yourself.* Reading, Mass.: Addison-Wesley Publishing Co., 1976.

A consumer's guide to medical care in the U. S.

Young, J. H. *The Medical Messiahs.* Princeton, N. J.: Princeton University Press, 1967.

This book is a fascinating history of medical quackery in the United States during the past century.

Chapter 3

Health Care and Protection

The problems of adequate health care for the population of the United States are increasing. These concerns include rising costs, the quality of care, and access to any sort of medical care.

In recent years, the cost of medical care has increased much faster than the consumer price index (see Figure 3.1). Health care costs are now rising at a rate double that of the overall cost of living. The amount of money spent each year by individuals and organizations on medical care is staggering. (See Table 3.1.) In 1974, a total of $94 billion—or $440 for each man, woman, and child—was spent on medical care in this country. By 1980, the cost per individual is expected to be between $700 and $800 annually. One response to this has been the Health Security bill sponsored by one hundred members of the House of Representatives in an effort to curb escalating medical and hospital costs.

Despite the tremendous inflow of funds, the medical care system in the United States is becoming less able to meet the needs of our citizens. There have always been some people who could not afford any sort of medical care, but that group is expanding to the extent that members of the middle class cannot always afford medical services. In addition, there is a shortage of physicians and other health care professionals, and of facilities to provide health care. Some problems can be met by the expansion of certain existing programs; the solutions for others have not yet been devised.

With the spiraling costs of medical care, some type of health insurance coverage is a necessity. Hospital care ranges from $75 to $150 daily, not including x-rays, drugs, doctors' fees, and other "extras." According to the National Health Survey, one out of every thirty families in the United States will face medical bills exceeding $5,000 in any given year. Few people can meet such costs themselves; they turn to insurance companies for protection.

Table 3.1 Total and per person national health expenditures, by source of funds, and percent of Gross National Product, selected fiscal years, 1928–1929 through 1971–1972. Source: Barbara S. Cooper and Nancy L. Worthington, "National Health Expenditures, 1929–1972," Social Security Bulletin, Vol. 36 (Jan., 1973), p. 5.

	Gross National Product[a] (in billions)	Health expenditures								
		Total			Private (Nongovernment)			Public (Government)		
Fiscal year		Amount (in millions)	Per capita	Per cent of GNP	Amount (in millions)	Per capita	Per cent of total	Amount (in millions)	Per capita	Per cent of total
1928–29	$ 101	$ 3,589	$ 29.16	4	$ 3,112	$ 25.28	87	$ 477	$ 3.88	13.3
1939–40	95	3,863	28.83	4	3,081	22.99	80	782	5.84	20.2
1949–50	263	12,028	78.35	5	8,962	58.38	75	3,065	19.97	25.5
1959–60	496	25,856	141.63	5	19,460	106.60	75	6,395	35.03	24.7
1965–66	719	42,109	211.64	6	31,279	157.21	74	10,830	54.43	25.7
1969–70	955	68,058	328.17	7	42,823	206.49	63	25,235	121.68	37.1
1971–72	1,096	83,417	394.16	8	50,560	238.90	61	32,857	155.25	39.4

[a] Gross National Product is the total value of all goods and services produced in the U.S.A. during that year.

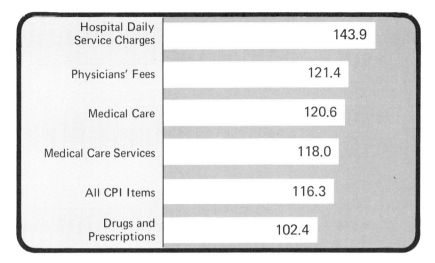

Hospital Daily Service Charges	143.9
Physicians' Fees	121.4
Medical Care	120.6
Medical Care Services	118.0
All CPI Items	116.3
Drugs and Prescriptions	102.4

FIGURE 3.1   *Increase in medical costs compared to increase in consumer price index, 1970 (1967=100). Source: U.S. Department of Labor, Bureau of Labor Statistics.*

Locating adequate medical protection or choosing among various programs is difficult for many people. Students may view concern over medical care and protection as a worry for the distant future. Many students are currently covered by their parents' policies or by programs offered by the university or college they attend. However, coverage under a parental policy usually ends when the person reaches age twenty-one and the school policy will run out upon graduation—in short, most individuals must choose some sort of medical protection.

VOLUNTARY HEALTH INSURANCE

Approximately 80 percent of American families are covered by some form of voluntary health insurance. There are six different types of coverage offered by Blue Cross/Blue Shield and other private companies.

(1) *Hospital expense protection.* This is the most popular type of coverage. It pays for part or all of one's hospital charges, which may include room and board, drugs, x-rays, laboratory tests, and other items. This type of protection usually covers a limited period of time, such as 30, 60, or 90 days.

(2) *Surgical expense protection.* This type of policy is often combined with hospital expense policies. It pays surgical expenses according to a predetermined fee schedule for each type of operation.

More people have hospital expense and/or surgical expense protection than general or comprehensive coverage, which acts in one way to make the health care situation worse. The individual and his doctor know that the patient's insurance will not pay for x-rays and other tests done in the doctor's office or on an outpatient basis. Thus, the doctor may admit the patient to the hospital needlessly, just so the insurance will cover routine diagnostic procedures. An otherwise healthy patient is then occupying an expensive hospital bed, requiring care from the staff and adding to the costs of the health care system.

(3) *General (regular) medical expense protection.* General medical coverage pays for part of all home or office visits and laboratory work, but does not cover surgery.

(4) *Major medical expense protection* is a type of policy most recently offered by insurance companies. It is now the fastest growing type of protection. It is designed to protect the individual against unusually large medical expenses. Such a policy may pay from 75 to 80 percent of costs ranging from $10,000 to $100,000 (after a deduction of $250 or $500 is paid by the policyholder).

(5) *Loss of income protection* pays cash benefits on a weekly or monthly basis to compensate a wage earner for loss of income resulting from sickness or injury.

(6) *Dental expense protection* is a type of coverage that has only recently been offered by insurance companies and is usually available for members of group plans. Such policies cover only necessary dental work (such as oral surgery).

The Insurance Dilemma

An insurance policy is a large investment, so the choice should be an informed one. Parents or close friends who have purchased policies may offer recommendations; a personal physician can provide good advice. Decide exactly what type of coverage you need before comparing different policies. You should be concerned with what hospitals are covered by the policy. Check the waiting period (the time that must elapse before you will be eligible for payment of benefits) of each plan, and find out the conditions under which any plan can be cancelled. If you are purchasing loss of income protection, be aware that payments of 50 percent of your salary are considered good. These points should be helpful in purchasing a voluntary insurance policy.

Although an individual may find a voluntary policy that is satisfactory, it is likely that he will still encounter problems with that coverage. Another possibility for health care protection and reliable medical treatment is the health maintenance organization.

HEALTH MAINTENANCE ORGANIZATIONS

Health Maintenance Organizations (HMOs) are becoming more prevalent in the United States. An HMO "assembles a number of health services under one roof for its enrolled members. Instead of charging a fee for each service, the HMO collects a lump sum in advance from subscribers (or their employers). That sum is to pay for comprehensive health care by the HMO's physicians. HMO, in short, is another name for prepaid group practice or group health."[1] Among the major HMOs today are the Health Insurance Plan (HIP) of Greater New York and the Kaiser Foundation Medical Care Program in the western states.

Dr. Sidney Garfield, one of the pioneers of the Kaiser Plan, advocates organizing HMO care around four centers of activity: (1) a screening center to separate those who are ill from those who are not; (2) a health maintenance center for immunization and other care of the well; (3) a center for the chronically ill; and (4) an acute care center. One advantage of this plan is that only in the latter two cases would the bulk of patient contact have to be with physicians, so that the problem of the shortage of doctors would be somewhat alleviated.

There are still some problems in the working of the HMOs, but for many people, health maintenance organizations are the answer to their health care worries. However, expanded voluntary coverage policies or HMOs are not, by themselves, the answer to our health care problems. One trouble with both of these programs is that many people cannot afford even the moderate rates of some HMOs, let alone the expensive premiums for a voluntary health policy. Some experts feel that a national health insurance plan may provide some answers, and steps have been taken in this direction.

GOVERNMENT PROGRAMS AND NATIONAL HEALTH INSURANCE

At the present time, there are two major federal programs of medical care—Medicare and Medicaid. In 1965, the federal government passed two amendments to the Social Security Act of 1935, Title 18 and Title 19; Title 18 established Medicare, a health insurance program for the elderly, and Title 19 established Medicaid, a health care assistance program for various parts of the population.

[1] "HMO's: Are They the Answer to Your Medical Needs?" *Consumer Reports,* 39, (October 1974) 756, cited in McTaggart and McTaggart, *Health Care Dilemma,* p. 139.

Medicare   The Medicare program has two parts: a basic compulsory hospital insurance plan (Part A) and a voluntary program of medical insurance (Part B).

Part A is financed mainly by social security deductions. Anyone who was sixty-five or older before January 1, 1968 is covered by Part A; people who turned sixty-five after this date must be eligible for Social Security or Railroad Retirement benefits to be covered. The benefits of Part A include partial payments for hospital and nursing home care and for home health care.

Part B is financed by monthly premiums paid by the individual and matched by the federal government. Anyone over sixty-five can sign up for this part of the program. Part B pays part of the costs of doctors' services, out-patient hospital care, x-rays, diagnostic tests, physical therapy, and other medical services and supplies.

Medicare thus does help the elderly with their medical bills at a period in their lives when they may be faced with large medical expenses and a decreasing ability to pay them. However, the program limits its coverage with various exclusions and does not cover many of the costs these people must pay.

Medicaid   Medicaid is a federal and state program of medical assistance. Coverage under this program may vary from state to state, but basically those eligible for benefits are the "medically needy," including blind, aged, and disabled people and children under twenty-one. Medicaid may pay the monthly premiums of Part B of Medicare for needy people over sixty-five. Among the costs covered by Medicaid are in-patient and out-patient hospital care, nursing home care, doctors' fees, x-rays, and laboratory services.

Medicaid also has problems. Its coverage varies greatly from state to state, and each state administration defines differently the "medically needy" or those who are eligible. Many physicians and institutions are unwilling to participate in the program. And as medical costs continue to rise, coverage becomes less comprehensive and less adequate.[2]

A National Health Insurance Program?   Because of the problems with all the existing programs, many experts have turned to the idea of a national health care plan. The National Health Planning and Resources Development Act of 1974 set the stage for a national health insurance program.

[2] Aubrey C. McTaggart and Lorna M. McTaggart, *The Health Care Dilemma*, 2d edition, Boston: Holbrook Press, 1976, p. 267.

Experts hope that the National Health Planning Act will help to place a ceiling on medical costs. They believe it will cut down unnecessary surgery by requiring doctors to justify the need for such expensive operations as open-heart surgery and organ transplants. Yet even with a national health insurance plan, there is no guarantee that we will be assured of quick access to a reliable source of medical care twenty-four hours a day, seven days a week.

CONCLUSION

Obviously, health care and protection are not at an acceptable level at the present time. Improvements are being made, but many of them will take a long time before they become effective solutions. There are some things that both health care professionals and health care consumers can do to alleviate this situation.

Our health care system is designed almost entirely for the person who has already been stricken by illness. Little emphasis is placed on *keeping* people healthy. Today's acute illness care contributes little to improvement in overall health of any individual or the nation as a whole. The major function of such care is to relieve immediate symptoms and increase patient satisfaction.[3] One positive step would be for doctors and other medical care professionals to concentrate more on preventive medicine.

One of the greatest improvements in health will come from actions taken by the individual to maintain his own well-being. Programs concerned with understanding good nutrition, exercising and keeping fit, and reducing alcohol, drug, and tobacco intake are becoming increasingly important.[4] Health education and health care programs today should stress preventive medicine—learning how to live healthier lives.

[3] R. J. Haggarty, "The Boundaries of Health Care," *Pharos,* 1972, pp. 106–111.
[4] W. B. Belloc and L. Breslow, "Relationship of Physical Health Status and Health Practices," *Preventive Medicine,* 1972, pp. 409–421.

FURTHER READINGS

Knowles, John, ed. *Hospitals, Doctors, and The Public Interest.* Cambridge, Mass.: Harvard University Press, 1965.

Edited by the director of one of the better-managed urban hospitals and outspoken advocate of health care reform, this work provides the serious student with comprehensive coverage of the specific aspects of this national issue.

Lewin, Stephen. *The Nation's Health.* New York: Wilson, 1971.

A series of articles concerned with adequacies and inadequacies of the American health care system.

Nolen, William A. *Surgeon under the Knife.* New York: Coward, McCann & Geoghegan, 1976.

Story of a surgeon who finds himself a patient rather than the doctor. Powerful story of his heart attack and recovery and his misadventures in a hospital are all here.

Schaller, Warren E. and Carroll, Charles R. *Health, Quackery & the Consumer.* Philadelphia: W. B. Saunders Co., 1976.

A complete coverage of the whole area of health care, quackery, and consumer health protection.

2

MAN'S SOCIAL EMOTIONAL ENVIRONMENT

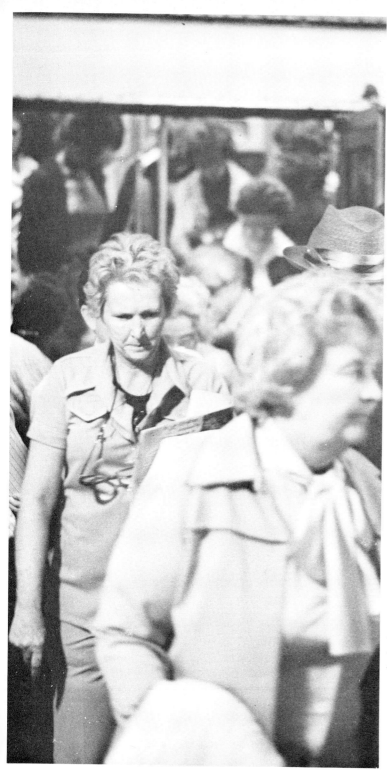

Turning and turning in the widening gyre
The falcon cannot hear the falconer
Things fall apart; the center cannot hold.

William Butler Yeats
The Second Coming

Chapter 4

Concepts of
Positive
Mental Health

In any given culture, good mental health, or what constitutes acceptable or desirable behavior, is defined in varying ways by those in the health professions and other members of the society. Some definitions of mental health stress the ability to work effectively;[1] Abraham Maslow stressed the ability to be creative in his definition.[2] B. F. Skinner, in *Walden Two,* sees mental health as consisting of happiness, productivity, and security.[3] Many views concentrate on the self-concept: Carl Rogers feels that successful adjustment requires the achievement of self-actualization—the expression of the highest potentialities of which a person is capable.[4] Marie Jahoda stresses accurate self-perception and self-knowledge in her definition.[5] Gordon Allport gives greater weight to moral values, meaningful commitments, and social responsibility.[6]

Thus, while there is widespread consensus that people require certain conditions for the development of psychological balance,

[1] S. W. Ginsburg, "The Mental Health Movement: Its Theoretical Assumptions," in R. Kotinsky and H. Witmer, eds., *Community Programs for Mental Health,* Cambridge, Mass.: Harvard Univ. Press, 1955, pp. 1–29.
[2] Abraham H. Maslow, ed., *Motivation and Personality,* New York: Harper, 1954.
[3] B. F. Skinner, *Walden Two,* New York: Macmillan, 1948.
[4] Carl R. Rogers, *On Becoming a Person,* Boston: Houghton Mifflin, 1961.
[5] Marie Jahoda, "Toward a Social Psychology of Mental Health," in Kotinsky and Witmer, *Community Programs,* 296–322.
[6] Gordon Allport, *Personality and Social Encounter,* Boston, Mass.: Beacon Press, 1964.

there is disagreement on a basic definition of mental health and the ways in which it is expressed. This leads to problems in deciding who should impose what mental health standards on other members of society.[7] However, in searching for a meaningful and useful definition of mental health, there are certain criteria generally viewed as important by most professionals.

FACTORS IN POSITIVE MENTAL HEALTH

Marie Jahoda has established a list of certain factors felt by many professionals to be important in developing positive mental health. These criteria are: attitude towards self, degree of self-actualization, personal integration, personal autonomy, perception of reality, and environmental mastery.[8]

Attitude toward Self (The Self-Concept)

Important to the development of a positive self-concept or attitude toward self are the development of self-esteem and of a sense of identity or self-knowledge.

Maintaining and if possible enhancing self-esteem is essential to successful coping behavior and positive mental health. Healthy self-esteem includes preserving a positive self-image (i.e., how one perceives oneself) and an inner assurance that one can do the things necessary for a satisfying life. A person with low self-esteem does not cope well in the face of a challenging situation. "No adaptive strategy is likely to be any good that is careless of the level of self-esteem."[9]

There are external and internal sources of self-esteem. The way others judge us and our own inner sense of competence in dealing with the environment are both important.[10] A child's self-esteem depends in great part on external sources. Children learn self-esteem when they feel valued for themselves and their accomplishments— by parents at first, and later by friends, teachers, and others. As children mature and become more independent, they learn the inner sources of self-esteem and gain satisfaction and a growing self-concept that no longer depends entirely on the opinions of other people.

[7] For those who would like to follow up this concept, read the works of R. D. Laing, epecially *Self and Others* and *The Divided Self,* and Thomas S. Szasz, *The Myth of Mental Illness.*
[8] Marie Jahoda, *Current Concepts of Positive Mental Health,* New York: Basic Books, 1958.
[9] Robert W. White, "Strategies of Adaptation: An Attempt at Systematic Description," in G. V. Coelho et al., eds., *Coping and Adaptation: Interdisciplinary Perspectives,* New York: Basic Books, in press.
[10] Robert W. White, *The Enterprise of Living: Growth and Organization in Personality,* New York: Holt, Rinehart & Winston, 1972, p. 398.

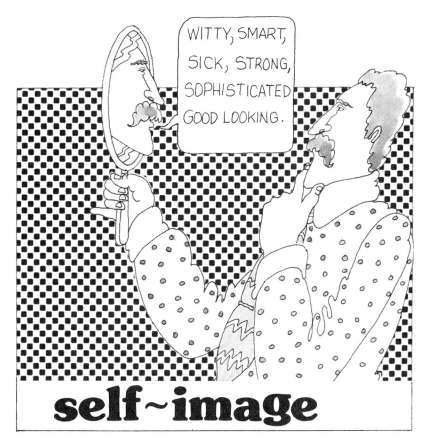

FIGURE 4.1 *How we see ourselves, how we feel about ourselves, how we think others see us is what we call our self-image or self-concept. This concept of self has a great deal to do with how we interact with others and how we live our lives.*

As a child matures, then, he develops a self-concept based on his own perceptions and those of others. He develops a sense of self-identity. Ideally, his own perception of himself and the perceptions of others are realistic and in harmony with his true personality. The person with a healthy self-concept thus has an *integrated self-identity*. (See Figure 4.2.) However, sometimes a person suffers from what is called self-alienation. He may see himself as being entirely different from what he is. In this case, he has not achieved an integrated self-concept. (See Figure 4.3.)

Part of the maturing process, then, involves developing a reasonable self-concept. Some people may always suffer from a negative self-concept for various reasons. (See Figure 4.4.) How can one learn

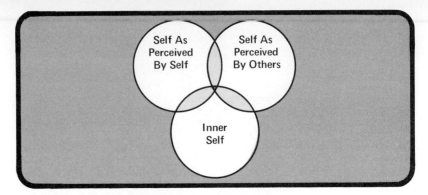

FIGURE 4.2   *The integrated self.*

to develop a positive sense of self? Carl Rogers has suggested a number of steps to "becoming a person."[11] These include:

1. *Rejection of facades.* The ability to reject being what one is not.
2. *Rejection of submissiveness.* The ability to reject being what one *ought* to be and *ought* to become.
3. *Rejection of cultural expectations.* The ability to evaluate the worth of one's cultural socialization.
4. *Movement away from trying to please others.* The ability to do what one feels is most natural to his own self.
5. *Movement toward being a "person" in flux.* The ability to be cognizant of fluid potentialities, not fixed goals.

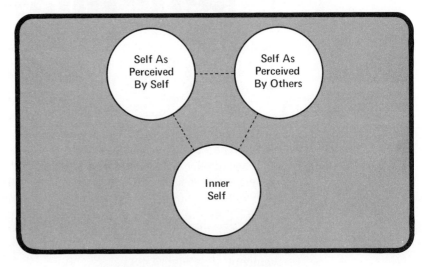

FIGURE 4.3   *The self that is not integrated.*

[11] Rogers, *Becoming a Person*, pp. 163–198.

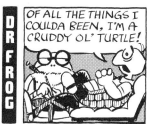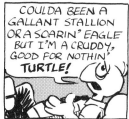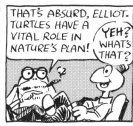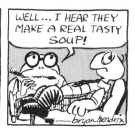

FIGURE 4.4

6. *Movement of completeness of self.* The need to realize that one must possess a personality consistent with itself.
7. *Movement toward being open to experience.* The need to avoid blotting out thoughts, perceptions, feelings, and memories that may, at times, be unpleasant.
8. *Movement toward acceptance of others.* The ability to accept others as they are and not as you would like them to be.
9. *Ability to trust.* The ability to trust and accept one's selves.

In essence, Rogers says that an individual with a healthy personality, the "fully functioning person," can present himself to others as he truly is at each moment. Such an individual does not try to misrepresent his beliefs or feelings, but instead is able to say what he thinks or express what he feels and accept the consequences of doing just that without being ashamed of who and what he is.

Richard Wright has expressed this concept:

> For a long time I toyed with the idea of writing a novel in which a Negro, Bigger Thomas, would loom as a symbolic figure of American life, a figure who would hold within him the prophecy of our future. . . .
>
> The more I thought of it the more I became convinced that if I did not write of Bigger as I saw and felt him, if I did not try to make him a living personality and at the same time a symbol of all the larger things I felt and saw in him, I'd be reacting as Bigger himself reacted; that is, I'd be acting out of *fear* if I let what I thought whites would say constrict and paralyze me.

As I contemplated Bigger and what he meant, I said to myself: "I must write this novel, not only for others to read, but to free myself of this sense of shame and fear."[12]

The Body Concept

The beliefs and ideals an individual feels in relation to his body—his body concept—play an integral role in the development of his self-concept or self-identity. A person who is mentally healthy usually accepts his body; a less mentally healthy person is more likely to have a negative body concept along with his negative self-concept.

For reasons which are not completely understood—they may include inadequate gratification of certain needs, too much or too little stimulation, parents who are unable to foster the child's efforts at individuation, or constitutional factors—some persons have been unable to meet and master these developmental tasks. Although these individuals may demonstrate a degree of maturity in other mental functions, they have become arrested at a developmental stage which does not enable them to establish a stable self-representation nor a stable body image. While they may be able to hold together under optimal circumstances, certain stresses or traumata may be sufficient to initiate a pathological regression. Such a regression reverses many of the developmental strides so that the individual must face anew the task of self-recognition, self-nonself differentiation, and body boundary determination. He senses that his grasp of self is weakening, and this generates anxiety. Whatever unity of self he has achieved, he fears, will now disintegrate. He sees himself beginning to fragment, and the common expression "I'm falling apart" is all too often literally precise.[13]

In this country especially there are several factors that may lead an individual to develop a negative body concept. Americans place great emphasis on youth and physical beauty. In many European countries overweight people are considered attractive, while in the United States, one must be almost underweight to be socially acceptable. This emphasis on appearance is seen in beauty contests, television and in advertisements in every communications medium.

[12] Richard Wright, "How Bigger Was Born," in Abraham Chapman, ed., *Black Voices: An Anthology of Afro-American Literature,* New York: New American Library, 1968, pp. 551–552.
[13] Thomas J. Luparello, "Chronic Illness, Conflict, and the Self: For Some, Illness Pays," *Medical Insight,* February 12, 1974.

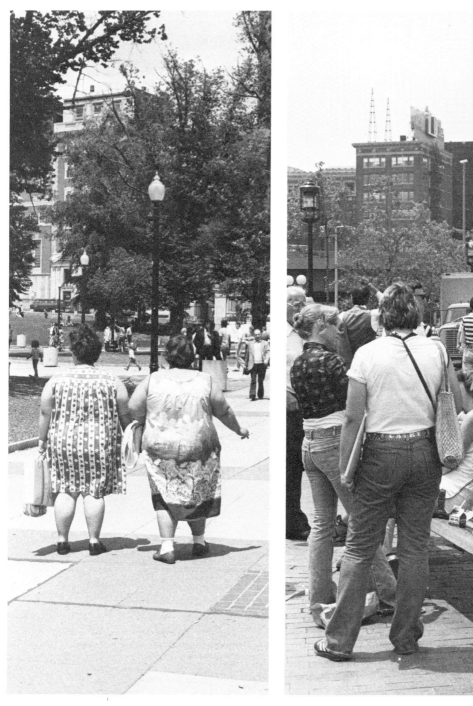

FIGURE 4.5   *Do these pictures reflect healthy body concepts?*

If a person in our society does not conform to society's concept of the ideal body, he or she may have problems in relationships with peers. This is especially true of teenagers, for adolescence seems to be a period when physical appearance is critical. This is unfortunate since this is also a period of great importance to the development of the self-concept.[14]

Usually, the first impression one receives from others is a visual one. Thus, an attractive person has less difficulty in gaining friends and socializing with the opposite sex than an unattractive person. The end result may mean an unnecessary amount of worry and anxiety simply because one does not conform to this cultural concept of the ideal face and body. A healthy acceptance of one's body can result from doing one's best to enhance his functioning and appearance. This makes acceptance and enjoyment of the qualities one has an easier task for self and others.

Self-Actualization

Abraham Maslow defined a self-actualizing person as one who is always striving to realize his inner potentialities to the fullest. In this process, he must satisfy a hierarchy of needs. According to Maslow, the seven basic needs are physiological or primary needs, security or safety needs, love or belonging needs, ego or esteem needs, self-actualization needs, cognitive needs, and aesthetic needs. (See Figure 4.6.) These needs must be approached in sequence; that is, a person must achieve fulfillment of the needs at the bottom of the hierarchy before he can strive for fulfillment of those higher up. For example, a person who is having difficulty satisfying his primary needs will not be concerned with satisfying his aesthetic needs; i.e., a person who is starving will not want to appreciate the beauty of a painting. Once the individual has satisfied certain lower, basic needs he can pursue higher goals leading to greater self-actualization and mental health.[15]

Personal Integration

The degree of personal integration is a third important factor in determining positive mental health. Jahoda defined three aspects of this integration: the balance of psychic forces in the individual, a unifying outlook on life, and resistance to stress.[16]

Balance of psychic forces means the healthy person is one whose level of consciousness is effective enough to permit the greatest discharge of primitive urges in a socially acceptable manner, and

[14] See the material on anorexia nervosa, a related problem, in Chapter 7.
[15] Those who are interested in researching this topic in greater depth should read Maslow's *Motivation and Personality* and other works.
[16] Jahoda, *Positive Mental Health.*

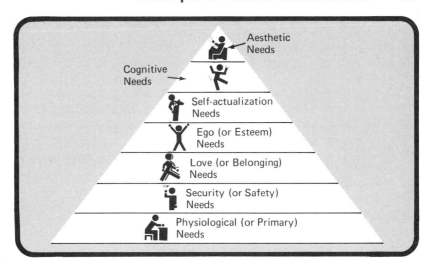

FIGURE 4.6 *The lines separating the groupings of needs in Maslow's pyramid are solid to show that, like climbing a ladder, one must gratify primary needs (take the first step) before other needs become functional, i.e., the person who is starving cannot worry about the societal consequences of stealing food.* Source: *A. H. Maslow,* Motivation and Personality, *New York: Harper & Row, Publishers, 1954.*

there is a balance between the conscious and unconscious. With this healthy balance, one has a certain degree of flexibility.

A *unifying outlook on life* does not refer to one's ability to verbalize his or her philosophy of life; it includes all aspects of personality that constitute inward unity. The ability to achieve this unifying phliosophy of life ultimately allows the individual to feel there is meaning and significance in living.

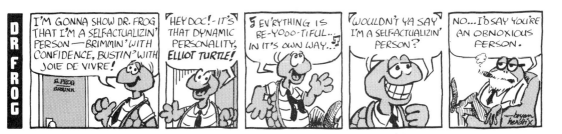

FIGURE 4.7

Resistance to stress is being able to cope with the stress of everyday living and any additional problems that may arise without excessive disruption. The healthy individual has enough ego strength to satisfy his needs, either by meeting them directly, or by finding a suitable sublimation for them. Episodes of emotional distress are inevitable, but they can be a stimulus to seeking information, preparing for change, buffering against loss, and opening new options.

Personal Autonomy

Personal autonomy is the degree of independence an individual achieves in regulating his own life. A person may be closely involved with one or more other people, but if he has a healthy degree of personal autonomy, he will maintain the independence of his personality and remain a significant person with individual characteristics. Albert Schweitzer maintained this autonomy while relating to the needs and emotions of many people: "I am life affirming itself in the midst of other lives affirming themselves."[17]

Perception of Reality

Jahoda found that of all these criteria, the perception of reality and environmental mastery were most frequently selected as determinants in mental health by the authorities consulted. An individual's perception of reality is quite important in his achievement of mental well-being.

One's reality perception should be compatible with evidence and logic and with the reality perceptions of others. Maslow found that one of the characteristics of an individual in the lifelong process of attaining self-actualization is that he has an efficient perception of reality and a comfortable relationship with it. He can detect what is real and authentic and gravitate toward it. Furthermore, he does not divide reality and unreality into mutually exclusive compartments; rather, he knows and appreciates the facts of existence without minimizing the importance of imagination, fantasy, dreams, and fiction.[18]

Environmental Mastery

A final criterion in the determination of mental health is environmental mastery. Jahoda listed six qualities necessary for environmental mastery: (1) the ability to love; (2) adequacy in love, work, and play; (3) adequacy in interpersonal relations; (4) efficiency in meeting situational requirements; (5) capacity for adaptation and adjustment; and (6) efficiency in problem solving.

The ability to love includes the ability to love both self and others. People who love themselves are people who also love others.

[17] Albert Schweitzer, *The Philosophy of Civilization,* New York: Macmillan Publishing Co., 1963.
[18] Maslow, *Motivation and Personality.*

Erich Fromm is criticized by traditional psychotherapists for his emphasis on self-love, which they feel is in opposition to loving others; yet, in *The Art of Loving,* Fromm says explicitly that people who do not love themselves cannot love others.[19] Adequacy in love, work, and play is being able to find enjoyment in family, work, and recreation; adequacy in interpersonal relations is the ability to get along with others.

Efficiency in meeting situational requirements means that the individual can cope with and tolerate well the demands of his environment. The capacity for adaptation and adjustment means that the individual has worked out an arrangement between himself and reality. Adjustment requires that the individual attain a satisfactory relationship between his environment and himself and between his needs and his interests. Finally, efficiency in problem solving means that the individual can both identify his problems and work on them directly.[20]

FURTHER READINGS

Harris, Thomas A. *I'M OK—YOU'RE OK: A Practical Guide To Transactional Analysis.* New York: Harper & Row, 1969.

A very easy reading book on the work of Dr. Eric Berne which clarifies the principles of Transactional Analysis.

Jourard, Sidney M. *The Transparent Self.* New York: D. Van Nostrand Co., 1971.

Explores the implications of a new premise: man can attain health and fullest personal development only insofar as he gains courage to be himself with others.

Lowen, Alexander. *The Betrayal of the Body.* London: Collier Books, 1967.

The author discusses the fact that bodily pleasure is a vital source of emotional fulfillment through body awareness and the recovery of a gratifying mind-body relationship.

Maslow, Abraham H. *Religions, Values, and Peak-Experiences.* New York: The Viking Press, 1970.

One of the foremost spokesmen for the Third Force movement in psychology, Abraham Maslow, here articulates one of his prominent theses: the "religious" experience is a rightful subject for scientific investigation and speculation and, conversely, the "scientific community" will see its work enhanced by acknowledging and studying the species-wide need for spiritual expression which, in many forms, is at the heart of "peak experiences" reached by healthy, fully functioning persons.

Pirsig, Robert M. *Zen And The Art of Motorcycle Maintenance.* New York: Bantam Books, 1974.

A book about feeling and caring, about what we are and the quality of our lives. The story of a father and son on the road and their story of self discovery.

---

[19] Erich Fromm, *The Art of Loving,* New York: Harper Colophon Books, 1956.
[20] Jahoda, *Positive Mental Health.*

Chapter 5

Coping with
Stress and Anxiety

STRESS AND ANXIETY

Almost every day brings some problems with which we must cope or situations that call for decision making. Most people react to difficult situations by feeling stress. There are various kinds of stress, classified by degree and duration.[1] Mild stress—lasting from seconds to hours—can be caused by missing a train, minor criticism, public appearances before large audiences, unexpected guests, or other lesser problems of daily life. Moderate stress, which can last from hours to days, may stem from disturbing factors such as overwork, temporary absence of a spouse, or some other relatively minor emotional problem. Severe stress—lasting for weeks, months, even years—could be precipitated by the death of a loved one, financial reverses, chronic illness, or the prolongation of an "intolerable situation."

A stressful situation, then, is one that imposes on an individual demands for adjustment.[2] Stress may be *external* (caused by environmental factors), *internal* (arising primarily out of the physical and/or emotional state of the individual), or a combination of the two.

Internal stress can result from an inability to satisfy a need or desire because of inhibitions, conflicts, or fear of the consequences. It may be caused by inner conflicts and self-doubt, concern about responsibility or about the future, or worries about being accepted and loved. Severe internal stress can represent a more serious threat to the personality than external stress, for severe internal stress

[1] D. L. Dodge and W. T. Martin, *Social Stress and Chronic Illness,* Notre Dame, Ind.: University of Notre Dame, 1970, pp. 60–61.
[2] M. Goldenson, *The Encyclopedia of Human Behavior: Psychology, Psychiatry and Mental Health,* Garden City, N.Y.: Doubleday, 1970, p. 1263.

may create dangerous emotional tension and accompanying behavioral disorders.

One of the symptoms of stress is anxiety. Anxiety reactions may involve shortness of breath, rapid heartbeat, dryness of mouth, loss of appetite, or insomnia. These reactions are actually the body's way of mobilizing itself to deal more effectively with danger, in what is called the "fight-or-flight" syndrome. The physical changes occur because of the increased adrenalin released by the glands in reaction to a stressful situation.

Conflict

Conflict is one of the major causes of stress. Kurt Lewen, an eminent psychologist, has developed a field theory of four kinds of conflict an individual may encounter. These four types are called approach-approach, avoidance-avoidance, approach-avoidance, and double approach-avoidance.[3]

> The terms *approach* and *avoidance* must not be understood simply as "going towards" or "away from" a stimulus in a spatial sense. Thus "rage," when it goes over into attack, is an "avoidance" response, even though it involves "going towards" something. *Avoidance* must be defined in terms of its objectives —to discontinue, to remove or escape from a certain type of stimulation and not in terms of its overt characteristics. Attack has as its objective removal of the source of stimulation in the same way that withdrawal does. *Approach* must also be defined functionally—i.e., it is any activity the objective of which is to continue, maintain, or pursue a certain kind of stimulation.
>
> *Source:* Michael Argyle, *British Journal of Social and Clinical Psychology,* 1962.

In an *approach-approach* conflict, the individual must choose between two equally desirable situations. An example of this would be the girl who is dating two boys. One may be good-looking, strong, athletic, and popular; the other may be studious, reliable, sympathetic, and understanding. She must weigh the advantages of each relationship.

An *avoidance-avoidance* conflict arises when the individual must choose between two undesirable alternatives. For example, a boy may no longer enjoy dating a certain girl, but he is afraid to break off their relationship for fear of hurting her. He no longer wants to date her, but neither does he want to cause her great unhappiness.

[3] Kurt Lewen, *A Dynamic Theory of Personality,* New York: McGraw-Hill, 1935.

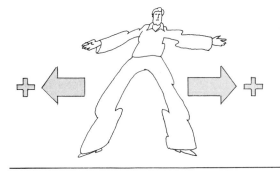

Approach-Approach: Here the individual is attracted by two equally desirable goals. His conflict is he cannot decide which one is best.

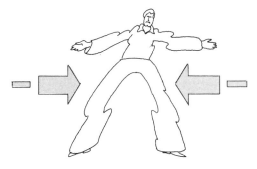

Avoidance-Avoidance: Here the individual is faced with two unpleasant alternatives. People caught in this situation usually react by vacillating — they move one way just a little, then the other.

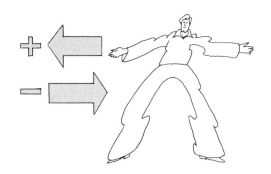

Double Avoidance-Approach: Here the individual is both attracted and repelled by the same situation or goal. An example is the "delightful scoundrel". . . the charmer you can't help but like, but certainly wouldn't want to marry!

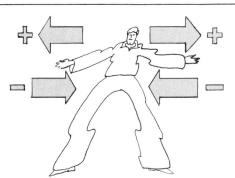

Approach-Avoidance: Everybody can think of the situation in which they wanted to do something but felt that it was wrong. Most often this has to do with family conflicts such as "You can take the car as long as you do not drive it too fast!"

FIGURE 5.1   *Ways of dealing with conflict.*

In an *approach-avoidance conflict,* the individual is confronted with a situation that is both attractive and repellent at the same time. Sexual conflicts often involve approach-avoidance responses. A girl may desire sexual intercourse with her boyfriend, but she has been brought up to feel that nonmarital sex is wrong. A boy may find masturbation pleasurable but he experiences guilt feelings because of the attitude of his parents toward this act.

A double *approach-avoidance* conflict involves two situations that each have positive and negative values. For example, a woman may want to have children and then spend a great deal of time with them, but she also enjoys her career. The children may stand in the way of her career for several years, but her career may not allow her to spend much time with her children. Each alternative is both desirable and undesirable.

COPING WITH STRESS AND ANXIETY

Individuals vary considerably in the extent to which they can tolerate stress and anxiety. A situation that one person finds extremely stressful may cause only mild anxiety in another individual. These variations in response and tolerance levels may be determined by genetic makeup, individual experiences, or the individual's internal perspective. Coping depends ultimately on the way problems are perceived.

Stress Tolerance

When danger threatens, the input and impact of warning messages may vary from one individual to another. In 1971, a Civil Defense warning system alarm was accidentally set off. Although the warning of impending disaster was received by radio stations all over the nation, most did not broadcast it to their listeners. Their reaction was a mixture of apathy and denial of the situation. Those radio stations that did warn people were besieged with telephone calls from listeners asking if the warning were authentic.

Thus, when a warning of impending disaster was received, the first response of many people was to deny the message or to have it verified. Then a check was made on the authority of the transmitter and truth of the warning. Many people tended to discount the authenticity of the warning, rationalizing it as a mistake.

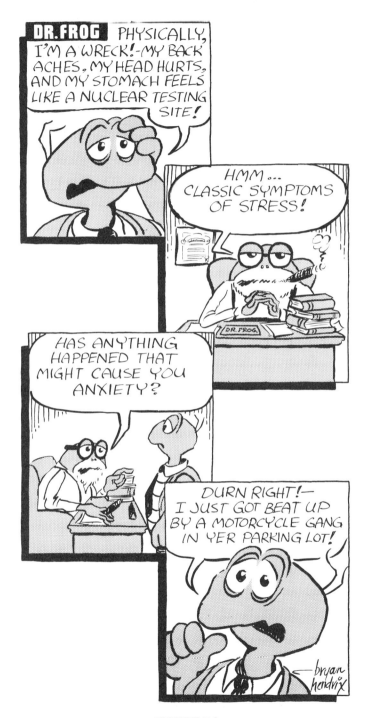

FIGURE 5.2

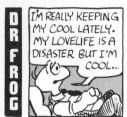 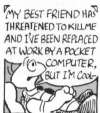 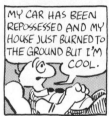 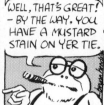 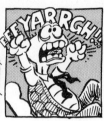

FIGURE 5.3

Mild or moderate stress actually can be helpful. Learning to handle stress is an essential component of the coping process. Just as exposure to small doses of certain noxious agents can prevent physical illness (e.g., a typhoid shot contains the typhus bacteria), exposure to relatively moderate stressful situations helps to build coping mechanisms. An individual must learn to mobilize his responses and resources. The degree of stress is the crucial factor—while moderate stress can motivate the individual to positive response, severe stress can be incapacitating.

Each person reacts to anxiety differently. Fifty "normal" men and women were asked to relate how they respond to anxiety-producing situations in their lives.[4] Their answers covered a broad range from: "There is a sense of uncertainty about the future" and "I try to stop thinking of the situation and try to think of other things" to "There's tension across my back," "I have no appetite," "I have a gnawing feeling in the pit of my stomach." No matter how anxiety is defined, each of us has two alternatives: to cope with anxiety and accept it as a signal ("I am feeling anxious now") or to become overwhelmed and helpless in the face of mass stimulation ("I always feel anxious").

The "fight-or-flight" reaction is a positive response. At an optimum level of anxiety, the individual can become increasingly vigilant, experiencing greater awareness of external events and a greater ability to cope with danger. Although increased vigilance and

[4] M. Lader and I. Marks, *Clinical Anxiety,* New York: Grune and Stratton, 1971, pp. 1–2.

sensitivity occur at higher levels of anxiety, the ability to differentiate the dangerous from the trivial is reduced. As anxiety mounts, the individual becomes less capable of mastering it. His behavior loses spontaneity and flexibility. The inability to cope may lead to depression or traumatic[5] or neurotic[6] anxiety. It is not the anxiety itself but the way we handle it that constitutes the difference between emotional sickness and health.

Defense Mechanisms   One of the most common ways of dealing with stress and anxiety is the use of *defense mechanisms*. These may be the easiest way of dealing with problems, but they are clearly not the most positive response. In moderation, they can be helpful modes of adjustment, but when they become the dominant modes maladjustment is indicated. All defense mechanisms involve self-deception. The price of persistent self-deception is likely to be a weakened capacity to adapt or deal with various situations. If the use of defense mechanisms is the consistent response to a problem, attention is distracted from the anxiety-provoking situation, obscuring it and making its eventual solution more difficult.

Among the most common defense mechanisms are:

1. *Repression* involves unconsciously banning from memory traumatic, dangerous, or embarrassing thoughts, events, and impulses. Repression can vary in degree from a relatively simple type of forgetting to pathological conditions. Repressors reveal long latencies in perceiving threat, they tend to deny failure, they either deny or are unaware of their anxiety, and they show tendencies to forget disturbing events.
2. *Regression* is a defense whereby the personality returns to earlier modes of behavior. The events most significantly related to regression seem to involve threats to security.
3. *Denial* is one of the most primitive of the defense mechanisms and one frequently used by children or severely disturbed adults. In denial, the individual rejects an intolerable reality by denying its existence.
4. *Fantasy* is a common form of escape, since everyone likes to daydream. Some daydreaming is normal and even beneficial or positive. An excessive reliance on fantasy can lead to increasing immobilization and incapacity to cope with the environment.
5. *Phobia* is an excessive and unreasonable fear of some object or situation. Usually the phobia represents a displacement from the stimulus that first aroused the fear.
6. *Amnesia* is an inability to recall past experiences. It is considered to be a defense mechanism since the act of forgetting is motivated by a need to shut out painful experiences.

[5] R. R. Grinker, *Archives of General Psychiatry,* November 1959, p. 537.
[6] M. Rosenberg, "The Association between Self-Esteem and Anxiety," *Psychiatric Research,* Great Britain: Pergmon Press, 1952, p. 137.

7. *Displacement* transfers emotions from one object, activity, or situation to another.
8. *Introjection and identification* both involve unconscious imitation of the attributes and qualities of another person. When a child has introjected the attributes of a parent, we say that he has identified with the parent; this process usually occurs at an early stage of development and is basic to healthy adjustment.
9. *Projection* is perceiving in others those weaknesses that the victim feels are his own.
10. *Rationalization* is one of the most common and harmless of the defense mechanisms. Rationalization is a way of fooling ourselves by substituting "good" reasons for "bad" ones in order to make our behavior more ethical or acceptable than it really is. We seek to excuse our failure by placing blame on circumstances that are outside our control.
11. *Sublimation* involves repressing the expression of an impulse in its original form and allowing it to emerge in a socialized manner so that it can be gratified without disapproval. Sublimation has a quality of maturity since it enables a person to meet reality rather than to flee from it.
12. *Reaction formation* constitutes developing the very behavior against which the individual is defending himself.
13. *Compensation* is a method for handling our deficiencies by "making up" for them in some way. Compensation may be direct or indirect. Direct action attempts to get at the source of the inferiority and remove it; sometimes the source of frustration cannot be removed by direct action—substitution is a form of indirect compensation.

✓ Selye's General Adaptation Syndrome

In 1936 Hans Selye published a major paper on stress and the human body. He coined the term "stress syndrome" in developing his concept of a General Adaptation Syndrome (GAS).

Selye discussed a three-stage action-reaction process, which could lead to stress-produced physiological illness. In the *alarm reaction stage,* the body sounds an alarm as a reaction to stress. If the stress lasts long enough, the body reaches the *stage of resistance,* in which it attempts to restore homeostasis (stability or balance) by making adjustments to meet the changes in the environment. In this stage, the ability to withstand the stressful situation is the strongest. After days or weeks, the final *stage of exhaustion* may occur. There may be a general breakdown of the adaptation process, resulting in damage to the body; there is little resistance to infectious organisms.[7]

[7] Hans Selye, *The Physiology and Pathology of Exposure to Stress,* Montreal: Acta, 1950, or the less technical *The Stress of Life,* New York: McGraw-Hill, 1956.

Illness Caused by Stress

If one's adaptation and tolerance levels are high, he is better equipped to deal with the tension produced by stress. Those with low levels may develop functional disorders. These disorders may have physical symptoms, but when they are produced by psychological stress, they are termed *psychosomatic disorders.* These are most likely to occur in a person at the resistance stage in the stress syndrome.

Minor problems caused by tension may be headaches, skin eruptions, temporary insomnia, or loss of appetite. More severe disorders that may be psychosomatic or psychophysiological are gastrointestinal problems such as ulcers or colitis, migraine headaches, respiratory ailments, and cardiovascular disorders.

RESPONSES TO STRESS AND ANXIETY

Some individuals have little difficulty in coping with their lives. Others may become moderately or severely depressed and serious mental illness may result. Some people view suicide as the only answer to their problems.

Depression

Depression is the leading mental illness in the United States today. According to Dr. Gerald Klerman, Professor of Psychiatry at Harvard, one out of every eight Americans will, at some time during his life, suffer from a depression serious enough to require psychiatric help. More disturbing is evidence that depression is spreading most rapidly among the nation's young people. Some psychiatrists discern a pervasive apathy among American youth, produced they believe by frustration over values, crime, corruption in government, and environmental problems.

Although depression is one of the most prevalent and serious of illnesses, it is one of the least understood. The term depression is really a catch-all; like some clinical labels, it embraces a whole family of disorders. To quote Dr. Ronald Fieve, Chief of Psychiatric Research at New York State Psychiatric Institute:

> In spite of all of our scientific efforts, to this day no agreement exists as to diagnosis, epidemiology, classification, cause, or effective therapies for this illness. The only area of agreement in depression is that it is ubiquitous and universal, and that it appears to be part of the human condition, ranging from a normal mood change to a qualitatively different psychiatric and medical state.

Everyone has highs and lows in mood. A grief reaction to a serious loss is a normal part of the human personality. Upsetting situations naturally result in depression. Physicians become concerned when these feelings are so intense and pervasive that they interfere with everyday living. Depressed people often cannot perform the most routine tasks: dressing, eating, even getting out of bed in the morning or talking may become an effort. Passivity and withdrawal are the most common symptoms of depression.

Types of Depression

Psychiatrists have long debated just when depression sets in and how it is triggered. In an attempt to impose some order on the problem, they have divided depression into two categories: endogenous and exogenous.

Endogenous depression originates within the body. Manic-depression and the involutional melancholy of menopausal women and middle-aged men are classified as endogenous. *Exogenous* depression is triggered by outside events. People suffering from exogenous depression usually show evidence of a long-standing neurotic personality disorder. In particular, their "ego strength" appears impaired because of habits established early in childhood and persisting into adulthood.

It is encouraging that despite all the controversy over diagnosing and understanding the illness, once identified, depression is one of the most treatable of all mental disorders.[8]

Psychosis and Neurosis

Psychiatry no longer recognizes any clear-cut division between normal and abnormal behavior. However, behavior is generally considered abnormal when it severely interferes with one's ability to function in society.[9] Abnormal behavior can be classified as either *neurotic* or *psychotic*. Neurotic behavior is closer to the normal end of the spectrum than is psychotic behavior. A neurotic may be aware of his problems and may be able to contribute to his recovery whereas psychotic behavior is far more serious and affects all aspects of the individual's personality. A psychotic person has lost some or all contact with reality.

The major symptom of neurosis is anxiety. Its various forms represent classes of habits used by neurotic individuals to reduce their anxiety and thereby live with it. In general, no matter what form his symptoms take, the neurotic finds life difficult, and others may find living with him difficult.

[8] See "Coping with Depression," *Newsweek,* January 8, 1973, pp. 51–54.
[9] Sigmund Freud, *An Outline of Psychoanalysis,* New York: Norton, 1949.

Table 5.1 *Comparison of Neurotic and Psychotic Disorders in Terms of Primary Characteristics. Source:* A. A. Schneiders, *Personal Dynamics and Mental Health,* New York: Holt, Rinehart and Winston, Inc., 1965, p. 308. Reprinted by permission of the publishers.

Neuroses	Psychoses
Reactions less severe	Reactions much more severe and disturbing: disruptive in character
Less pervasive, involving only several areas of personality	Extremely pervasive; tend to involve the whole personality
Fairly good contact with reality	Generally poor contact with reality; may involve total abandonment of reality
Emotions fairly flexible: little impoverishment	Considerable emotional debilitation; often seriously diminished or abolished altogether
No intellectual deterioration; some impairment	Often serious intellectual deterioration or impairment
Generally fairly good insight: capacity to be objective regarding self	Generally lacking in insight; little understanding of difficulty
Not incapacitated; able to live in society	Incapacitated; often dangerous to self and society
Seldom require hospitalization	Require hospitalization

The psychotic presents an altogether different picture. Where the neurotic finds life difficult and may be incapacitated in some respects, the psychotic has lost his normal behavioral controls. He may actually be dangerous to himself and others.

As with neurosis, the forms of psychotic disorders reflect the particular adjustment mechanisms normally used to deal with life's stresses. There are some milder forms of psychoses, but there is usually a severe breakdown of normal adult or even neurotic adjustment patterns. The adjustments used are primitive, often child-like.

Though there are no sharply defined distinctions between neurotic and psychotic disorders, Schneiders, in his *Personal Dynamics of Mental Health,* has made comparison of generally observed differences. These are shown in Table 5.1.

Suicide   Some people who find they are failing to cope with their problems turn to suicide as the ultimate answer. Twelve out of every 100,000 people in the United States take this "final step" each year. If hidden and otherwise unrecorded suicides were included, this rate would probably double. More deaths are actually suicides than those in which the victim has left a note. Some of these are what Dr. Edwin Shneidman of the Los Angeles Suicide Prevention Center calls "subintentioned suicides"—deaths that occur from overindulgence in drink and drugs, from reckless driving, or from untreated illness. Many experts see a "hidden death wish" being carried out in such careless behavior that leads to a fatality.

In all countries more men than women kill themselves, though the past decade has seen an increase in the number of female suicides in this country. Suicide rates increase with age, which follows from the fact that the threat of ill health is one of the most common reasons for suicide.

Why?

". . . there are accidental suicides," writes Karl Menninger, "there are suicides which are substitutes for murder, there are suicides which are a cry for help, and suicides which are miscarriages of an attempt to get oneself rescued. But some suicides are also expressions of total despair and ruthlessly directed at one's own self-annihilation."[10]

Emile Durkheim, generally regarded as the father of suicide research, related all suicides to the individual's degree of societal integration. He found three major categories of suicides: the altruistic, the egoistic, and the anomic. Altruistic suicides are committed by people who have completely subordinated themselves to their social identities (e.g., the Kamikaze pilots). The egoistic group consists of those individuals whose lives have no structure because of their tenuous links to society; they have lived an almost hermetic existence. Anomic suicides are committed by those individuals who have suddenly become detached from the needed structure of their lives because of events around them (the Great Depression, a death of a loved one). Sociological factors that contribute to the suicide rate in the United States are: war and postwar adjustment, economic depressions, religious and social disorganization.

Suicide is often difficult to comprehend. The increase over the past decade of suicides by young people is one fact that is especially difficult to explain.

Suicide and the College Student

Suicide is the second leading cause of death (after accidents) among college students. In any given year, approximately 1,000 college students actually commit suicide; another 9,000 attempt it; and 100,000 threaten it. Richard Seiden feels that these statistics, showing suicide to be increasing as a major cause of death, are misleading.

[10] Karl Menninger, *Man against Himself,* New York: Harcourt, Brace & Co., 1938.

Spotting the Potential Suicide

Both patients are obviously depressed. But their symptoms vary considerably. Patient A complains of chronic tiredness, indecisiveness, and an inability to get anything done. Patient B is nagged by a sense of failure and a lack of satisfaction.

Which of the two is more likely to commit suicide? According to a report by psychologists Aaron T. Beck and David Lester, it's B. In a study of 254 attempted suicides, the two found feelings of guilt, hopelessness, failure, self-hate, and suicidal wishes to be the most commonly expressed sentiments.

Other depressives, they note, complain of listlessness, irritability, and loss of libido and exhibit such psychological symptoms as weight loss and fatigability. But rarely, if ever, do they express feelings of hopelessness or extreme guilt.

A. T. Beck and D. Lester "Components of Depression in Attempted Suicides." Journal of Psychology, *(Nov.) 1973.*

He attributes the prominence of suicide to a "mortality shift." Improvements in sanitation, medical care, and pharmacology have all but eliminated many infectious diseases as causes of death, so that the position on the scale of violent deaths and suicide has risen.[11]

Seiden has discovered some dominant characteristics of college students who attempt to commit suicide:

- Many students who commit suicide lack any involvement with other students (or professors). He cites the example of a student who had died eighteen days before he was found in his room.
- Married teenagers have a higher risk of suicide than nonmarrieds. (This applies not just to college students.)
- Most students who commit suicide have a prior psychiatric history.
- There is no evidence for a causal connection between adolescent drug use and suicide.
- High achievers have a higher incidence of suicide.
- Early loss or absence of a parent is extremely important as a precursor to suicide.
- Realistic stresses (e.g., final exams, etc.) are not as important as they may first appear to be in precipitating suicidal behavior.[12]

Another cause that has been found is the fear of emotional illness. "In case after case among those attempting self-destruction, the reason given for the act has been a variation of the refrain,

[11] Richard H. Seiden, "The Problem of Suicide on the College Campuses," *Journal of School Health,* May 1971, p. 243.
[12] Ibid.

. . . thought I was going crazy; tried to kill myself so I wouldn't go crazy; did not want to lose my mind,' and so on.''[13]

Disappointment in love or problems with sexual relations are other important factors in suicide attempts by college students, especially women. Because parents exert intense pressure on their daughters to conform to social codes of premarital chastity, sexual relationships seem to carry a disproportionate load of guilt for many female students. To some, suicide seems the only way out.

SEEKING HELP

Most of us, at one time or another, face problems with which we feel we need help. We may be able to work out the solutions ourselves or with the advice of a friend; sometimes counselling is necessary. The tragic cases are those people who need help but do not seek it, because they feel they don't need it or because they think getting help is only for "crazy people."

Transcendental Meditation

Transcendental meditation is enjoying widespread popularity as a method of relieving tension and anxiety. This technique involves two periods of "quietness" (about twenty minutes in length) each day, in which the meditator frees his mind of all thoughts by concentrating on a special repeated word (or *mantra*).

Scientific research has shown that during the meditation period the body attains the deepest possible state of rest, a state far deeper than sleep. This profound rest eliminates accumulated tension and anxieties that often remain even after sleep. Doctors have long realized the relationship between tension and disease, and TM has been shown to lower high blood pressure, and contribute to overall physical and mental well-being.

The technique of TM is easily learned in a few short periods of instruction. It can then be practiced at almost any time or place, without any special setting, preparation, or lifestyle. There are various experts or groups offering training in transcendental meditation (in which each person is assigned his *mantra*). One of the researchers of transcendental meditation, Dr. Herbert Benson, a cardiologist at Harvard Medical School, has published a "self-help" book. The technique he employed for relaxation and meditation can be easily learned from his text, *The Relaxation Response*.

---

[13] Louis I. Dublin, *Suicide: A Sociological and Statistical Study,* New York: Ronald Press, 1963, p. 24.

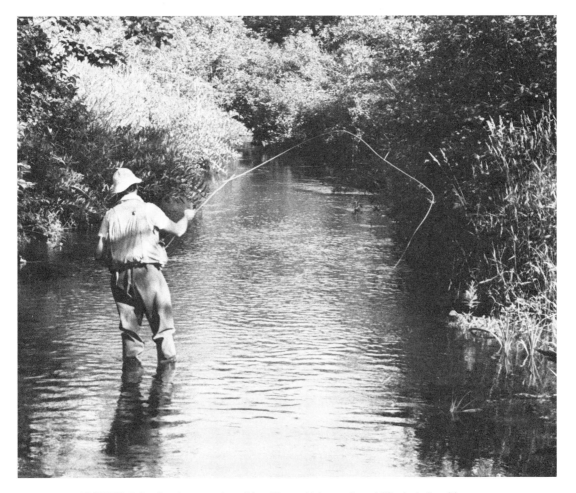

FIGURE 5.4 *Such normal and healthy outlets as the ability to talk with some-one are sometimes difficult to come by. For everyone certain activities become a form of self-therapy.*

Helping Yourself   Sometimes you can change life conditions; other times you can only adapt to them. There are many ways of learning to cope.

Only trial and error will teach you how much you can take—how many courses, deadlines, competitions, or roles (such as student, lover, worker, socialite). Pare away excess—try not to do what you don't want to do, and don't do what you don't have to do. Try to deal with anxiety realistically when it occurs—if you're afraid you're going to flunk, then study harder or drop the course. Put off going out if you don't feel up to it. Postpone a visit from parents if it is causing you anxiety. Space your time so that you can do those things well that you want to do. Exercise more—it is a better stress defense than sleep. Get involved with those activities that you enjoy most and bring you the greatest reward. Pills or alcohol are *not* the answer to stress.

There are an increasing number of books and programs aimed at self-help. Some of these are worthwhile, while others may be worthless. Some are of value to some individuals but do not apply to other types of people. *Escape from Stress* by Kenneth Lamott discusses several techniques for coping with the problems of anxiety. Transcendental meditation and yoga are increasingly popular methods of learning to relax. (See box for a fuller description of transcendental meditation.) Meeting with other people in group sessions can be a solution for some of your problems and theirs.

Helping Others   The recent trend toward discussion or personal growth groups to increase self- and other-awareness is an encouraging one. *Anyone* has the capacity for becoming a helping person. Carl Rogers, who was among the first to conceive of the psychotherapy relationship as one of mutual trust and respect, states:

> I believe the quality of my encounter is more important in the long run than is my scholarly knowledge, my professional training, my counseling orientation, the techniques I use in the interview. In keeping with this line of thought, I suspect that for a guidance worker also the relationship he forms with each student—brief or continuing—is more important than his knowledge of tests and measurements, the adequacy of his record keeping, the theories he holds, the accuracy with which he is able to predict academic success, or the school in which he received his training.[14]

When you are placed in the role of a counselor, an attitude of firmness and common sense is usually the most helpful. Be kind, but not overly so; in other words, discuss problems realistically. Your friend will learn to trust you if you seem to present an honest evaluation; if you are overly optimistic, he may feel you are lying or being evasive.

The individual struggling with a crisis situation may often send out messages such as these:

> "I feel hopeless, and nothing or nobody can help." At this point, the one thing the person may need most is a significant relationship with someone else.

[14] Carl R. Rogers and Barry Stevens, *Person to Person,* New York: Pocket Books, 1972, p. 86.

- "I'm a failure." This is a statement from depression; other signs may indicate the severity of the depression.
- "I feel terribly guilty and ashamed." This is another aspect of depression. Much of the guilt here is not true guilt, but rather the "if only . . ." variety. In very few cases is the individual truly at fault, but a depressed person cannot see this.

You may reach a point when you feel you are no longer able to help the person. Know when to refer him to someone more qualified than you. Remember, though, that the individual turned to you as a special person, and reassure them that you will continue to stand by them.

Professional Help   There are various qualified people offering different types of professional counseling. Some types of therapy are more productive for a specific individual than others.

Types of Therapy

There are many techniques employed in therapy, from psychoanalysis to group therapy. The major types (with some overlap) are described here:

- *psychotherapy* is a general term for the treatment by a qualified individual of a patient's mental disturbances
- *psychoanalysis* is a type of therapy first practiced by Sigmund Freud. It concentrates on the patient's subconscious mind, using techniques such as dream analysis and free association. It is usually a lengthy process, involving several meetings weekly over a period of years. Psychoanalysis is a very specific type of treatment that is only beneficial for a small number of patients
- *behavior therapy* is concerned with modifying behavior problems through various techniques rather than concentrating on the inner motivations of the patient
- *gestalt therapy* was originated by Fritz Perls. It is an approach opposite to Freudian psychotherapy and analysis, as it deals with the patient's present reactions and feelings rather than past influences and motivations
- *expressive therapy* uses Freud's free association technique. The therapist creates a permissive atmosphere but plays an indirect role in the therapeutic process
- *creative therapy* uses creative activity to achieve adjustment
- *directive therapy* is a technique in which the therapist takes an active role by helping to uncover conflicts and giving interpretations and directive guidance
- *nondirective therapy* places the major responsibility for the direction of a therapy on the patient
- *group therapy* assists the individual in achieving conflict resolution and orientation through a process of interaction with other individuals

- *multiple therapy* involves more than one therapist working with one patient
- *psychodrama* or *role playing* lets the patient act out his problems to gain more insight into these problems, his relationships with others, and his self-concept
- *drug therapy* involves the use of tranquilizers or stimulants, usually together with another form of psychotherapy
- *shock therapy* may use insulin or electric current for shock to make the patient receptive to psychotherapy. It has been replaced by drug therapy except in extreme cases

Most therapists or counseling groups use a combination of these techniques. Sometimes the specific technique used is determined by the nature of the patient's personality and problems; in other cases the therapist concentrates on one type of therapy.

Types of Therapists

The major experts in therapy are the psychiatrist, psychoanalyst, psychologist, the psychiatric social worker, and the psychiatric nurse.

The *psychiatrist* is an M.D. who specializes in the diagnosis, care, and treatment of patients suffering from emotional disorders. He must spend three years in residency training in a hospital where mental illness is treated, and two additional years of specialty experience; he must be licensed by the Board of Psychiatry and Neurology of the American Medical Association, the American Psychiatric Association, and the American Neurological Association. He may use various methods of treatment, including drug therapy.

The *psychoanalyst* is usually an M.D. with extensive training in the area of psychoanalysis. He must undergo analysis as part of his training.

The *psychologist* is an individual without a medical degree who has done postgraduate work in human behavior or mental disorders. He may have an M.A. or a Ph.D.; a *clinical psychologist* must have a Ph.D. The clinical psychologist has had training in areas such as personality dynamics, learning, psychometrics, neurology, mental hygiene, and/or clinical therapy. He cannot use drug or shock therapy, but applies psychological testing, diagnostic, and treatment procedures. He is licensed by the American Psychological Association.

The *psychiatric social worker* has an M.A. in social work with concentration and training in psychology. He has done field work in a mental hospital, clinic, or family service agency and works in one of these areas.

A *psychiatric nurse* is a registered nurse with additional training and experience with emotionally disturbed patients.

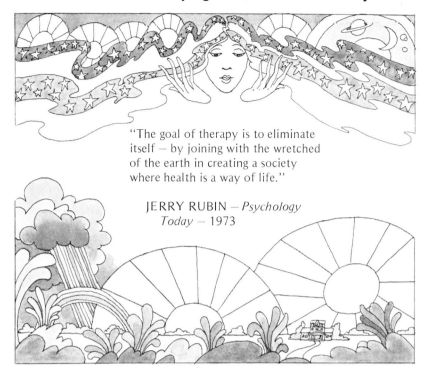

"The goal of therapy is to eliminate
itself — by joining with the wretched
of the earth in creating a society
where health is a way of life."

JERRY RUBIN — *Psychology
Today* — 1973

FIGURE 5.5

Where To Find Help

Information on where to find help can be obtained from many places.
Most public schools and almost all colleges and universities have
counselors who can provide help or suggest further sources of treatment. Community mental health centers may offer counseling or
recommendations for therapists.

Beware the Quacks

All states require medical doctors to be licensed, but not all states
set up standards for those offering various counseling services. This
lack has led some experts to focus attention on quackery within the
mental health profession.

Dr. Roger D. Freeman, a psychiatrist associated with Temple
University, says there is no easy way to spot a quack, but a prospective patient should be suspicious of therapists who:

> offer to provide services for which their training and experience
> are clearly inadequate

- make excessive claims without good evidence (caution is typical of the honest professional)
- are unwilling to consider that results might be caused by factors other than therapy
- claim without evidence that their treatment is more "natural" than others and that they are treating not merely symptoms, but basic causes

SUMMARY

No one of the therapies, groups, situations, or activities may be held up as "the way to happiness." As the late Alan W. Watts, a devotee of Zen, Episcopal priest, and lay psychologist said:

> Since there is no real "way" to *satori* (enlightenment or self-realization), the way you are following makes very little difference . . . If you really want to spend some years in a Japanese monastery, there is no earthly reason why you shouldn't. Or if you want to spend your time hopping freight cars and digging Charlie Parker, it's a free country.
>
> *In the landscape of Spring there is neither better nor worse;*
> *The flowering branches grow naturally, some long, some short.*[15]

FURTHER READINGS

Brennecke, John H. and Amick, Robert G. *The Struggle for Significance.* Beverly Hills, Calif.: Glencoe Press, 1971.

This book gives the individual student and casual reader some idea of the importance of life and of living it fully, experimentally, excitingly.

Frankl, Viktor E. *Man's Search for Meaning.* New York: Washington Square Press, Inc., 1963.

In this book, Dr. Frankl develops his theory of *logotherapy,* which, according to Frankl ". . . makes the concept of man into a whole . . . and focuses its attention upon mankind's groping for a higher meaning in life."

Lowen, Alexander. *The Betrayal of the Body.* London: Collier Books, 1967.

The author discusses the fact that bodily pleasure is a vital source of emotional well-being. The book charts a new course toward emotional fulfillment through body awareness and the recovery of a gratifying mind-body relationship.

Lynd, Helen Merrill. *On Shame and the Search for Identity.* New York: Harcourt, Brace & World, Inc., 1958.

This book probes into the complex and still unexplored phenomenon of understanding one's self and one's relation to others and to society.

[15] Alan W. Watts, *The Joyous Cosmology,* New York: Pantheon, 1962, pp. 106–110.

Martin, Lealon E. *Mental Health/Mental Illness.* New York: McGraw-Hill Book Co., 1970.

A main theme of this book is the author's positive concept of mental health and its overriding importance for the individual and for society.

Reutenbeek, Hendrick M. *The Individual and the Crowd: A Study of Identity in America.* New York: Mentor Book, 1964.

The author explores the problem of achieving individual identity in a culture in which one must function as a member of the group.

Schultz, William. *Joy.* New York: Grove Press, Inc., 1967.

A description of the ways one can bring joy into his life without the use of drugs.

Szasz, Thomas S. *The Myth of Mental Illness.* New York: Dell Publishing Co., 1961.

Szasz presents the theory that mental diseases do not exist in the same sense in which bodily diseases exist.

Other Readings

Axline, Virginia. *Dibs: In Search of Self.*

Cantril, Hadley. *Reflections on the Human Venture.*

Dethier, Vincent. *To Know a Fly.*

Green, Hannah. *I Never Promised You a Rose Garden.*

Hesse, Hermann, *Siddhartha.*

Lorenz, Konrad. *King Solomon's Ring.*

3

PHYSICAL WELL-BEING

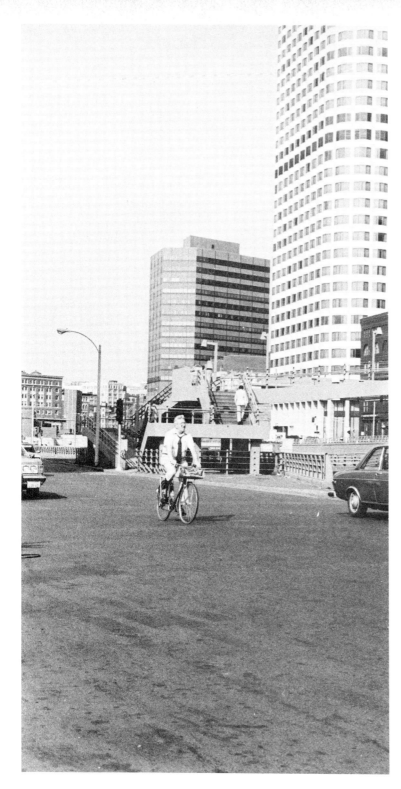

Now I see the secret of
making the best persons.
It is to grow in the open air
and to eat and sleep with
the earth.

Walt Whitman

Chapter 6

Maintaining
Physical Well-Being

Recently Americans have shown an upsurge of interest in achieving and maintaining physical fitness. The President's Council on Physical Fitness, set up by President John F. Kennedy, was an important agency in developing and spreading this interest in the early 1960s. The Council publicized research showing just how poor the physical condition of most Americans was. Our technological society emphasizes riding instead of walking, sitting in front of the television instead of exercising—in short, avoiding any form of exertion. Fortunately, many people have begun to realize the problems in both physical and mental well-being that lack of exercise can cause.

EXERCISE AND GOOD HEALTH

Inactivity can lead to or aggravate a variety of physical disorders. Thrombophlebitis (an inflammation of the veins) is one such disorder; atherosclerotic vascular disease is another. Atherosclerosis is reaching almost epidemic levels in the highly technological cultures of the world; research by a New York insurance group found inactivity and sedentary living to be the primary causes of this rise.[1]

Lack of exercise can make the skeleton atrophy, shrink the size of the muscles, and lead to a loss of strength. Insomnia and overweight are often caused by the sedentary lifestyles of many people; the primary elements in any weight loss program are lower calorie intake and a regime of regular physical exercise. (See Chapter 7.)

By exercising regularly, an individual can not only hope to avoid many of these problems, but he can also gain many other positive

[1] "Despite Studies, Framingham Eats, Smokes, and Rides," *Medical Tribunal Report,* May 22, 1974, pp. 1, 12.

Physical Fitness

According to the President's Council on Physical Fitness and Sports, the American sedentary way of life constitutes a serious national health problem, particularly for the 45 percent of all American adults who never exercise. Studies have reported that regular exercise can lower the serum triglycerides, reduce the clinical manifestations of heart disease, improve the efficiency of the heart and circulation, and reduce blood pressure levels in individuals with hypertension.

Last year's Prevention Theme stressed the importance of physical fitness and encouraged places of work to provide facilities and time for employees to participate in individual and group physical fitness activities.

The experience of the President's Council confirms that such on-the-job programs of regular, vigorous physical exercise can make an important contribution to the health, well-being, and productivity of working people while reducing the human and financial cost of physical degeneration. There has been an encouraging growth of such programs in public agencies and private companies throughout the country.

Since authority exists for Federal agencies to promote and maintain the physical fitness of their employees, the PHS strongly supports the Council's recommendation that "all branches and departments of the Federal Government provide their employees with time and facilities for regular, vigorous physical activities."

Source: Forward Plan for Health, U.S. Department of Health, Education, and Welfare, Public Health Service, August 1976.

benefits. In general, one looks and feels better when he is physically fit. Daily exercise helps metabolic processes, conditions the lungs to process more oxygen with less effort, strengthens the heart, improves muscle tone and reaction time, and increases the size of the blood vessels, thereby lowering blood pressure. Women usually experience specific benefits, such as less menstrual discomfort or irregularity and fewer backaches.[2] Furthermore, complications in labor are less common and delivery is less difficult for women who have kept themselves physically fit.[3] Exercise also allows one to work off some of the daily tensions, helping to improve mental and emotional health.

[2] Women who exercise regularly do not need to, nor should they, discontinue their activities during menstruation.
[3] G. J. Erdelyi, "Women in Athletics," Proceedings of the Second National Conference on the Medical Aspects of Sports, AMA, Washington, D.C., 27 November 1960.

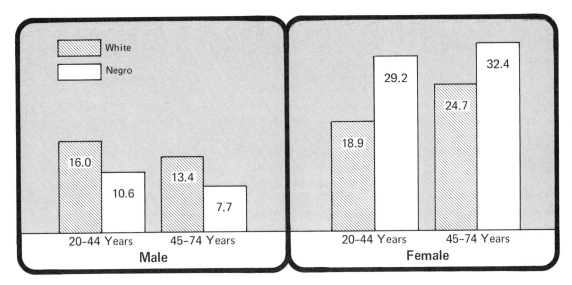

FIGURE 6.1 *Percent of obese adults by sex, age, and race, 1971–72. Source: National Center for Health Statistics, Health and Nutrition Examination Survey.*

PHYSICAL EXERCISE

There is no one best type of exercise although some activities such as swimming, provide better conditioning for all parts of the body than others, such as volleyball. A varied program, which may include calisthenics, jogging, walking, and sports, is usually best. Variety means that more parts of the body will be affected, and variety will also help the individual to stay interested in achieving and maintaining physical fitness. The individual should enjoy the exercise program itself as well as its benefits.

To receive any improvement in physical well-being, the individual should engage in some form of exercise every day or at least several times a week. Those who exercise only on weekends, for example, are receiving little or no benefit and in fact may be endangering their health. Too much exercise after prolonged periods of inactivity can prove harmful or even fatal—shoveling snow once or twice a winter without any other form of exercise can put strain on an older person's heart and possibly cause a heart attack.

How To Exercise   The three key variables in any exercise program are amount, intensity, and pace. Initially, any regimen should be sufficiently low in amount and intensity to fit the individual's degree of tolerance. For those in poor physical condition, tolerance should be determined by a physical examination. Anyone over thirty should have a physical exam before beginning an exercise program. It is important to know your physical capacity.

Any program should begin with short periods of exercise, possibly only several times each week, working up to longer periods every day. The individual should warm up to the strenuous exercise and cool down gradually afterwards. Four or five minutes of stretching muscles and bending joints at the beginning of each session are important; simple calisthenics, running in place, or running and walking alternately are good ways to loosen up. Then, towards the end of any session of strenuous exercise, the individual should slow down by decreasing the speed and intensity of his exertions, perhaps ending up with a few minutes of walking.

After two to three weeks of regular exercise, some improvement in physical fitness should be noticeable, with a measurable difference after four to six weeks.

One important fact to remember when taking a shower after an exercise session is that very hot water temperatures dilate the blood vessels of the skin and may cause faintness.

Types of Exercise

As mentioned earlier, some types of exercise may benefit all parts of the body while other forms may focus on only certain areas or systems. Only those exercises that significantly increase the flow of blood through the heart and large skeletal muscles will increase cardiovascular fitness and, consequently, overall fitness.

Jogging requires nearly continuous movement of the arms and legs. The resulting rhythmic tensing and relaxing of these muscles aids the flow of blood through the heart and muscles. Bicycling, swimming, and rhythmic calisthenics are also good activities in this sense.

Other types of exercise are less helpful in improving the efficiency of the heart, leading to increased fitness. Both weight lifting and isometric exercise (tightening muscles against fixed objects) cause the muscles affected to contract or tense up. The pressure squeezes the blood vessels, slowing down the flow of blood instead of speeding it up. Thus, such static muscular activity can actually cause an undesirable rise in blood pressure. This kind of exercise can therefore be harmful or even fatal to someone who is hypertensive (has high blood pressure), whereas the dynamic forms of exercise such as jogging can be helpful by actually lowering blood pressure.[4]

[4] Norman M. Kaplan, "Changing the Hypertensive's Life Style," *Practical Psychology for Physicians,* January 1975, p. 48.

> **Exercise for Women and Men**
>
> The apparent differences in strength and endurance between men and women may be at least as much a function of training and lifestyle as of physiology. Not only are the strength and the endurance capacity of some female athletes superior to that of untrained males, but strength in the lower extremities, relative to lean body weight, is higher in the trained female than in the trained male. The endurance capacity, relative to lean body weight, of the trained female distance runner closely approximates that of a male runner.
>
> However, the far greater androgen levels in males may account for their greater ability to proliferate muscle and achieve a relatively higher lean body weight than females. Women who exercise do not overdevelop their muscular systems. The hormonal difference may explain the difference in actual athletic performance of male and female athletes competing in the same event.
>
> *Source:* G. J. Erdelyi, "Women in Athletics," Proceedings of the Second National Conference on the Medical Aspects of Sports, AMA, Washington, D.C., 27 November 1960.

SUGGESTED EXERCISE PROGRAMS

Those who have not been exercising regularly and are now beginning have several choices. Jogging, swimming, or bicycling have all been mentioned as recommended forms of exercise. Any varied program of simple calisthenics is also good for acquiring and maintaining physical fitness, either used as a complete regimen in itself or in combination with other forms of exercise. Two popular conditioning programs today are Kenneth Cooper's Aerobics and the Royal Canadian Air Force's Exercise Plans.

Aerobics   "Aerobics" was designed by Dr. Kenneth Cooper, a major in the U.S. Air Force. His premise is that effective functioning of all muscles depends on an adequate supply of oxygen. (The term "aerobic" means "living, active, or occurring only in the presence of oxygen.") Since oxygen intake begins at the lung surfaces, all fitness and endurance depend on a sequence of events starting there.

How to Read and Record Your Heart Rate

The action of your heart is the best gauge of your physical fitness. An accurate record of your heart rate (beats per minute) under various conditions over a period of time will enable your physician to gauge your progress. Accordingly, you'll need to learn to take your pulse under these conditions:

» At rest, for example, when you first awaken in the morning, before rising or exercising

» After a specific period of exercise, as directed by your physician

» After you have performed your regular work for a specific period, as directed by your physician

Taking your pulse is, for these purposes, the same as counting the number of times your heart beats per minute. Don't be concerned that your heart rate seems fast at one reading or slow at another; many factors, including sex and age, affect the heart rate under various circumstances. To get an accurate measurement for your physical fitness program, follow the simple steps below:

1.   Experiment a bit and select the best body site to take your pulse. In some sites the pulse is prominent at rest; in others, after exercise. The best locations are typically at the wrist, just below the base of the thumb; at the neck, just over the collar line and to the right or left of the windpipe; and at the inside of the elbow, just above the skin crease.

Aerobics offers both testing and conditioning. Before beginning the program, the individual determines the greatest distance he can comfortably cover in twelve minutes by running and walking. *The New Aerobics* then presents a scale for rating oneself according to age and sex. (*Aerobics for Women* has specific charts for women.)

The individual then follows a program designed to increase his heart beat during exercise to a rate of about 150 beats per minute (compared to the average resting pulse rate of 72 or 80 beats per minute). (See the above box on how to read your heart rate.) Throughout the "training program," the crucial part of the workout is the length of time one stays at the target zone for heart rate. As the individual gains in physical fitness, he must increase the vigor of the exercise program to make further progress.[5] (This is true of any exercise program.)

[5] Kenneth H. Cooper, *Aerobics,* New York: Bantam Books, 1968; Cooper, *The New Aerobics*, New York: Bantam Books, 1970.

(Continued)

2.   When taking your pulse at rest, simply count the number of pulsations for a full minute, using a watch with a second hand for accuracy.

3.   *Immediately* after exercise count the beats for the first 10 seconds *only;* then multiply this number by six to get a per minute reading. Don't try to take your pulse during exercise, but start *immediately* after the prescribed exercise. The reason for this is that the heart rate rapidly slows after the stress of exercise; in fact, the faster it slows the more fit you are, as a rule. If you do take a full minute's count, you'll notice a significant difference in the number of heartbeats during the first 10 seconds of the minute and the last 10 seconds.

4.   One of the reasons for testing your heart rate is to find out what normal work activity does to your heart. Select an activity that is ordinary and usual—both in the stress it creates and the muscular power it requires. Take a resting pulse count just before doing the activity, then take a post-activity count for 10 seconds and multiply by six.

5.   Write down the count of your pulse immediately after taking it. Keep a small notebook for the purpose, and enter the date, time, and kind of reading (resting, postexercise, postwork) for each count.

Source: Patient Care, March 15, 1974. © Copyright, 1974, Miller and Fink Corp. Darien, Conn. All rights reserved.

Royal Canadian Air Force Exercise Plans

The Royal Canadian Air Force has designed two sets of exercise plans for physical fitness: the XBX Plan for women and the 5BX Plan for men. These exercise plans consist of sets of basic calisthenics. They were designed specifically for simplicity, in that they can be done almost anywhere and take only eleven or twelve minutes a day. The goal is overall physical fitness, with maximum functioning of the cardiovascular and cardiorespiratory systems.

The individual's specific program is determined by age. Each person starts with a number of fairly easy exercises and progresses through levels in which the exercises increase in number and difficulty. The program explains the specific area affected by each exercise, with the overall results of increased muscle tone, increased muscular strength, increased muscular endurance, increased flexibility, and the increased efficiency of the heart.[6]

[6] *Royal Canadian Air Force Exercise Plans for Physical Fitness,* New York: Pocket Books, 1975.

FURTHER READINGS

Hittleman, Richard. *Yoga.* New York: Bantam Books, 1973.

A four-week exercise program through the use of yoga.

Johnson, Perry B., ed. "Fact and Fancy," *Journal of Health, Physical Education and Recreation.* 39:10, (November-December, 1968) pp. 25–33.

This special series of articles provides, in addition to useful information concerning exercise, some fascinating insights into the efforts of dedicated professionals to be rigorously objective about their own cherished field of endeavor.

Kauz, Herman. *Tai Chi Handbook.* Garden City, N.Y.: Dolphin Books, 1974.

The ancient Chinese art of Tai Chi explained and demonstrated in words and photographs—showing the rhythmic co-ordination, balance, and harmony with nature developed by the practice of this relaxed mental-physical exercise.

Levy, Janine. *The Baby Exercise Book.* New York: Pantheon Books, 1975.

A guide on how to aid a child's growth through exercise.

Morehouse, Laurence E. and Miller, Augustus T. *Physiology of Exercise.* St. Louis: The C. V. Mosby Co., 1971.

This standard work should prove attractive to the advanced undergraduate who desires a deeper understanding of this topic; the organization of the chapters makes it easy to examine specialized aspects of the exercise phenomena.

Chapter 7

Nutrition
and Health

"You are what you eat." The truth of this simple statement is seen daily in our society, from the martini-drinking businessman who suffers from cirrhosis of the liver to the unhappy, overweight teenager living on pizza and soft drinks. Some people have followed good eating habits since childhood, others may need to *learn* how to eat wisely. However, developing good eating habits is not difficult.

MEETING THE BODY'S NEED FOR FUEL

To stay healthy one must balance the input of chemical nutrients into the body. The body needs large quantities of certain nutrients and lesser amount of others. Some nutrients are stored in the body, if the basic requirements have been met, while the excess of others is eliminated.

A healthy person will take in only as many *calories* (the heat or energy units provided by various foods) as he needs. Calories are provided by three types of substances: proteins, carbohydrates, and fats. These substances are made usable by the body through the process of digestion. The energy provided is then used for muscular activity, which accounts for one-half of the average daily expenditure of energy, and for all the other activities the body performs to maintain life and health. Some of these substances are digested and stored if all the calories consumed are not burned.

There are three other substances the body needs: minerals, vitamins, and water. In the following paragraphs we will examine each of these six substances in relation to maintaining health through good nutrition.

Protein

Protein is composed of amino acids. There are twenty-three amino acids, some of which can be synthesized by the body. However, there are eight amino acids that the body cannot synthesize, and these must be taken from the protein in the food one eats. These essential amino acids are valine, isolucine, methionine, phenylalanine, leucine, lysine, threonine, and tryptophane.[1]

Protein is the most abundant organic compound in the body. It is especially important in the processes of growth and lactation. Protein is not stored in the body as a reserve, so it is important for the individual to take in an adequate amount of protein each day (approximately 68 grams or 2¼ oz.) The protein consumed that is not necessary for the repair, manufacture, or maintenance of vital body components provides a source of energy.

If a person eats meat, milk and/or cheese, and eggs every day, his protein need is probably well met. The Nutrition Society has found that, "In general, any calculated requirements for amino acids by humans over one year can be met by a much lower level of dietary protein than is actually consumed by people in Western cultures and by most other people whose diet is not severely limited by poverty."[2]

People who do not consume enough protein at any one period or throughout their lives may experience a greater susceptibility to infection and suffer from fatigue and irritability; they may recover more slowly from disease, and any wounds or burns will heal more slowly. Other problems resulting from protein deficiency include liver disorders, anemia, impaired antibody production, and edema.

Protein deficiency in infants and children has serious consequences. *Kwashiorkor* is a protein deficiency disease common among infants and young children in Indochina, the Near East, much of Africa, and parts of South America, as well as in severely deprived areas of the United States. The child may exhibit apathy, loss of appetite, anemia, nutritional edema, and pigmentation change. Such protein deficiency can slow growth and cause severe mental retardation. This disease is a serious problem for underdeveloped nations today.

Carbohydrates

The term *carbohydrate* refers to sugars, starches, and cellulose. The major function of carbohydrates is to provide energy for cell life and growth. Approximately 50 percent of the body's energy needs are provided by carbohydrates.

[1] For children there are ten essential amino acids.
[2] Carpenter et al. "Problems in Formulating Simple Recommended Allowances of Amino Acids for Animals and Man," *The Proceedings of the Nutrition Society,* 30, No. 1, May 1971, p. 6.

Diet and Tooth Decay

What you eat has a significant effect on the health of your teeth. Foods heavy in sugar can promote tooth decay and gum disease. Sugar combines with plaque, a sticky colorless film of harmful oral bacteria that constantly forms on the teeth, and produces acids, which in turn attack the tooth enamel and lead to decay. Experiments have shown that most people who eat lots of sweets get three to four times as many caries [cavities] as those who eat very few.*

Vitamin D is also important to the health of your teeth. Calcium is necessary for the production of strong teeth. Since vitamin D facilitates the absorption of calcium from the small intestine, it is important for pregnant women to make sure they get enough vitamin D so that the fetus will be well supplied. Adequate vitamin D in an infant's diet is crucial for the development of good teeth.

* Lou Joseph, "Foods and Drinks that Will Cause You the Fewest Cavities," *Today's Health,* October 1973, pp. 41–43.

Carbohydrates are consumed as simple or compound sugars and as starch. Both compound sugars and starches (which are actually long chains of simple sugar units) are degraded by the body in digestion into simple sugar units. Then all simple sugars (except glucose) are further converted by the liver into glucose, which is the only form of carbohydrate that can be used by the body for energy.

The body stores some carbohydrates in the liver and the muscles, in the form of glycogen. Glycogen is ready for immediate release into the blood stream when the blood sugar level becomes too low.

The excess ingested carbohydrates (those that are neither used immediately for energy nor stored as glycogen) are converted into what are called triglycerides and stored as fatty acids in fat tissue. About 85 percent of the original potential energy in glucose is stored this way, and can be used by the body for energy when it is needed.

The body burns up carbohydrates much more efficiently than protein and fat, so the simple sugars are used for energy before either of these other nutrients. Thus, protein is spared for the important function of providing energy for cell maintenance, and fats can be used as some of the structural components of the body.

Fats   Fats are the third important source of energy for the body. Fats can be stored in the body, like carbohydrates, as a nutritional and energy reserve. Body fat is by far the greatest nutritional reservoir in man. Most food consumed in greater amounts than is immediately needed by the body is converted to fatty acids and stored in the appropriate tissues.

Much of the structure of the cellular cytoplasm is made up of fat. Depot fat also provides thermal insulation and protection from mechanical shock. The fat reservoirs are continually drawn upon by the body and the fat delivered to the liver, which is the main site of fatty acid breakdown and synthesis.

Vitamins   Vitamins are needed only in small or "trace" amounts, but are very important for bodily function. Vitamins and enzymes both work to help various chemical reactions take place in the body. Thus vitamins are considered co-enzymes. In many cases vitamins are catalysts, meaning they start a necessary reaction or part of a reaction that would otherwise not take place.

Table 7.1 lists the most important vitamins and their sources, and describes the effects of deficiency or total absence of each vitamin.

Minerals   Trace amounts of various minerals are also essential to good health. Among the necessary minerals are calcium, chloride, chromium, cobalt, copper, fluoride, iodide, iron, magnesium, manganese, phosphorus, potassium, sodium, and zinc. Many essential minerals are retained indefinitely and recycled in the body, so that a few millionths of an ounce often fills the daily requirements. Calcium and phosphorus are exceptions because growing children and expectant mothers need them in substantial amounts for bone and teeth formation.

Iron, zinc, and chromium are needed to form hemoglobin for oxygen transport and to use oxygen in tissue respiration. Iodine is necessary for the formation of the thyroid hormones, which regulate the bodily processes. Sulfur is required for the synthesis of many important proteins (amino acids). Sodium, potassium, and magnesium all help to regulate body fluids. Each essential mineral works in some important process. Table 7.2 lists the most important minerals, their functions, sources, and daily requirements.

Water   Water is involved in a great number of the functions of the body. Water makes up from 40 (in an obese individual) to 70 (in a very thin person) percent of the body weight, and is so important that a loss of less than 20 percent of the body's water can result in death.

Table 7.1 *Vitamin Function.*

VITAMIN A

FUNCTIONS:
1. Promotes tissue formation.
2. Increases blood platelets.
3. Promotes growth and feeling of well-being.
4. Promotes appetite and digestion, especially in children.
5. Essential to the health and integrity of epithelial tissue and its resistance to infection, notably of eyes, tonsils, sinuses, air passages, lungs, and gastrointestinal tract.

RESULTS OF DEFICIENCY:
1. Loss of appetite.
2. Retardation of growth and development.
3. Physical weakness.
4. Susceptibility to disease of the eyes (night blindness, corneal ulcers), ears (otitis media), kidneys.
5. Interferes with reproduction by failure of ovulation in the female and temporary injury to the semeniferous epithelium in the male.
6. Secondary anemia.
7. Excessive growth of lymphoid tissue.
8. Dullness or perversion of special senses.
9. Formation of kidney stones.
10. Cystitis, gastritis, sinusitis, bronchitis.

RESULTS OF ABSENCE
1. Xerophthalmia (eye inflammation and ulcers).
2. Cessation of growth.
3. Failure of appetite and digestion.
4. Sterility of both sexes.

MOST RELIABLE SOURCES:
Whole milk, butter, cheese, egg yolk, cod liver oil, thin green leafy vegetables, yellow corn, yellow sweet potatoes, carrots, spinach, green beans, peas, bananas, and fish oils.

VITAMIN B₁ (Thiamine)

All cooked foods are deficient in this nerve and brain nourishing element depending on the degree of heat and the time the food is exposed to the heat.

FUNCTIONS:
1. Increases appetite.
2. Promotes digestion.
3. Promotes growth by stimulating metabolic processes.
4. Protects body from certain nerve and brain diseases.
5. Increases quantity and improves quality of milk during lactation. Mothers who do not have enough milk usually lack Vitamin B.
6. Stimulates pancreatic secretions, including insulin.
7. Necessary to maintenance of thyroid and adrenal glands.
8. Necessary to normal function of anterior pituitary.

RESULTS OF DEFFICIENCY:
1. Impairment of appetite and digestion.
2. Loss of weight.
3. Loss of vigor.
4. Constipation.
5. Emaciation.
6. Subnormal temperature.
7. Pathological enlargement and functional disorders of the thymus, adrenals, pancreas, testes, ovaries, spleen, heart, liver, kidneys, stomach, thyroid, brain, and anterior pituitary.
8. Various manifestations referable to the nervous system, leading to paralysis of groups of muscles.
9. Tendency to diabetes. (Probably the major cause.)
10. Tendency to nervous disorders.
11. Tendency to disorders of alimentary mucosa.
12. Tendency to thyroid disorders.
13. Reduces hemoglobin.
14. Loss of sexual potential because of anterior pituitary.

RESULTS OF ABSENCE:
1. Beri-beri (paralysis of certain groups of muscles).
2. Peripheral and other forms of neuritis.
3. Atrophy of certain lymphoid tissues throughout the body.

MOST RELIABLE SOURCES:
Whole grain cereals, peas, beans, raw fruits, buttermilk, corn, cabbage, spinach, egg yolk, honey, and yeast.

VITAMIN B₂ (Riboflavin)

FUNCTIONS:
1. Necessary to growth and development.
2. Necessary to normal calcium metabolism and erythrocyte formation.

Table 7.1 (continued)

RESULTS OF DEFICIENCY:
1. Underdevelopment.
2. Cataract of the eye and other calcium deposits.
3. Pellagra.
4. Abnormally slow regeneration of erythrocytes —secondary anemia.

MOST RELIABLE SOURCES:
Cereal germ, brewer's yeast, eggs.

VITAMIN B$_6$ (pyridoxine)

FUNCTIONS:
1. Essential for amino acid metabolism.
2. Essential for functioning of cells.

RESULTS OF DEFICIENCY:
1. Skin lesions.
2. Nerve inflammation.
3. Anemia.

MOST RELIABLE SOURCES:
Fish, vegetables, molasses, yeast, liver, whole grains, kidneys, meat, wheat bran and germ.

VITAMIN B$_{12}$ (Cyanocobalamin)

FUNCTIONS:
1. Essential for production of red blood cells.
2. Essential for normal growth.
3. Essential for nerve functioning.

RESULTS OF DEFICIENCY:
1. Penicious anemia.
2. Retarded growth.
3. Disorders of nervous system.

MOST RELIABLE SOURCES:
Liver, beef, pork, organ meats, eggs, milk.

VITAMIN C

FUNCTIONS:
1. Essential to the health and integrity of endothelial tissues.
2. Cooperates with B in nutrition of thyro-adrenal system.
3. Is essential to oxygen metabolism.
4. Cooperates with D in regulation of calcium metabolism.
5. Promotes leucocytic and phagocytic activity.

RESULTS OF DEFICIENCY:
1. Tendency to bruise easily, producing "black and blue" spots in skin.
2. Loss in weight.
3. Physical weakness.
4. Shortness of breath.
5. Rapid respiration.
6. Rapid heart action.
7. Tendency to hemorrhage.
8. Reduced hemoglobin and tendency to certain types of anemia.
9. Hypertrophy and reduced secretion of adrenals.
10. Hypertrophy or morbid secretion of thyroid (toxic goiter).
11. Decrease in weight of spleen, liver, stomach, and intestines. B deficiency a cooperating factor in this.
12. Necrosis of pulp of teeth. Most cases of tooth decay are due to Vitamin C deficiency.
13. Friability of bones.
14. Swelling and redness of gums.
15. Tendency to disease of blood vessels and heart.
16. Tendency to peptic and duodenal ulcers.

RESULTS OF ABSENCE:
1. Scurvy.

MOST RELIABLE SOURCES:
Green peppers, oranges, lemons, tomatoes raw or canned (without the addition of soda), bananas and other raw fruits, sprouted grains, green leafy vegetables, potatoes, unpasteurized milk, liver, and raw cabbage.

Vitamin C is not stored in the body. A fresh supply must be had every day.

VITAMIN D

FUNCTIONS:
1. Controls calcium equilibrium and regulates mineral metabolism.

RESULTS OF DEFICIENCY:
1. Rickets.
2. Deformity of bones in children.
3. Defective development of teeth.

Vitamin D, the only dangerous vitamin, causes arteriosclerosis in overdosage and premature symptoms of senility.

MOST RELIABLE SOURCES:
Cod liver oil and other fish oils, egg yolk, whole milk, and spinach. Exposure of naked skin to sunshine or ultraviolet light. Few foods contain Vitamin D. Nature expects the animal to get this vitamin from the sunshine by the short wave length rays changing the ergosterol in the skin into Vitamin D.

Table 7.1 (continued)

VITAMIN E

FUNCTIONS:
1. Necessary to reproduction—in both male and female.
2. Probably concerned in the metabolism of calcium and magnesium by increasing their diffusibility in the tissue fluid and increasing the mineral nutrition to the nervous and muscular tissues. This action also prevents the formation of calcium deposits in blood vessel walls, tendency to arterial hypertension, and loss of motility of eye lens.

RESULTS OF DEFICIENCY:
1. Sterility. Deficiency causes permanent and irreparable injury to the semeniferous epithelium in the male, temporary sterility in the female.
2. Mysterious pains in soft tissues, nervous system and muscles.

3. Tendency to cerebral hemorrhage.
4. Tendency to arthritis.
5. Loss of accommodation in lens and iris of the eye.
6. Dermatitis, eczema, urticaria.

MOST RELIABLE SOURCES:
Whole grain cereals (whole wheat, whole corn, etc.), milk, lettuce, watercress, and raw fruits.

VITAMIN K

FUNCTIONS:
1. Essential for blood clotting.

RESULTS OF DEFICIENCY:
1. Slow blood clotting.
2. Anemia.

MOST RELIABLE SOURCES:
Spinach, eggs, liver, cabbage, tomatoes.

Water is found within and among the cells, where it forms a medium for the various chemical reactions, such as digestion. Water conducts heat efficiently and so serves to maintain uniform body temperature (evaporation of water from the skin acts as a cooling mechanism for the body to avoid overheating). Water also acts as a cushion to protect body organs and as a lubricant in joint, synovial, and central nervous system fluids. Water is needed in the lungs for breathing. It is also a transport for many substances throughout the body.

THE SOURCE OF GOOD HEALTH: FOUNDATION FOODS

How do you know what and how much to eat in order to be taking in the right amounts of the essential nutrients? One basis for establishing a healthy diet has been determined by the National Academy of Science/National Research Council with what are called Recommended Dietary Allowances (RDAs). Table 7.3 shows the list these organizations drew up. RDAs are estimates of the amounts of essential nutrients that the average adult must consume in order to be reasonably assured that his daily physiological needs are met. The estimates are somewhat high, because they were intended to meet the needs of a heterogeneous population; that is, the recommendations are high enough to meet the needs of those adult individuals with the highest requirements.

Table 7.2 *Minerals**

Mineral	Primary Function in Man	Food Source	Daily Requirement
Calcium (Ca)	Building material of bones and teeth; regulation of body functions: heart muscle contraction, blood clotting	Dairy products, leafy vegetables, apricots	Men: .8 grams Women: .8 grams
Phosphorus (P)	Combines with calcium to give rigidity to bones and teeth; essential in cell metabolism; serves as a buffer to maintain proper acid-base balance of blood	Peas, beans, milk, liver, meat, cottage cheese, broccoli, whole grains	Men: .8 grams Women: .8 grams
Iron (Fe)	Component of the red blood cell's oxygen and carbon dioxide transport system; enzyme constituent necessary for cellular respiration	Liver, meat, shellfish, lentils, peanuts, parsley, dried fruits, eggs	Men: 10 mg. Women: 18 mg.
Iodine (I)	Essential component of the thyroid hormone, thyroxin, which controls the rate of cell oxidation	Iodized salt, seafood	Men: 140 mg. Women: 100 mg
Sodium (Na)	Regulates the fluid and acid-base balance in the body	Table salt, dried apricots, beans, beets, brown sugar, raisins, spinach, yeast	Men: 10–15 grams Women: 10–15 grams
Chloride (Cl)	Associated with sodium and its functions; a component of the gastric juice hydrochloric acid; and chloride ion also functions in the starch splitting system of saliva	Same as sodium	Men: 10–15 grams Women: 10–15 grams
Potassium (K)	Component of the system that controls the acid-base and liquid balances; is probably an important enzyme-activator in the use of amino acids	Readily available in most foods	

Mineral	Function	Food sources	Recommended amount
Magnesium (Mg)	Enzyme-activator related to carbohydrate metabolism	Readily available in most foods	Men: 400 mg. Women: 350 mg.
Sulfur (S)	Component of the hormone insulin and the sulfur amino acids; builds hair, nails, skin	Nuts, dried fruits, barley and oatmeal, beans, cheese, eggs, lentils, brown sugar	?
Manganese (Mn)	Enzyme activator for systems related to carbohydrate, protein, and fat metabolism	Wheat germ, nuts, bran, green leafy vegetables, cereal grains, meat	?
Copper (Cu)	The function of copper has not been fully resolved although it is known to function in the synthesis of the red blood cell and the oxidation system of the body	Kidney, liver, beans, Brazil nuts, wholemeal flour, lentils, parsley	?
Zinc (Z)	The function is unknown although it is a component of many enzyme systems and is an essential component of the pancreatic hormone insulin	Shellfish, meat, milk, eggs	?
Cobalt (Co)	A component of the vitamin B_{12} molecule	Vitamin B_{12}	?
Fluorine (F)	Essential to normal tooth and bone development and maintenance; excesses are undesirable	Drinking water in some areas	1 part per million in drinking water

99

* Several trace minerals—chromium, silenium, nickel, molybdinum, vanodium, and tin—are now known to be required in very small amounts by experimental animals (studies have not been done on man). Their distribution in food varies considerably, depending in part on the composition of the soil in which plants are raised.

Source: Values are taken from *Recommended Dietary Allowances*, 7th ed. Washington, D.C.: National Academy of Sciences Publication 1694, 1968.

Table 7.3 *A Table of Vital Nutrients*

The U.S. Food and Drug Administration's Recommended Daily Allowances (RDAs), listed here, represent the estimated amounts of nutrients the average healthy person needs daily to stay healthy. Because nutrient requirements for individuals are not known, these quantities are weighted on the high side, the FDA says; many adults need only two-thirds to three-fourths of these established amounts, and children need only about one-half.

RDAs, stated in grams (g.), International Units (IU), milligrams (mg.), and micrograms (ug.):

	Adults and Children Over 4 years	Infants and Children Under 4 Years
Protein	65 g.*	28 g.*
Vitamin A	5,000 IU	2,500 IU
Vitamin C	60 mg.	40 mg.
Thiamine	1.5 mg.	0.7 mg.
Riboflavin	1.7 mg.	0.8 mg.
Niacin	20 mg.	9.0 mg.
Calcium	1.0 g.	0.8 g.
Iron	18 mg.	10 mg.
Vitamin D	400 IU	400 IU
Vitamin E	30 IU	10 IU
Vitamin B_6	2.0 mg.	0.7 mg.
Folacin	0.4 mg.	0.2 mg.
Vitamin B_{12}	6 ug.	3 ug.
Phosphorus	1.0 g.	0.8 g.
Iodine	150 ug.	70 ug.
Magnesium	400 mg.	200 mg.
Zinc	15 mg.	8.0 mg.
Copper	2 mg.	1.0 mg.
Biotin	0.3 mg.	0.15 mg.
Pantothenic Acid	10 mg.	5 mg.

* If an individual's protein intake comes primarily from high-efficiency-protein foods such as milk and milk by-products, the RDA for protein is 45 g. for adults and 20 g. for infants.

There are four basic food groups of foundation foods that should be consumed (along with adequate amounts of water) to meet these nutrient requirements and maintain a healthy body. These are the dairy group, the meat group, the vegetables and fruit group, and the bread and cereals group. The box on page 101 shows why each group is especially important.

Dairy Group   Skimmed, dry, or whole milk can be used to meet the daily requirements for dairy foods. Cheese, ice cream, and other dairy products can be used to supplement the milk intake. However, in the process of making cheese, some vitamins are lost, so that cheese

Dairy Foods Help To:
· Build strong bones and healthy teeth
· Build and repair all body tissues
· Promote growth and provide energy
· Keep muscles active and nerves calm

Vegetables & Fruits Help To:
· Keep skin healthy
· Maintain normal eyesight
· Build resistance to infection
· Provide "cementing" material that holds body cells together

Meat Group Helps To:
· Build strong and agile muscles
· Make healthy blood and all body tissues
· Promote growth and provide energy

Breads & Cereals Help To:
· Promote growth and body building
· Create a good appetite
· Provide energy

does not have the full nutritive content of milk. Ice cream does contain the full nutritive value of milk, but not on a comparable volume basis; that is, there will be fewer nutritive values in a cup of ice cream than in a cup of milk.

The average adult should have two glasses of milk a day. Children need three to four glasses; teenagers, four or more; pregnant women, four or more; and nursing mothers, at least six glasses. One ounce of hard cheese or one-half cup of cottage cheese supplies the same amount of calcium as two-thirds of a glass of milk, and one-quarter of a pint of ice cream supplies the same amount as one-quarter cup of milk. Milk values other than calcium are found in variable amounts in these other dairy foods.

Meat Group   The meat group is the protein group, including foods that supply animal *and* vegetable protein. The sources for these proteins are meat, fish, or poultry; eggs and cheese; and dry legumes, lentils, peas, beans, and nuts.

Everyone should have two or more servings daily from this group. A serving of meat, fish, or poultry equals 2 to 3 ounces after cooking and does not include bones or fat. Two eggs, 2 ounces of cheese, 1 cup of cooked beans, or 4 tablespoons of peanut butter would also each equal a serving.[3]

[3] There is some debate over the effects of eating many foods high in cholesterol, such as eggs and steaks. Some people feel a high cholesterol diet can cause heart attacks or arteriosclerosis in any adult male, while others believe there are many factors involved in each case. Someone worried about cholesterol could eat fewer eggs and concentrate on foods such as fish for their protein intake.

Vegetables and
Fruit Group

The vegetables and fruit group has three subdivisions: the dark green vegetables, the deep yellow vegetables, and the vegetables and fruits that are high in vitamin C. Both dark green and deep yellow vegetables are high in vitamin A. Dark green vegetables are beet greens, broccoli, chard, collard greens, cress, kale, mustard greens, spinach, and turnip greens; deep yellow vegetables are carrots, pumpkin, winter squash, and yams. Vitamin C fruits and vegetables include oranges, grapefruit, cranberries, raw cabbage, strawberries, and melon.

Everyone should have four or more servings from this group daily. A serving equals one-half cup vegetables or fruit; half a medium grapefruit or cantaloupe, or a medium orange, apple, or other whole fruit. Since the body does not store vitamin C, it is important to eat a food rich in this vitamin every day. Dark green and deep yellow vegetables should be eaten at least every other day. Other fruits and vegetables, such as potatoes and bananas, are also important.

Bread and
Cereals Group

The last basic food group is the bread and cereal group, with three subgroups: enriched flour, whole grains, and restored grain. Enriched flour is white flour to which specific amounts of iron, thiamine, riboflavin, and niacin have been added. Whole grains are those that retain the germ and the outer layers, with the nutrients stored therein. Restored grains are those that have lost the nutrients in processing but they have been replaced in appropriate amounts.

The average individual needs four or more servings of bread and cereals a day. A serving equals one slice of bread; one ounce of ready-to-eat cereal; or one-half to three-quarters cup cooked cereal, grits, macaroni, noodles, or rice. Be sure that the breads and cereals consumed are either enriched, whole grain, or restored. Macaroni, spaghetti, noodles, and rice, for example, contribute toward the daily requirement only if they are enriched.

Changing
Requirements

The requirements listed above in the RDAs and described under the food group sections are usually the requirements for an average healthy adult. Food requirements vary, of course, with a person's size and with their energy level. The requirements also change at different periods in one's lifetime. At some times the healthy individual needs more than the suggested serving amounts, while at other times he may need less.

Infancy and Early Childhood

Because of rapid growth and development during the early phase of life, the energy requirements are higher (relative to weight) during childhood than they will be throughout life. Milk is the most important food for the infant or young child, but milk alone will not provide an infant with all the necessary nutrients. Particularly if the child is bottle-fed, additional vitamins are necessary. Vitamins A, C, and D are the most important. Today, milk is usually fortified with vitamins A and D; however, the pediatrician will prescribe the specific amount of a vitamin supplement for the child. Iron deficiency is common in infants, so this may be added to the vitamin preparation.

Adolescence

There is a marked acceleration of growth in adolescents preceding their attainment of sexual maturity. The adolescent thus must have adequate protein, minerals, and vitamins to support this period of growth, as well as enough calories to provide energy. A diet emphasizing these special needs is important.

Pregnancy

The pregnant woman must be sure to eat enough "building" foods for good development of the fetus, as well as follow a good overall diet to keep herself healthy. She needs extra protein, minerals, and vitamins, and enough calories for the necessary weight gain and to provide energy.

The physician should prescribe the specific weight gain and increased calorie intake for each individual, based on her activities, her frame, and her general physical condition. An average recommended weight gain is about twenty to twenty-five pounds. The pregnant woman should gain only a little in the first trimester (first three months), gradually reaching the desired weight over the last six months.

If a woman has been well-nourished before pregnancy and eats well during pregnancy, she can expect the following benefits:

- a generally healthy pregnancy
- few or no complications
- safe delivery
- good health after childbirth
- a better chance to nurse successfully

The fetus has a chance for healthy growth and development, and the baby should have better health during early infancy.

Advanced Age

The growth of the average individual "slows down" as he ages, so an older person has fewer energy requirements than a younger one. The individual should be aware of his lessening requirements, including a lowered calorie intake. He should be eating smaller amounts of the basic foods, but an individual of any age needs adequate protein, calcium, and vitamins.

OBESITY AND HEALTH

For various reasons, including ignorance of good eating habits, over 25 percent of the population of the United States can be considered obese. Obesity is a major health problem in this country.

Patterns of   Some obese people did not have a weight problem until ado-
Obesity   lescence or even later in life; others have always been overweight. What causes obesity?

Childhood Obesity

Some obesity may begin in a child's first year. Overfeeding a baby may cause him to become passive and inactive, and the unused calories turn into fat. Many researchers now believe that fat cells developed early in life can create a lifetime of weight problems.

The most useful thing any parent can do about childhood obesity is to prevent it. If the individual acquires good eating habits when he is young, he is far less likely to have diet problems when he is older. It is easier to learn to eat a healthy balanced diet when young than to have to relearn eating patterns later.

Adolescent and Adult Obesity

Other factors may produce obesity in adolescence or adulthood. Teenagers often consume mostly starchy foods, with resultant health problems. Poverty can also be a factor in obesity—potatoes and bread are much cheaper than meat and fresh vegetables. Furthermore, if a person has not learned good eating patterns in childhood, he may never be aware of what he should be eating for the amount of exercise he gets. Obesity may sometimes be caused by metabolic or other physiological problems. Some people gain weight because of stress or other emotional problems.

There are other causes of obesity, but at this time all the factors that determine obesity are imperfectly understood. However, health professionals are definite on the dangers of obesity and the health problems it can cause.

**Obesity and
Health**

The obese person carries an unnecessary burden, which places strain on his body's systems and can lead to health problems of varying severity. The obese person may become breathless just from climbing stairs. Obesity places a continual strain on the cardiovascular system. Carrying excess weight for an extended period of time is wearing on the knee and ankle joints and can cause bad posture, leading to severe back problems.

In addition, excess fat makes even the most routine surgical procedures more difficult and increases surgical risk. Obesity causes serious complications in gallbladder disease and diabetes, and is an added problem for those with asthma, putting further strain on the already-overburdened heart and lungs. Extreme obesity can even disturb brain function by compromising adequate oxygen supply to the lungs and hence to the brain.

There is every reason for an overweight person to want to reduce. In its booklet *Obesity and Health* (compiled by a panel assembled by the Heart Disease Program of the Public Health Service Division of Chronic Disease), the U.S. Department of Health, Education and Welfare presents a long list of conditions that are relieved or possibly avoided altogether by a loss of excess weight: "angina pectoris, hypertension, congestive heart failure, intermittent claudication (lameness), varicose veins, rupture of the intervertebral discs, osteoarthritis, and other bone and joint disease."[4] A thin person has the possibility of much greater health than an overweight person.

**Who Is
Overweight?**

It is usually obvious when someone is obese. It is not always obvious, however, that a person is carrying around fifteen or twenty pounds of unnecessary weight. How do you tell if you need to lose weight?

The American Medical Association recommends the "pinch test" to determine whether or not one is overweight. This is done by grasping the flesh just above the waist between the thumb and the tip of the forefinger. If there is more than a one-inch thickness, the individual probably needs to lose some weight. He should con-

[4] U.S. Dept. of Health, Education and Welfare, *Obesity and Health,* U.S. Public Health Service Publication 1485, Washington, D.C.: U.S. Govt. Printing Office.

sult established standards of weight for height, age, and sex. A figure that is more than 10 percent over the established standard is considered overweight. Table 7.4 provides recommended weights for men and women.

Table 7.4 *Desirable weights for men and women aged 25 and over* (in pounds according to height and frame, in indoor clothing)*

Height		Small frame	Medium frame	Large frame
Men				
Feet	Inches			
5	2	112–120	118–129	126–141
5	3	115–123	121–133	129–144
5	4	118–126	124–136	132–148
5	5	121–129	127–139	135–152
5	6	124–133	130–143	138–156
5	7	128–137	134–147	142–161
5	8	132–141	138–152	147–166
5	9	136–145	142–156	151–170
5	10	140–150	146–160	155–174
5	11	144–154	150–165	159–179
6	0	148–158	154–170	164–184
6	1	152–162	158–175	168–189
6	2	156–167	162–180	173–194
6	3	160–171	167–185	178–199
6	4	164–175	172–190	182–204
Women				
4	10	92– 98	96–107	104–119
4	11	94–101	98–110	106–122
5	0	96–104	101–113	109–125
5	1	99–107	104–116	112–128
5	2	102–110	107–119	115–131
5	3	105–113	110–122	118–134
5	4	108–116	113–126	121–138
5	5	111–119	116–130	125–142
5	6	114–123	120–135	129–146
5	7	118–127	124–139	133–150
5	8	122–131	128–143	137–154
5	9	126–135	132–147	141–158
5	10	130–140	136–151	145–163
5	11	134–144	140–155	149–168
6	0	138–148	144–159	153–173

* Adapted from Metropolitan Life Insurance Co., New York. New weight standards for men and women. *Statistical Bulletin* 40:3, Nov.–Dec., 1959.

Anorexia Nervosa

Recently, a disease called anorexia nervosa has become increasingly common in the United States. This disease, which has been defined as "the relentless pursuit of thinness through starvation" occurs mostly in teenage girls, who are usually bright and very ambitious. It is extremely rare in males.

The victim develops a morbid fascination for anything to do with food while struggling to lose more and more weight. The patient's perceptions of her body's shape and needs become distorted, so she may believe she is obese when she is actually dangerously underweight. Symptoms include extreme constipation, depression, complete absence of menstrual periods, and an inability to feel hunger or tiredness. Serious complications such as the collapse of circulation may occur, and death is a possibility.* Treatment usually involves a psychiatrist as well as other physicians, and may take months or more.

* Hilde Bruch, *Eating Disorders,* New York: Basic Books, 1974.

Losing Weight   Treatment for obesity is largely empirical, often unsatisfactory, and frequently frustrating. Nevertheless, overweight people can lose weight and enjoy the benefits of greatly increased health.

Very simply, weight is determined by an individual's caloric intake-output balance. Energy output is equally as important as calorie intake. In fact, some researchers believe that the significant reason for some people being fat while others are thin is not so much what they eat, but how many calories they burn.[5] Thus, the two components of a successful weight-reduction or weight-control program are regular physical exercise and a program of *moderation* in eating.[6] People are always trying to find a quick and easy way to lose weight, but the only real way is just to eat less. Individuals on a diet need all the essential nutrients as much as anyone, and the best way to get all the essential nutrients is to eat foods from the four basic groups discussed earlier. Fad diets may in fact be dangerous to one's health. Unless a person develops good eating habits, he will just regain all the weight he loses. A person interested in permanently losing weight must develop a healthy pattern of adequate, but not excessive, nutrition intake.

[5] Carl C. Seltzer and Frederick J. Stare, "Obesity: How It Is Measured, What Causes It, How To Treat It," *Medical Insight,* July-August 1973, pp. 10–28.
[6] Ibid.

Various authorities (the American Medical Association, Harvard University, and the Public Health Service) feel that the best way to lose weight is to eat fewer calories and exercise more. They recommend the caloric balance or caloric "checking account" approach. The individual must be aware of the calorie count of the food he eats and set up a meal plan according to the calories he needs while reducing and those he needs to maintain his desired weight once

Table 7.5 *Food and Nutrition Board, National Academy of Sciences—National Research Council Recommended Daily Dietary Allowances,*[1] *Revised 1973. Designed for the maintenance of good nutrition of practically all healthy people in the U.S.A. (Source: Food and Nutrition Board, National Academy of Science—National Research Council, Recommended Daily Dietary Allowances, 1973).*

	(years) From Up to	Weight (kg)	(lbs)	Height (cm)	(in)	Energy (kcal)[2]	Protein (g)	Vitamin A Activity (RE)[3]	(IU)	Vitamin D (UI)	Vitamin E Activity[3] (UI)	Ascorbic Acid (mg)
Infants	0.0–0.5	6	14	60	24	kg x 117	kg x 2.2	420[4]	14,400	400	4	35
	0.5–1.0	9	20	71	28	kg x 108	kg x 2.0	400	2,000	400	5	35
Children	1–3	13	28	86	34	1300	23	400	2,000	400	7	40
	4–6	20	44	110	44	1800	30	500	2,500	400	9	40
	7–10	30	66	135	54	2400	36	700	3,300	400	10	40
Males	11–14	44	97	158	63	2800	44	1,000	5,000	400	12	45
	15–18	61	134	172	69	3000	54	1,000	5,000	400	12	45
	19–22	67	147	172	69	3000	54	1,000	5,000	400	15	45
	23–50	70	154	172	69	2700	56	1,000	5,000		15	45
	51+	70	154	172	69	2400	56	1,000	5,000		15	45
Females	11–14	44	97	155	62	2400	44	800	4,000	400	10	45
	15–18	54	119	162	65	2100	48	800	4,000	400	11	45
	19–22	58	128	162	65	2100	46	800	4,000	400	12	45
	23–50	58	128	162	65	2000	46	800	4,000		12	45
	51+	58	128	162	65	1800	46	800	4,000		12	45
Pregnant						+300	+30	1,000	5,000	400	15	60
Lactating						+500	+20	1,200	6,000	400	15	80

[1] The allowances are intended to provide for individual variations among most normal persons as they live in the United States under usual environmental stresses. Diets should be based on a variety of common foods in order to provide other nutrients for which human requirements have been less well defined. See text for more-detailed discussion of allowances and of nutrients not tabulated.

[2] Kilojoules (KJ) $= 4.2$ xkcal.

[3] Retinol equivalents.

[4] Assumed to be all as retinol in milk during the first six months of life. All subsequent intakes are assumed to be one-half as retinol and one-half as β-carotene when calculated from international units. As retinol equivalents, three-fourths are as retinol and one-fourth as β-carotene.

he has reached it. Table 7.5 lists caloric intake for various weights, and there is a calorie chart on page 360.

A Sensible Diet

A strongly recommended diet plan (*Consumer Guide* gives it its highest rating) is Dr. Norman Jollife's Prudent Diet. The diets in the following list are modifications or adaptations of Dr. Jollife's plan and are equally recommended:

- New York Department of Health Diet
- Weight Watchers' Diet
- Diet Watchers Diet
- Diet Workshop Diet
- *Redbook's* Wise Woman's Diet

Water-Soluble Vitamins						Minerals					
Fola-cin[6] (µg)	Nia-cin[7] (mg)	Ribo-flavin (mg)	Thia-min (mg)	Vita-min B[4] (mg)	Vita-min B[12] (µg)	Cal-cium (mg)	Phos-phorus (mg)	Iodine (µg)	Iron (mg)	Mag-nesium (mg)	Zinc (mg)
50	5	0.4	0.3	0.3	0.3	360	240	35	10	60	3
50	8	0.6	0.5	0.4	0.3	540	400	45	15	70	5
100	9	0.8	0.7	0.6	1.0	800	800	60	15	150	10
200	12	1.1	0.9	0.9	1.5	800	800	80	10	200	10
300	16	1.2	1.2	1.2	2.0	800	800	110	10	250	10
400	18	1.5	1.4	1.6	3.0	1200	1200	130	18	350	15
400	20	1.8	1.5	2.0	3.0	1200	1200	150	18	400	15
400	20	1.8	1.5	2.0	3.0	800	800	140	10	350	15
400	18	1.6	1.4	2.0	3.0	800	800	130	10	350	15
400	16	1.5	1.2	2.0	3.0	800	800	110	10	350	15
400	16	1.3	1.2	1.6	3.0	1200	1200	115	18	300	15
400	14	1.4	1.1	2.0	3.0	1200	1200	115	18	300	15
400	14	1.4	1.1	2.0	3.0	800	800	100	18	300	15
400	13	1.2	1.0	2.0	3.0	800	800	100	18	300	15
400	12	1.1	1.0	2.0	3.0	800	800	80	10	300	15
800	+2	+0.3	+0.3	2.5	4.0	1200	1200	125	18+[8]	450	20
600	+4	+0.5	+0.3	2.5	4.0	1200	1200	150	16	450	25

[5] Total vitamin E activity, estimated to be 80 percent as σ-tocopherol and 20 percent other tocopherols. See text for variation in allowances.

[6] The folacin allowances refer to dietary sources as determined by *Lactobacillus case:* assay. Pure forms of folacin may be effective in doses less than one-fourth of the RDA.

[7] Although allowances are expressed as niacin, it is recognized that on the average 1 mg of niacin is derived from each 60 mg of dietary tryptophan.

[8] This increased requirement cannot be met by ordinary diets; therefore, the use of supplemental iron is recommended.

This basic diet is recommended by several health groups, including the American Heart Association, because it takes into account all the latest findings on the role food plays in high blood pressure, heart disease, and stroke.

The basic principles of the Prudent Diet are these:

· reduced calories
· reduced total fat intake
· increased polyunsaturates
· reduced dietary cholesterol
· adjusted carbohydrate intake (carbohydrates derived from grain, fruits, and vegetables instead of sugar)
· reduced salt intake
· stabilized protein intake

The most sensible diet contains a large proportion of protein, moderate amounts of fat (with polyunsaturated fat predominant), and a minimum of carbohydrates (with little sugar), since protein is the most important food category.[7] The body needs less fat and carbohydrates; however, it does need certain amounts of both, so beware of diets that eliminate one or both of these food categories almost entirely. The list of additional readings in the box on pages 112–13 includes some diets that are *not* recommended.

SOME COMMON NUTRITIONAL MYTHS

The areas of nutrition and diet have long been exploited by food faddists and quacks. In addition, "old wives' tales" predominate on this subject. As mentioned above, there are many diets which guarantee quick and easy weight loss, when there is actually no way to achieve this. A major area of confusion is the recent health food movement. Other food faddists propose they have found the one food that will not only keep people healthy, but will also act as a cure-all.

The Natural Foods Movement   In recent years interest in "natural" or "organic" foods has spread to many segments of the population. There is some basis to the claims made by the strong supporters of this movement, but there are also many fallacies taken as truth. Part of the problem has

[7] "Food Is More than Just Something To Eat," Prepared for the U.S. Department of Agriculture and Health, Education and Welfare in cooperation with the Grocery Manufacturers of America and the Advertising Council. This publication may be received at no charge by writing Nutrition, Pueblo, Colorado 81009.

been lack of adequate definition of the organic, natural, and health foods.

In 1971, Harvard University's Department of Nutrition offered the following definitions:

> *Health foods* are those that promote health. We maintain that all edible foods are health foods when properly used as part of a balanced diet, whether they are purchased in a neighborhood grocery store, a supermarket, or a so-called health food store.
>
> *Natural foods* are those that have no substances (nutritive or non-nutritive) added during processing. They are foods with "no additives."
>
> *Organic foods* are organic because they are all made up of compounds containing carbon—protein, fat, carbohydrate, and vitamins. Generally, organic foods are grown in soil with organic fertilizers and grown without chemical pesticides.

Many of the foods and vitamins found in health stores are really no different from those in neighborhood grocery stores—except that they are more expensive. The consumer should learn to read labels and lists of ingredients so as to know what he is buying, and to compare the content of "health" foods with "regular" foods.

Some people are concerned about foods grown with pesticides or foods that have chemical additives; some of their concern in valid. The Food and Drug Administration allows many food additives to be used even though they have received no prolonged testing for safety. This policy often results in certain products being taken off the market and condemned as unsafe—after people have been buying the product for many years. One example is Red Dye #2, which is used in both foods and cosmetics; recently it was investigated as a possible carcinogen (cancer-producing agent) and has now been banned. However, some additives, especially preservatives, are necessary in the preparation of certain foods. The wisest course for the consumer is to be aware of the ingredients in the foods he eats and to be cautious about excesses.

Another fear is that modern food processing and storage methods remove vital nutrients from foods. This is true to some extent: for example, vegetables may lose some vitamins in the canning process, and converted rice has fewer nutrients than whole grain rice. However, some problems are now being alleviated by enriching the foods or restoring their original nutritive values.

RECOMMENDED READINGS

Normal Nutrition:

Chaney, M.S. and Ross, M.L., *Nutrition,* Houghton Mifflin Co., 1971.

Deutsch, R., *The Family Guide to Better Food and Better Health,* Creative Home Library, 1971.

Leverton, R., *Food Becomes You,* Iowa Press, 1969.

Martin, E., *Nutrition in Action,* Connally and Brown, 1971.

National Academy of Sciences, *Recommended Dietary Allowances,* 7th Ed., 1968.

Stare, F., *Eating for Good Health,* Cornerstone Library, 1969 (Paperback or Hardcover), Doubleday.

Infant and Child Care:

Fomon, S. J., *Infant Nutrition,* W. B. Saunders Co., 1967.

Spock and Lowenberg, *Feeding Your Baby and Child,* Pocket Books, Inc., 1968.

Teenagers:

McWilliams, M., *Nutrition for the Growing Years,* Wiley, 1967.

Mature Years:

Institute of Rehabilitation, New York University Medical Center, *Mealtime Manual for the Aged and Handicapped,* Simon & Schuster, 1970.

About Food Fads:

Deutsch, R., *Grass Lovers,* (novel) Doubleday, 1962.

Deutsch, R., *Nuts Among the Berries,* Ballantine, 1967 (Paperback).

Tatkon, D., *The Great Vitamin Hoax,* The Macmillan Company, New York, 1968.

Wyden, P., *The Overweight Society,* Morrow, 1965.

Young, J., *The Medical Messiahs,* Princeton University Press, 1967.

A Study of Health Practices and Opinions, Accension No. PB 210–978, National Tech. Info. Services, Springfield, VA 22151, 1972.

Weight-Control:

Mayer, J., *Overweight,* Prentice-Hall, Inc., New Jersey, 1968, (Paperback).

Schoenberg, H., *Cookbook for Calorie Watchers,* Good Housekeeping Books, 1972.

Wyden, P., and Libien, L., *The All-in-One Diet Annual,* Bantam Books, New York, 1970, (Paperback).

Heart Disease:

Blakeslee and Stamler, *Your Heart Has Nine Lives,* Prentice-Hall, 1966.

Keys and Keys, *Eat Well and Stay Well,* Doubleday, 1963.

Payne and Callahan, *The Fat and Sodium Control Cookbook,* Little Brown, 1966.

Depleted Soil

Another myth currently propagated is that foods grown in the United States suffer in nutritional content because of depleted soils and lead to malnutrition because of vitamin deficiencies. Research on soil has shown that the nutritional value of crops grown in the United States is not significantly affected by the soil in which they are grown. Rather, it is the *quantity* of crops produced per unit area that is affected by the nutrient value of the soil.

NOT RECOMMENDED

Abehsera, *Cooking for Life,* Avon, 1972.

Abehsera, *Zen Macrobiotic Cooking,* Avon, 1970.

Atkins, *Dr. Atkins' Diet Revolution,* McKay, 1972.

Alexander, *Good Health and Common Sense,* Crown, 1960.

Bailey, *Vitamin E—Your Key to a Healthy Heart,* ARC Books, Inc., 1971.

Bieler, *Food Is Your Best Medicine,* Random House, 1965.

Cameron, *The Drinking Man's Diet Cookbook,* Bantam, 1969.

Clark, *Stay Younger Longer,* Devin-Adair, 1961.

Davis, Adelle, (any book).

Donaldon, *Strong Medicine,* Doubleday, 1961.

Elwood, *Feel like a Million,* Pocketbooks, Inc., 1965.

Glass, *Live to Be 180,* Taplinger, 1962.

Hauser, Gayelord, (any book).

Jacobson, *Eater's Digest,* Anchor-Doubleday, 1972.

Jameson and Williams, *The Drinking Man's Diet,* Cameron, 1964.

Jarvis, *Folk Medicine: A Vermont Doctor's Guide to Good Health,* Holt, 1958.

Jarvis, *Arthritis and Folk Medicine,* Fawcett, 1962.

Keller, *Healing with Water,* Award Books, 1968.

Kirschner, *Live Food Juices,* Kirschner, 1960.

Kloss, *Back to Eden,* Lancer, 1971.

Kordel, *Eat and Grow Younger,* McFadden, 1962.

Lappe, *Diet for a Small Planet,* Friends of the Earth/Ballantine, 1971.

Lindlahr, *Calorie Countdown,* Prentice-Hall, 1962.

Longgood, *The Poisons in Your Food,* Simon and Schuster, 1960.

Mackarness, *Eat Fat and Grow Slim,* Pocketbooks, Inc., 1962.

Marsh, *How to Be Healthy with Natural Foods,* ARC Books, Inc., 1969.

Martin, *Low Blood Sugar: The Hidden Menace of Hypoglycemia,* ARC Books, Inc., 1970.

Netzer, *The Brand-Name Calorie Counter,* Dell, 1969.

Nyoiti, *You Are all Sanpaku,* University Books, Inc., 1965.

Ohsawa, *Zen Macrobiotics—The Art of Longevity and Rejuvenation,* Ignoramus Press, 1966.

Rose, *Faith, Love and Seaweed,* Prentice-Hall, 1963.

Rosenburg, *Eat Your Way to Better Health,* Bobbs-Merrill, 1961.

Twitchell, *Herbs: The Magic Healers,* Lancer, 1971.

Wade, *Helping Your Health with Enzymes,* ARC Books, 1966.

Wade, *Magic Minerals,* ARC Books, 1971.

Weiner, *Get Your Health Together,* Lancer, 1971.

West, Ruth, (any book).

Winter, *Beware of the Food You Eat,* Signet, 1971.

Winter, *Poisons in Your Food,* Crown, 1969.

Source: Medical Opinion, December, 1972, p. 16.

Special Diets

There are various diets that are supported by members of the health food movement or by certain (often religious) groups. Among these are the different forms of vegetarian diets and the macrobiotic diets.

A moderate vegetarian diet excludes meat but not dairy products and possibly not fish. As long as the vegetarian makes sure he is

Uses and Safety[a] of Some Food Additives

Additive	Function	Safety[b]	Examples of use
Adipic acid	Acidulant	Safe	Fruit drinks, gelatin desserts
Agar	Thickener	Safe	Frostings, ice cream
Algin, sodium alginate	Thickener	Unknown	Ice cream, cheese spreads
Ascorbic acid (vitamin C)	Preservative anti-oxidant	Safe	Frozen fruits, yogurt
BHA (butylated hydroxy-anisole)	Preservative, anti-oxidant	Questionable	Shortening, vegetable oil, cereal, convenience foods
BHT (butylated hydroxy-toluene)	Preservative	Questionable	Same as BHA
Calcium propinate	Preservative in baked goods	Safe	Baked goods
Calcium stearoyl-2-lactylate	Emulsifier		Baked goods; dried egg whites
Carageen (carraghee-nan)	Thickener	Safe for adults, questionable for babies	Milk drinks, ice cream
Carboxymethylcellulose	Thickener	Safe	Ice cream, pie filling, diet foods
Citric acid	Acidulant	Safe	All fruit drinks, gelatin
Dextrin	Thickener	Safe	Candy, powdered mixes
Dextrose	Sweetener, browning agent	Safe	Bread, soft drinks
Dimethylpolysiloxane	Antifoaming, anti-splattering agent	Safe	Vegetable oil, wine, gelatin
Disodium guanylate	Flavor enhancer	Safe	Soup mixes, canned stews
Disodium inosinate	Flavor enhancer	Safe	Same as disodium guanylate
EDTA (ethylenediamine tetraacetic acid)	Preservative, sequestrant	Safe	Salad dressing, pickles, canned vegetables
Fumaric acid	Acidulant	Safe	Pudding, gelatin, soft drinks
Glycerol (glycerin)	Moisturizer, softener	Safe	Candy, baked goods
Glycerol lactopalmitate	Emulsifier, surfactant	Safe	Cake mixes, convenience foods
Glyceryl monooleate	Emulsifier	Safe	Baked goods, pudding
Guar gum	Thickener	Unknown	Pudding, salad dressing
Gum arabic	Thickener, anticrystalization agent	Unknown	Cake mixes, ice cream
Hydroxylated lecithin	Emulsifier	Unknown	Baked goods, margarine
Hydroxymethylcellulose	Thickener	Safe	Ice cream, pie filling
Lactic acid	Acidulant preservative	Safe	Frozen desserts, soft drinks

(continued)

Additive	Function	Safety[b]	Examples of use
Lactostearin	Emulsifier	Safe	Cake mixes
Lecithin	Emulsifier, antioxidant	Safe	Margarine, chocolate, ice cream
Mannitol	Sweetener, moisture inhibitor	Safe	Chewing gum, diet food
Mono- and diglycerides	Emulsifiers	Safe	Baked goods, candy, margarine
Monosodium glutamate (MSG)	Flavor enhancer	Causes discomfort in sensitive people; general safety questioned	Soup mixes, canned stews, soups
Polysorbate 60, 65, 80	Emulsifiers	Safe	Nondairy coffee creamers, frozen desserts
Potassium bromate	Aging flour	Safe	Flour
Potassium citrate	Buffer	Safe	Imitation fruit juices
Potassium sorbate	Preservative	Safe	Cheese, jelly mayonnaise
Propylene glycol	Moisturizer, solvent	Safe	Candy, soft drinks, marshmallows
Propylene glycol alginate	Thickener	Unknown	Frozen desserts, cheese spreads
Propyl gallate	Preservative, antioxidant	Questionable	Cereal, instant potatoes, vegetable oil
Sodium ascorbate	Preservative, antioxidant	Safe	Frozen fruits
Sodium citrate	Acidulant, antioxidant, sequestrant	Safe	Drink mixes
Sodium benzoate	Preservative	Safe, not tested for teratogenicity	Fruit juices, salad dressing, preserves
Sodium erythorbate	Preservative, antioxidant, gives red color to meat	Unknown	Bologna, frankfurters
Sodium nitrite and nitrate	Preservative, gives red color to meat	Questionable	Frankfurters and pork products
Sodium silicoaluminate	Anticaking agent	Safe	Salt, dessert topping mixes
Sodium sulfite	Prevents discoloration	Safe	Fruit juice, maraschino cherries
Sorbic acid	Preservative	Safe	Cheese, baked goods, mayonnaise
Sorbitol	Moisturizes, sweetener	Safe	Chewing gum, candy, soft drinks
Sorbitan monostearate	Emulsifier	Safe	Chocolate, frostings
Tregacanth	Thickener	Unknown	Salad dressing

[a] Information from (6). [b] Safe; has been subjected to full range of tests with no ill effects noted; unknown, has not been fully tested; questionable; although not proved harmful, ill effects noted in some animal studies.

Source: Chemistry, May 1974.

ingesting enough protein, from mainly vegetable sources, this diet should keep him as healthy as a person following a diet that includes meat. In fact, the vegetarian may even be healthier in that he is avoiding certain high-cholesterol foods. A more restricted vegetarian diet avoids dairy products as well as meat, fish, and poultry. A person following this type of diet must be sure to get enough protein from other foods.

A macrobiotic diet, unlike a vegetarian regime, can prove dangerous to health and can even be fatal. This diet concentrates heavily on grains, eventually to the point that brown rice is the only food allowed. This type of diet does not provide enough vitamins and minerals in its early stages, and provides almost no nutrition in its most extreme stages.

Curing Disease with Foods or Vitamins

It is true that improper diet can cause certain nutritional disorders, such as scurvy which is caused by a lack of vitamin C. There are other diseases caused by a specific lack of an important nutrient, and poor nutrition in general can lead to a weakening of the body's defenses, increasing susceptibility to disease.

However, there have recently been many claims made by authorities, reputable and otherwise, that are still largely unsubstantiated. Devotees of megavitamin therapy feel that massive doses of vitamins can not only prevent but also can cure disorders ranging from mental illness to cancer. One widespread belief, originally promulgated by Nobel Prize winner Dr. Linus C. Pauling, is that large amounts of vitamin C can prevent common colds. This claim is not supported by scientific research, although there recently has appeared some evidence that vitamin C may at least ameliorate the symptoms of a cold, though it may not prevent it.

Table 7.6 shows some of the recent claims made about various vitamins. Some of these claims may prove to be true, but most are as yet unsubstantiated. In fact, massive doses of certain vitamins (e.g., vitamin A) can prove harmful to your health.

WORLD HUNGER

Malnutrition and famine occur in many parts of the world today, and the fear of inadequate nutrition and food supplies increases as the population grows.

The spectre of diminishing food supplies is becoming an increasing reality:

- Stocks of grain have hit an all time low since the end of World War II.
- Food prices have reached new highs, and this increase threatens serious hardship for many people already spending most of their budget on food.
- Less of the cheaper protein foods, which normally supplement grain diets, is available.
- Fertilizer and energy shortages are reducing food production in certain areas and increasing food prices.[8]

Responsible officials have publicly stated that there is no way to help the starving people.[9] There is no easy solution to be offered. If we are to avoid worldwide hunger, a monumental effort, both scientific and political, must be made to improve both the production and distribution of food.

Table 7.6

VITAMIN and recommended daily allowance for adults	RECENT CLAIMS
A 5,000 International Units	Prevents some cancers; protects against air-pollutants
B₁ (Thiamine) 1.5 milligrams	Anti-depressant; reduces craving for certain drugs
B₃ (Niacin) 20 milligrams	Stabilizes manic-depression; relieves schizophrenia
B₆ (Pyridoxine) 2 milligrams	Overcomes fatigue; helps relieve Parkinson's disease
B₁₂ (Cobalamin) 6 micrograms	Aids in treatment of neuritis, neuralgia and psoriasis
C 60 milligrams	Prevents colds; relieves back pains; lowers cholesterol
D 400 International Units	Promotes general well-being
E 30 International Units	Promotes healthy skin, overcomes impotence, increased fertility

[8] "We the Undersigned . . . ," *The UNESCO Courier,* July-August 1974, p. 4.
[9] See Philip Handler, President, National Academy of Sciences, "Let Nature Take Its Course," *Science News,* 2 November 1974, p. 278.

FURTHER READINGS

Bruch, Hilde. "Psychological Aspects of Obesity," *Medical Insights,* July-August 1973.

Engel, Mary and Rudolph, Mae. "Let's Talk About Good Foods," *Family Health,* July 1970.

"Good Food for Good Health," *Family Health,* June 1971.

Harris, T. George. "Affluence, the Fifth Horseman of the Apocalypse: A Conversation with Jean Mayer," *Psychology Today,* January 1970.

Hegsted, D. Mark. "The Recommended Dietary Allowances for Iron," *American Journal of Public Health,* April 1970.

Lee, D. "Food and Human Existence," *Nutritional News,* June 1962.

Setizer, Carl and Mayer, Jean. "An Effective Weight Control Program in a Public School System," *American Journal of Public Health,* April 1970.

Seltzer, Carl C. and Frederick J. Stare. "Obesity: How It Is Measured, What Causes it, How To Treat It," *Medical Insights,* July-August 1973.

White, Philip S. *Let's Talk About Food,* Chicago: American Medical Association, 1968.

White, Philip S. and Rynearson, Edward. "The Dangers in Diet Advice," *Medical Insights,* July-August 1973.

4

SEXUAL AWARENESS

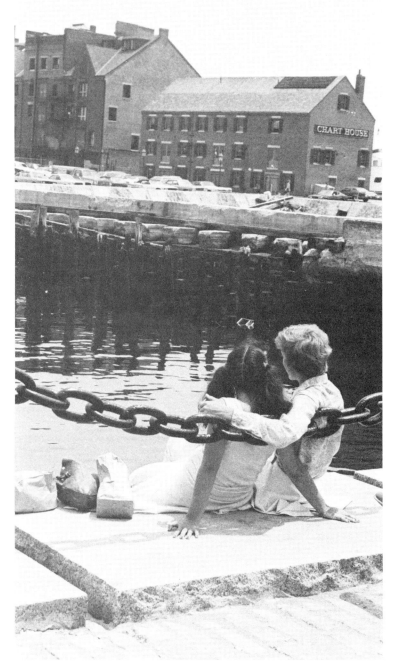

The omnipresent process
of sex, as it is woven into
the whole texture of our
man's or woman's body,
is the pattern of all the
process of our life.

Havelock Ellis
The New Spirit

Chapter 8

Healthy Sex and Sexuality

Sex and sexuality are of more concern in the United States today than almost any other topic. Almost any magazine or conversation is likely to include a reference to the subject. There is a new openness in discussion of all aspects of sex and sexuality.

CHANGING SEXUAL ATTITUDES

Some see this new openness about sex as being very positive. Others, including Rollo May (the author of *Love and Will*), feel that this trend may create greater internal anxieties and guilt feelings for many people. Yet sex and sexuality are an integral part of the life of the healthy individual.

Young people are especially eager to learn facts and attitudes about sex. However, they may get little or no information from their parents because of moral attitudes, ignorance, confusion, or fear. Schools have only recently begun to provide sex education. Any discussions in church groups of sex and sexuality may be more concerned with questions of immorality.

Many of these problems have historical roots. Most religions have traditionally viewed sex only in terms of procreation; thus sex was seen as being necessary and certainly not as a source of pleasure. Sex apart from procreation is as much a sin in the eyes of certain religions today as it was in the early days of the American colonies. Times are changing, however. The use of contraceptives to free sex from the threat of unwanted pregnancy, and the advent of antibiotics to treat venereal diseases have made it possible to have sex for pleasure. Today most doctors and sexologists feel that sex, if agreed upon as acceptable by the individuals involved, is a healthy and positive outlet.

Sexual Behavior in the Seventies

The basic change in sex and sexuality in the past few decades seems to be a trend towards better interpersonal relationships. The new openness has helped people, in many cases, to discuss and define their feelings toward themselves and others.

Statistics from two different sexual surveys provide a view of specific changes in sexual behavior in the last few decades. In 1948 and 1953, Alfred Kinsey conducted intensive research into various aspects and attitudes of sexual behavior; in the early 1970s *Playboy* magazine commissioned a survey of a national sample of 2,000 adults by Hunt. Some of the contrasts are quite interesting.

Kinsey found that a little over half of the single males aged sixteen to twenty-five in his sample were engaging in premarital sex, while the *Playboy* survey shows that over three-quarters of the sample's single males aged eighteen to twenty-four were sexually active. The shift is even more impressive for women. Kinsey found that one-fifth of single women sixteen to twenty, and one-third of the single women sixteen to twenty-five surveyed had engaged in premarital sex, while in the *Playboy* sample, two-thirds of the single women eighteen to twenty-four had been sexually active.

The data also indicate that more and more people are breaking the "taboos" about various sexual practices, such as oral and anal sex. (Both of these acts are still labeled as "punishable crimes against nature" in many states, even if they involve married or consenting adults.) In Kinsey's survey, 15 percent of the high school educated married men and 43 percent of the college educated married men were found to have engaged in fellatio. In the *Playboy* survey, 54 percent of the high school graduates and 61 percent of the college graduates had engaged in oral sex (the figures are roughly equivalent for cunnilingus.) The *Playboy* survey found 49 percent of those over the age of fifty to have engaged in oral sex as opposed to Kinsey's figure of 26 percent, suggesting that the lessening of these taboos is taking place throughout the social structure, though at different rates.

Sexual Morality

A growing number of psychologists, sociologists, educators, religious leaders, and others are recognizing that sexual morality is relative. It cannot be regulated effectively by laws or through fear of pregnancy or venereal disease. Its focus is bound to change with time and attitudes. Already there has been a shift from a condemnation of the act of intercourse in certain circumstances to a consideration of the two persons involved in each individual situation.

New standards are replacing traditional ones. Greater emphasis is placed on individual decisions about sex, than on applying a constant, absolute response based on a vague "common standard." This emphasis on the individual's decision makes the development of healthy attitudes toward sex and sexuality especially important.

HEALTHY SEXUALITY

A healthy acceptance of one's emotions concerning sex and sexuality is an important part of one's maturation and development. The success or failure of sexual relationships may depend on how one relates to others as a sexual person, how one sees himself in sexual terms, and on the type of sexual communication that exists. The emphasis on the importance of sex and sexuality may make some people afraid, but the topic becomes less awesome with knowledge and experience. Honest sexuality will be beneficial to anyone involved in a relationship, and meaningful sexual communication conducted in a nondefensive, nondegrading, and nonexploitative manner will almost certainly lead to a more positive sexual understanding.

Some of the following points should be helpful for anyone striving for healthy attitudes toward sex and sexuality.

Be true to yourself. In sex as well as in life one must constantly attempt to be true to oneself. For example, if you do not agree with the philosophy of intercourse before marriage, then don't be swayed when others attempt to make you think and feel differently.

Learn to accept yourself. People who are unsure, unhappy, and detached from themselves are often seeking approval through others. This is easily done through sex. The woman who sleeps with one man after another *may* be looking for affection and love she does not even feel for herself. The same may be applied to a man who cannot establish a warm relationship with any one person he dates. People with healthy self-concepts find it unnecessary to use sex as reassurance.

Measure what you do against what you believe. A young college girl who came in for counseling stated that she was very unhappy because she was having intercourse with a particular guy. She liked the boy but was being pressured by him to indulge in intercourse. Further discussion disclosed that she had had intercourse with a number of other guys, starting in high school. It was only when she was able to recognize a pattern in her choice of sex partner (or dating partner) that she was able to see it was she, not her dates, who initiated the act. At that point the inconsistency between what she did and what she believed became visible.

Develop a sense of trust in self and others. If one thinks about the people he likes, he would probably find that those are also the people he trusts. Furthermore, the more one can trust himself, the more he can like himself. Trust enhances relationships, for it allows an individual to be his or her natural self. A healthy sexual relationship between two people depends on the degree of mutual trust. All will agree that being able to accept another's feelings and needs facilitates involvement in a meaningful relationship.

Sexuality is an ever-present phenomenon. One cannot separate himself from his sexuality. The way one acts, feels, and relates are all dependent to some degree on one's sexuality. For this reason an individual should learn to accept and enjoy his sexuality. It is not necessary to reject feelings of arousal, but individuals should learn to trust, direct, and enjoy those feelings.

Sex is enjoyable. This is not to endorse the "fun morality," but the point needs to be made that kissing and other forms of sexual activity can be fun. They are an expression of closeness between two individuals and closeness, if it is sincere and shared honestly, can be rewarding to both partners.

SOME FORMS OF SEXUAL EXPRESSION

Nonmarital Sex

"Nonmarital sex" seems to be a more sensible term than "premarital sex" in that not all sexual relationships between single people lead to marriage, nor are they intended to. Nonmarital sex may mean anything from kissing to sexual intercourse. Petting can be used to describe any sexual activity involving more than kissing but less than intercourse. For some couples who do not want to become involved in intercourse, petting sometimes can be the solution to the need for close emotional and physical contact. However, heavy petting can lead easily to intercourse.

Ira Reiss, a sociologist who has written extensively on sexual behavior, has suggested that much of our societal difficulty in dealing with sex stems from the lack of a uniformly accepted code of sexual behavior, especially nonmarital sexual behavior. Reiss has identified four major standards that can be applied to American society:[1]

> *Abstinence.* Those adhering to this belief feel that nonmarital intercourse is unacceptable for both sexes. A Gallup poll of several years ago found that abstinence was the standard endorsed by 64 percent of those they interviewed (73 percent women, 54 percent men). Since it has been repeatedly documented that the majority

[1] Ira L. Reiss, *Premarital Sexual Standards in America,* New York: The Free Press of Glencoe, 1960.

of both men and women violate this standard, one might wonder for whom they were endorsing it.

· *The double standard.* Under this philosophy, nonmarital intercourse is acceptable for the male but not for the female. A male who takes this position considers any woman who has had sexual intercourse unacceptable for marriage. This is the "It's all right for me, but I want my wife to be a virgin" philosophy.

· *Sex without affection.* This is the "anything goes" philosophy which allows both sexes complete freedom from commitment and responsibility. This standard has been, and continues to be, popular among only a small number, in contrast to the media-created picture of "rampant immorality" on college campuses. The philosophy becomes increasingly more common as one descends the socioeconomic scale.

· *Sex with affection.* This standard is that of permissiveness with some affection or emotional attachment involved. Such a standard promotes the acceptability of nonmarital intercourse for both males and females while clearly establishing the quality of the relationship as a precondition. Permissiveness with affection is predicted upon the acceptance of "person-centered" rather than "body-centered" coitus.

Many young people may seek a reasonable set of guidelines that will help them in their decision about nonmarital sexual intercourse. Dr. Willard Dalrymple suggested a number of such questions.[2]

· What are some of the qualities a warm, lasting relationship calls for, and how does one acquire or develop them?
· How is a mutual sense of human dignity, actual and potential, best preserved in a continuing relationship?
· Does such a relationship involve fidelity? Continuity?
· What does either partner see as crucial milestones on a possible journey to a lasting relationship?
· How many of these milestones have to do with physical relations, up to and including sexual intercourse?
· What happens when the partners decide to opt for a lasting relationship (marriage, or their idea of its equivalent)?
· Is the individual's respect for himself or his partner increased or diminished by a sexual relationship or the lack of it, once the above decision is made?
· Will it be easier or harder to create an ideal relationship later on if one has had previous sexual experience?
· Will a relationship be stronger and more lasting if the individuals have their first sexual experience with each other?
· How important is it to make public announcement of an engagement or to have a legal marriage ceremony?

[2] Dr. Willard Dalrymple, "Sex and the College Student," *University—A Princeton Quarterly,* Winter 1973.

Many people can answer these questions easily and without hesitation. These are people with a high degree of personal maturity and self-knowledge; they know who they are and what they want. These individuals have no doubts about guilt feelings over their sexual activities, for they believe in what they do. They have no need to use others to find out who they are.

Sexual Variations

What does the term "making love" mean? For some, making love means only sexual intercourse, but for others making love evokes the image of two people engaged in oral lovemaking, kissing, touching, anal intercourse, and many other types of interaction.

In essence, making love or sexual activity for pleasure may mean many things depending on your mood, sex, age, experience, and beliefs. An open definition of sex can be a true sharing of love and emotion in any act that is self-enhancing, beautiful, or whatever two people agree upon.

Differences in attitudes toward such sexual activities as oral or anal sex are common. Such differences do sometimes cause problems between sexual partners, and call for negotiations or compromise to resolve conflicting desires.

Oral Sex

The mouth is a source of sexual stimulation. People kiss each other without hesitation or condemnation, bringing the tongue into play as a stimulus to further excitement. So too do people orally excite their sexual partners by kissing and sucking the sexual organs during lovemaking.

Fellatio, oral stimulation of the male genitals, and *cunnilingus,* oral stimulation of the female genitals, are often used as forms of sexual arousal or foreplay for genital intercourse. These forms of sexual activity can be used to provide orgasm and are often used instead of genital intercourse as a stimulating and natural way for variety and experimentation in sexual activity.

Anal Sex

Anal sex can be defined very broadly as an oral, penile, or manual manipulation of the anal region for erotic purposes. Anal sex provides sexual satisfaction for various reasons. The erotic reflexes engendered by anal and vaginal stimulation are somewhat comparable (see Chapters 9 and 10 for a more detailed discussion).

Anal penetration as a coital position has advantages. It allows the male manual access to the female's clitoral and vaginal regions for additional stimulation. Some women find satisfaction in experiencing penetration in an anatomical orifice other than the vagina; anal sex as a novelty is arousing to many people. Also, many older women whose vaginas have been stretched by childbirth and age experience a lack of vaginal tone and sensitivity and therefore find anal sex more stimulating.

Homosexuality   There has been much speculation on the causes of homosexuality, its influence on society, and society's influence on it, but very little empirical research has been done in this area. This is partly because of the strong negative attitudes traditionally expressed in this society regarding homosexual behavior. Recently however the openness and tolerance that have been emerging in relation to all types of sexual expression have affected the views on homosexuality as well. Many old myths and stereotyped ideas have begun to disappear.

Each person is not necessarily completely heterosexual or homosexual. There are degrees, and many people who consider themselves heterosexual may have been involved in homosexual activities at some time in their lives. A homosexual can be defined as a person who prefers and experiences sex primarily with members of his own sex.

Homosexuality is no longer considered as a mental illness or deviance. In 1973 the American Psychiatric Association struck homosexuality from a listing in its *Diagnostic and Statistical Manual* and stated that "homosexuality shall no longer be listed as a mental disorder if the individual is not dissatisfied with homosexuality and if it does not regularly impair his or her social functioning." The APA also went on record as stating that homosexuals who are troubled by their condition should be characterized as persons with "a sexual-disorientation disturbance." A major upshot of the APA's action was a vigorous counterattack by those psychiatrists and psychoanalysts who thought the decision was wrong. A study cited in the *American Journal of Psychiatry* found that practicing homosexuals with few or no heterosexual interests are no more subject to conflicts or psychological disturbances than any other members of the society.[3] A recent study in Britain of a matched sample of homosexual and heterosexual women found that the lesbians were as well adjusted as the heterosexual women.[4]

The fact that any number of sexual acts (masturbation, oral, or anal sex) have been considered "abnormal" in the past shows how

[3] Saghir et al. "Psychiatric Disorders of Male Homosexuals," *American Journal of Psychology,* February 1970, p. 1079.
[4] Dr. Garfield Tourney, "Advising the Homosexual," *Medical Aspects of Human Sexualtity,* January 1973.

relative the terms "normal" and "abnormal" are in sexual matters. Attitudes about homosexuality are changing as attitudes are redefined and as the homosexual community becomes more active in its fight for recognition and rights.

SEX AND SEXUALITY IN LATER YEARS

"The aged are sexually underprivileged," contends Erik Pfeiffer (Associate Professor of Psychiatry at Duke Medical Center). He urges that older adults as well as the young should be included in this era of sexual liberation.

In our youth-oriented culture there still exists a prevailing attitude that old people are "beyond" sex. Widely held myths include the beliefs that older men and women lack sexual needs or desires and that after menopause, coital gratification lessens substantially because of physiological reasons.

Fortunately, some of these beliefs are now being reevaluated and the myths exploded. For example, sexual gratification in women may actually increase after menopause because the threat of a possible unwanted pregnancy no longer exists. Masters and Johnson have studied sex in the older male and found that the achievement of erection and orgasm may take longer and occur less frequently than in the younger male, but neither the desire nor the capacity are necessarily diminished by aging.

Masters and Johnson include extensive research on sex in older people in *Human Sexual Response* and *Human Sexual Inadequacy*. Their work and the research of others (such as Alex Comfort, in *A Good Age*) should help to include the old as well in this era of sexual awareness. People can feel "sexy" at any age.

LOVE AND LOVING

Sexual love is one type of love. There are many other types and many more definitions of love. One possible definition is that love is an interrelationship between two people that is greater than the sum of the two individuals in isolation.

Mature love is primarily giving rather than receiving. Erich Fromm stresses this active aspect of love rather than a passive aspect. He describes three types of loving: infantile love states "I love because I am loved"; immature love reasons "I love you because I need you"; and mature love means "I need you because I love you."[5]

[5] Erich Fromm, *The Art of Loving,* New York: Bantam Books, 1956, p. 34.

Burgess and Locke defined ten components of love which can be used to understand most types of loving.[6]

1. Sexual desire—the domain of biochemistry and physiology.
2. Physical attraction—social and personal discriminations of sex appeal.
3. Attachment—rapport through intimate association, mutual responsiveness.
4. Emotional interdependence—mutual fulfillment of basic personality needs.
5. Idealization—distortion of the other's image of lovers' dreams.
6. Companionship—common interest, mental interstimulation, and response.
7. Stimulation—adventure in new experiences together.
8. Freedom of communication and action—exchange of confidences, freedom to be oneself.
9. Emotional reassurance—mutual reaffirmation.
10. Status—pride of possession, mutual self-congratulation.

The interrelationship between love and sexual desire is very important but is sometimes difficult to define. People may use the excuse of love as a justification for what is actually casual sex. "Making love" has become an often inappropriate euphemism for having sex. Love is not present in all sexual relationships; indeed, Rollo May believes that "the Victorian person sought to have love without falling into sex; the modern person seeks to have sex without falling into love."[7] But in a loving relationship between two people, sex is usually quite important; e.g., problems in the sexual relationship lead to or may mean problems in other aspects of the relationship.

Other components—loneliness, communication, etc.—described by Burgess and Locke are more or less important in each loving relationship. The definition of love one decides upon is unimportant. What is important is that a person make a healthy choice, so that the loving relationship contains mutual gratifications, happiness, and possibilities for growth of each partner.

MARRIAGE AND DIVORCE

In 1963 Betty Friedan's *The Feminine Mystique* was published, attacking the ideals of marriage, motherhood, and the happy housewife which had been part of our culture for generations.[8] Since her docu-

[6] Ernest W. Burgess and Harvey J. Locke, *The Family from Institution to Companionship,* New York: American Book, 1953, pp. 322–326.
[7] Rollo May, *Love and Will,* New York: W. W. Norton & Company, 1969, p. 46.
[8] Betty Friedan, *The Feminine Mystique,* New York: Dell Publishing, 1963.

mentation of some of the results of these widely accepted concepts, traditional marriage has been seriously criticized and reexamined. There is even speculation as to how much longer traditional marriage will exist. William J. Lederer, Director of the Palo Alto Mental Health Institute, has found that:

- at least one-third of the couples married in 1972 ultimately will divorce
- of the couples who do not get divorced, at least 70 percent will live in considerable unhappiness[9]

Questions about the success of marriage focus on the institution of marriage itself as well as on its inability to survive in light of recent social developments such as changing sexual attitudes and the growing independence of women. Some moralists question whether individuals can now maintain the necessary virtues for a lasting and secure relationship. Other views hold that the institution of marriage has become outdated and is no longer appropriate for our society.

Wilhelm Reich wrote about "The Problem of Marriage" in *The Sexual Revolution,* which was published in 1945. He viewed marriage as a product of the time when some type of social contract was needed for the survival and protection of society's members. At the time he wrote, Reich believed that the economic dependence of women, though lessening to some degree, was still a reality.[10] Thus, marriage was still important in a culture of which this economic dependence by some members was a part.

Today, economic dependence of women is becoming less and less a fact in our society. A feminist paper distributed at a bridal fair at the University of Massachusetts underlines the changing attitudes toward woman's role in society and marriage:

> We are not here because we are opposed to the idea of marriage in itself. . . . We are opposed to the idea that from your wedding day forward, you should be dependent on your husband—that you need him to be responsible for you, for everything from your budget to your ideas. The only price you pay for this is a lack of your own identity, a lack of belief and confidence in yourself as a whole person, a lack of trust in your own judgment about things outside of the home; in short, the inability to fulfill your potential.

[9] William J. Lederer, "Putting Marriage on Camera," *New York* Magazine, 1973.
[10] Wilhelm Reich, *The Sexual Revolution,* New York: Farrar, Straus and Giroux, 1945.

> ### Anger is love?
>
> Not quite. But, some psychiatrists say that anger is closely related to love. They're both forms of communication and personal involvement. And for whom, after all, do we reserve our most intense anger? Those closest to us. Those who arouse the greatest expectations and disappointments. Therefore, these psychiatrists conclude, when anger is accompanied by clear communication, it's a sign of basic respect for the other person.
>
> If that's too far-fetched, consider this explanation by Dr. Daugherty: "Sometimes, anger can be fun. Once in a while, an argument—if it lasts only a short time and has some resolution—gets your adrenalin going. It can be the highlight of your day."
>
> If 'you don't buy that explanation either, you'll probably agree with this: Anger, especially when bottled up, is self-destructive. So don't play deaf and dumb. Relieve the angry patient's tension—and your own in the bargain.
>
> *Source: Practical Psychology For Physicians,* March 1975, p. 38.

Another factor that may be relevant to the status of marriage today is the rise of the nuclear family. The extended family—a unit of parents and children and other relatives, spanning several generations—has been largely replaced in the United States by the nuclear family—husband, wife, and children living together. Author and critic Marya Mannes writes: "I have come to believe that the small, single-family unit—whether urban or suburban—contributes to the death of marriage as we have known it and literally 'locks in' not only man and wife, but also child and parent, allowing neither to develop freely and fully as individuals."

Many other authorities still uphold marriage as a valuable and viable institution in our society. Yet it is evident, in view of the dissatisfaction shown by vociferous critics and the skyrocketing divorce rate, that changes must occur. Perhaps changes in the whole concept and role of marriage will not be necessary, but new attitudes and expectations are definitely needed.

Changing Attitudes and Expectations

Myths about marriage and the roles of husband and wife abound. The authors of *The Mirages of Marriage* contend that a marriage is doomed when these false ideals are acted upon; these writers attack these attitudes and expectations in an attempt to abolish them.

Many people believe that marriage is based only upon love. In fact, individuals marry for many different reasons: societal expectations, parental pressures, tradition, and loneliness. People without any real idea of love believe love to be the necessary basis for marriage and disguise their real reasons for marrying under a declaration of love.[11] Romantic literature often provides a false view of love and it may also lead to unrealistic expectations of marriage.

The best marital foundation will fail to support a marriage constructed with the materials of a dream. Authors Nena and George O'Neill have explored some of the common expectations of marriage and divided them into two categories, unrealistic ideas and realistic ideas.

Among the unrealistic expectations of marriage are:

·   It will last forever
·   It will bring you happiness, comfort, and security at all times
·   You will have constant attention, concern, admiration, and consideration from your mate
·   You will never be lonely again
·   Your mate belongs to you
·   Your mate would rather be with you than anyone else at all times
·   Your mate will never be attracted to another person
·   Your mate will always be true to you; fidelity is the true measure of your love

More realistic expectations of marriage include:

·   Each partner will change—and positive change can occur through conflict as well as through a gradual evolvement
·   You will share most things but not everything
·   You cannot expect your mate to fulfill all your needs or to do for you what you should be doing for yourself
·   The mutual goal is the relationship, not status or the house by the sea or children
·   Liking and loving will grow because of the mutual respect that your relationship engenders[12]

Foundations for a Good Marriage   In addition to reevaluating the myths and unrealistic expectations that surround marriage, there are other positive steps two people making a decision on marriage can take. The greater openness about sex and sexuality has extended into other areas as well, leading to greater communication in general.

Individuals considering marriage can make use of this openness by discussing their own ideas of marriage, including role expectations. The women's liberation movement is challenging many stereo-

---

[11] William Lederer and Donal D. Jackson, *The Mirages of Marriage,* New York: W. W. Norton & Co., 1968.
[12] Nena O'Neill and George O'Neill, *Open Marriage,* New York: M. Evans and Company, 1972.

typical ideas and replacing them with more open views. Among these are:

1. *A woman's place is in the home.* A woman's place is in the world —home, office, school, etc.
2. *Working women are unfeminine.* Working women are people.
3. *All women want to be married.* Some women and some men want to be married, some women and some men do not want to be married.
4. *Woman's true fulfillment comes through having children.* Woman's true fulfillment comes through whatever satisfies her expectations of herself.
5. *Cooking and cleaning are woman's work.* Cooking and cleaning are just plain work, and can be done by everyone.
6. *Women are instinctively better at raising children than men.* Some women or men may be better parents than others.
7. *Men are the breadwinners.* In some families women are the main wage earners, in some men are, and in others both are.

Role expectations should be clarified *before* marriage. Questions such as who will do the household tasks, who will handle the finances, who will care for the children, and so forth must be answered before the wedding, not afterwards.

Lederer's study on marriage and divorce also found that:

- People who have good marriages enjoy better health and live longer than those who have discordant marriages or who remain single.
- People who have good marriages usually experience a higher measure of economic comfort than those who have bad marriages.
- The children of parents who have good marriages are more inclined to have good marriages of their own. Generally they also have better health, a lower juvenile-delinquency rate, and a lower dropout level than the children of bad marriages.[13]

What defines the healthy relationship necessary for a good marriage? Sidney Jourard has suggested certain guidelines to consider before marriage:

1. The partners know each other to be distinctly individual.
2. Each finds more desirable traits than undesirable traits in the other.
3. Each feels concern for the happiness and development of his partner.
4. The partners actively behave in ways that promote this growth and happiness.
5. The partners can make themselves understood and known to each other: they communicate effectively.

[13] Lederer, "Putting Marriage on Camera."

6. Each makes reasonable demands on the other.
7. Both value and respect the autonomy and individuality of the other.[14]

These ideas should concern individuals before they marry, and they can also test their relationship periodically once they are married. If one (or more) criterion is missing, they should reevaluate their marriage and work on the trouble spots.

ALTERNATIVES TO TRADITIONAL MARRIAGE

Cohabitation and Trial Marriage

Cohabitation and trial marriage are becoming increasingly common among college students and other members of the population today. Some individuals may live with a member of the opposite sex in a long-lasting relationship but with no plans or expectations for marriage. Others may view their living together as a definite prelude to marriage if the arrangement is satisfactory.

Trial marriage is not a new concept. It was practiced by Peruvian Indians for more than four centuries. The first American to propose trial marriage was Judge Ben B. Lindsay, in 1927. Many other authors and experts including Robert Rimmer[15] have discussed trial marriage and advocated its use.

There are problems, however, and trial marriage is not for everyone. A number of individuals may feel insecure without a legal marriage certificate. One or both partners may worry that the other may leave when things get rough, feeling that they have made no real commitment. Perhaps this is more a reflection on the relationship involved than on the concept of trial marriage.

A second problem is that parents and others do not always view trial marriage or cohabitation as satisfactory arrangements. Couples who cannot declare their living arrangements publicly may feel guilty and resentful.

Many people do overcome the problems involved and are able to maintain a healthy relationship that sometimes leads to marriage. In addition to trial marriage, other alternatives to the traditional procedures of marriage are appearing.

[14] Sidney Jourard, *Personal Adjustment,* New York: The Macmillan Company, 1963, p. 358.
[15] See Robert Rimmer, *The Harrad Experiment,* Los Angeles: Sherbourne Press, 1966 and *The Harrad Letters,* New York: New American Library, Signet Books.

***New Types
of Marriage***

As early as 1924, Melvin M. Knight suggested that two people who were married but had no children be referred to as a "companionate," and that only a married couple with one child or more be called a "family." He recommended that a companionate should be dissolvable upon mutual consent after nine months of separation.[16]

Margaret Mead has proposed two kinds of marriage, or a two-step marriage. An *individual marriage* would involve a simple ceremony, limited economic responsibilities between the partners, and no children. Divorce, if desired, could be easily achieved. *Parental marriage* would follow individual marriage as a second step for couples ready to undertake the obligations of parenthood. The contract for this step would be more difficult to make and break; divorce would entail mutual continuing responsibility for the children.[17]

Vance Packard discusses a variation on trial marriage in *The Sexual Wilderness*. He stresses that this would in no way constitute the typical trial marriage (an arrangement he views as no more than unstructured cohabitation). He suggests that the first two years of marriage should be viewed as a confirmation period. After these two years, the couple could either dissolve the relationship or finalize the marriage document.[18]

Communal Living

Communal living is another concept with old historical roots that has gained popularity in recent years. The existence of communes can be traced through centuries, but the idea of communal living really caught on in the United States in the 1960s. First appearing mainly in New York City and the Haight-Ashbury district of San Francisco, these modern communes now exist all over California, New Mexico, Arizona, New England, and other parts of the country.

Variations of communes range from groups who believe only in sharing living quarters to those who raise children together or who all work together as well. Groups may consist of two married couples living together or may include single individuals of both sexes in numbers as great as one hundred. Some communes are based on religious beliefs shared by all, others include groups with little in common but a desire for group living. Some commune groups may reject the ideas of private property and defined relationships, sharing everything from money and personal possessions to sex; others live much more conservative or traditional forms of life. Some groups may practice asceticism, rejecting drugs, alcohol, and/or sex.

[16] Melvin M. Knight, "The Companionate and the Family," *Journal of Social Hygiene,* 10, 1924, pp. 257–267.
[17] Margaret Mead, "Marriage in Two Steps," *Redbook,* 1966, pp. 48–49.
[18] Vance Packard, *The Sexual Wilderness,* New York: David McKay, 1968, pp. 466–468.

Although some communes have lasted many years, Herbert A. Otto has found that commune dwellers, especially in the most unstructured groups, are transients who drift out of the commune to more conventional lifestyles after a few years. Otto listed four major reasons for the short life spans of many communes: disagreement over household chores or other work, interpersonal conflicts, problems associated with economic survival, and hostility from surrounding communities.[19]

Remaining Single   Although there are a wealth of books available on marriage, marital sex, and child rearing, works dealing specifically with the single person are rare. This is unfortunate, as over 10 percent of the American population remains single. There are four basic categories of single people: those who are single because of religious or altruistic reasons, those who are single but would like to marry, those whose circumstances dictate a single life (e.g., the severely mentally retarded), and those who have no desire to be married.

Our culture and its laws take a negative view of the unmarried person. Most people assume marriage is an answer and goal for everyone and feel sorry for anyone who is not married. There are numerous clubs and dating bureaus eager to marry off all single people. Healthy sexual outlets are often a problem for the single person in a society that has traditionally reserved legal, approved sex for married couples.

Changes must occur so that remaining single can be viewed as a positive alternative to marriage for those who want it. Equality and liberation for the single person are necessary.

[19] Herbert A. Otto, "Has Monogamy Failed?" *Saturday Review,* April 25, 1970, pp. 23–25+.

FURTHER READINGS

Amazon Expedition. New York: Times Change Press, 1973.

A lesbian feminist anthology.

Bohannan, Paul. *Love, Sex and Being Human.* Garden City, N.Y.: Doubleday & Co., Inc., 1970.

The author presents the point of view of the anthropologist who sees clearly the relatedness of the biological and social aspects of being human.

Fisher, Peter. *The Gay Mystique.* New York: Stein & Day Pub., 1973.

The myth and reality of male homosexuality.

Fromm, Erich. *The Art of Loving.* New York: Bantam Books, 1956.

This classic book explores the way in which love can be used to alter the whole course of life.

Kuten, Jay. *Coming Together—Coming Apart.* New York: Macmillan, 1974.

This book deals with the interplay of forces moving people toward and away from one another in love and sex.

Masters, William and Johnson, Virginia. *The Pleasure Bond.* Boston: Little Brown, 1974.

Deals with the problem of keeping alive the physical attraction that originally brought a couple together.

Chapter 9

Female Sexuality

HELMER: Before everything else you're a
                wife and mother.
NORA: I don't believe that any longer.
                I believe that before everything else
                I'm a human being, just as much as
                you are—or at any rate I shall try to
                become one.
                                —Ibsen, *A Doll's House*[1]

Physical differences between males and females begin before birth. Male or female genital differentiation begins between the sixth and tenth week of the development of the fetus. There is also some speculation that there may be sexual differences in the brain. Anthropologist Margaret Mead suggests that there are genetic predispositions to male or female types of behavior, citing such "cultural universals" as male dominance and aggressiveness or female submissiveness and maternal instincts.

Yet most experts now agree that it is society and our cultural training that define our sexual roles. What Margaret Mead sees as cultural universals may just be stereotypes that exist in great part because of acceptance and reinforcement. Some of these stereotyped ideas see a girl as being very talkative, tactful, gentle, aware of feelings in others, and unassuming, with a strong need for security. Boys are pictured as being very aggressive, independent, logical, direct, adventurous, self-confident, ambitious, and unemotional.[2] The

[1] Henrik Ibsen, "A Doll's House," in *The Collected Works of Henrik Ibsen,* vol. 7, translated by William Archer, New York: Charles Scribner's Sons, 1906, p. 147.
[2] Florence Howe, "Sexual Stereotypes Start Early," *Saturday Review,* 16 October 1971, p. 80.

women's movement is a major factor in showing these views to be only stereotyped ideas and, by spreading its belief in sexual quality and interchangeable social roles, is helping to bring about a change in attitudes and behavior.

> . . . talk about women's lib, or promoting mental health, or consciousness raising should encourage all of us to use our real experiences as mothers to move away from a world where individuals find it easier to adopt a cardboard, ready-made image than to create one. The mature person defines herself; she is not defined by others.[3]

FEMALE SEXUALITY

Present evidence indicates a greater increase in the number of women than in the number of men engaging in nonmarital intercourse before graduation from college. Contrasting with Kinsey's finding of fewer than 20 percent, recent reports estimate that nearly 50 percent of all undergraduate women have had nonmarital sexual relations. These changes in sexual behavior reflect an earlier introduction to dating and in increased acceptance of nonmarital sex within the context of a "meaningful relationship."

These more rational attitudes toward sex have not solved all the grievances and unhappiness of past centuries of women. It has been found that the pressure of boys' demands for nonmarital sex experience is a common cause of drug overdoses and other attempted suicides by girls thirteen and fourteen years old. These girls often suffer tremendous emotional pressures from their boyfriends at a time in their lives when they are not really ready to think about such things.

Another problem found by Dr. Judianne Densen-Gerber, a Manhattan psychiatrist, is that "The teenage girl hung up on the idea of female orgasm ends up by humiliating her masculinity-obsessed but usually inexperienced partner, leaving both disillusioned with sex as a cure for alienation."[4]

While the majority of undergraduate college women appear to cope satisfactorily with their sexual relationships, an increasing number are requesting counseling for problems caused by nonmarital sexual relationships, including depression, anxiety, or guilt (related to in part rigid or permissive upbringing), unhappy home life, ambivalence about nonmarital coitus, lack of sex education, intimidation by a

[3] Angela Barron McBride, *The Growth and Development of Mothers,* New York: Harper & Row, 1973.
[4] "Sex and Change," *Time,* 20 March 1972, p. 47.

boyfriend, and/or fear of sexual desires, or fear of permanent relationships.

University of Michigan psychologist Judith Bardwick feels that instead of allowing women to enjoy sex, the pill has replaced the fear of pregnancy with a fear of being used. "Far from giving young women the sexual license that men have so long enjoyed, the Pill has caused some women to resent male freedom even more," she states. "Far from alleviating anxiety over sexual use of the body, the Pill has exacerbated it."[5]

There are of course positive sides to the new freedom. Cornell psychiatrist James Masterson feels that social pressure to have sex sooner leads to early discovery and treatment of any sexual problems. Further, a succession of close involvements "may teach one to deal not only with the emotional potential for a close relationship, but also with the emotional problems of separation—two important keys to adjustment."[6]

There are many reasons for learning and knowing more about one's sexuality:

> We are not learning more about our sexuality in order to produce bigger and better spasms in orgasm. We are concerned about why women are encouraged to think about sex in such competitive, objectifying ways. We want to help ourselves and each other grow to be full people capable of open, loving relationships. And before we can really love another, we must learn to love ourselves. By looking carefully at our needs, by dealing honestly with our sexuality, we free up lots of energy for other satisfying work, activity, and living.[7]

FEMALE SEXUAL ANATOMY

The female genitals are both external and internal. The external genitalia, or *vulva,* includes the mons veneris, the labia, and the clitoris. The internal organs are the vagina, the uterus, the fallopian tubes, and the ovaries.

The External Organs   One of the most obvious features of a mature woman is the pubic hair, which grows from the *mons veneris* (mound of Venus)—

[5] Ibid.
[6] Masterson, James. *Focus: Human Sexuality* (Guilford, Conn.: The Dushkin Publishing Group, Inc., 1976.
[7] The Boston Women's Health Collective, *Our Bodies, Ourselves,* New York: Simon and Schuster, 1971, p. 23.

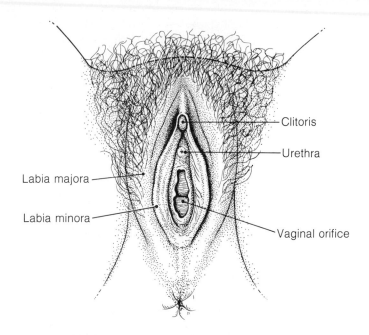

Clitoris

Urethra

Labia majora

Labia minora

Vaginal orifice

FIGURE 9.1   *The female external genitalia.*

the soft fatty tissue that covers the joint of the pubic bones—and extends over the *labia major,* or outer lips, of the vulva. The labia major surround the *labia minora,* or inner lips, which are delicate folds of skin not covered by any pubic hair. With sexual stimulation the inner lips swell and turn a darker color.

Between the labia minora is an area called the *vestibule* or "entrance". In the front part of the vulva area the labia minora forms a *hood* over the *clitoris.* The clitoris is the most sensitive part of the genitals. It is made up of erectile tissue and during sexual arousal it swells and protrudes from the hood. Below the clitoris is the *urethra,* or urinary opening, leading to the bladder.

Below the urethra is the vaginal orifice. Within the vaginal opening is the *hymen,* a thin membrane of varying size or shape. It may be broken by sexual intercourse, exercise, or insertion of tampons, so that a hymen that is not intact does not necessarily mean that the woman has had sexual intercourse. Even when a hymen becomes stretched by intercourse, folds of the membrane tissue remain.

The area of the vulva between the vaginal opening and the anus (rectal opening) is called the *perineum.* It forms a wedge of tissue separating the vagina and the rectum. In childbirth this tissue is stretched a great deal.

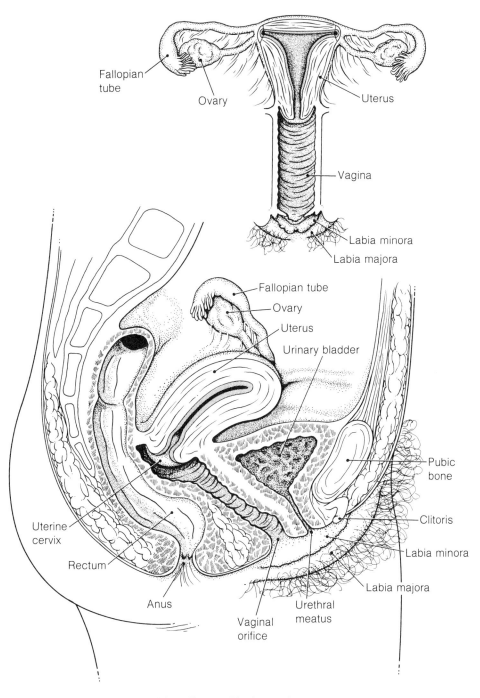

FIGURE 9.2 *The internal organs.*

The Internal Organs

The *vagina* is a muscular tube extending from the external genitals to the uterus. It is composed of an inner lining, which is soft, pliable, and moist, and an outer, thicker layer composed of muscle fibers. It lies between the bladder and the rectum and it is surrounded and protected by the strong muscles of the floor of the pelvis. The vagina has a remarkable self-cleansing capacity, and because of this, "cleansing" vaginal douches are usually unnecessary.

Above the vagina is the *uterus*, which is made up of the upper *body* (or fundus) and a lower neck, or *cervix*. The nonpregnant uterus is about the size of a fist and, unless pushed apart by a tampon or abnormal growth, its walls touch each other. Normally the uterus lies at a ninety degree angle to the vagina, above the bladder. As the bladder fills, the uterus may tip farther back, falling back into place when the bladder is emptied. About 10 percent of all women have a displaced uterus or one that is tipped backwards (a condition called retroversion).

Two small *fallopian tubes* (or *oviducts*, meaning egg tubes) extend out and back from the upper part of the uterus. They are about four inches long and they connect the uterus with the *ovaries*. The outer end of each fallopian tube is fringed, or *fimbriated.*

The ovaries are small and almond shaped. They have two functions: the development of eggs, and the production of ovarian hormones, estrogen and progesterone.

OVULATION AND MENSTRUATION

The ovaries are filled with a large number of what are called *ovarian follicles* (or sacs), each containing an unripened egg. When a female is born, her ovaries contain around 200,000 immature egg follicles, but only about 400 of these follicles will mature and produce a ripe egg. The immature follicles ripen at a rate of about one every twenty-eight days, maturing into a *graaffian follicle.* The graafian follicle ruptures to expel the egg (or *oocyte*) that is then swept into the fallopian tubes. The discharge of the ripened egg or *ovum* from the ovary is called *ovulation*.

Ovulation usually alternates between the two ovaries, each producing an egg every other month. However, this is not always the case and one ovary may produce an egg for several months in succession. Both ovaries may produce an egg in the same month—if these eggs were fertilized, fraternal twins would result.

Once the mature egg has been expelled from the ovary, it is swept up by the fimbriated ends of the fallopian tubes. The fimbria contain multiple cilia (hairs) that create a strong current in the minute amount of fluid that surrounds the ovary and fallopian tube, carrying the egg into the oviduct. Because there is no direct link between the ovary and the fallopian tube, the role of the fimbria in the process of ovulation is a vital one.

The walls of the fallopian tubes are composed of an outer layer of muscle and an inner lining membrane covered with hairlike projections. These projections are continuously in a swaying, sweeping motion that helps to send the ovum down toward the uterus; they may also aid sperm in coming up the fallopian tube to reach the egg.

If there are viable sperm in the fallopian tube, a spermatozoan may penetrate the egg and conception or fertilization takes place. Whether or not conception occurs, the egg is swept down the oviduct over a period of three or four days, finally reaching the uterus.

The uterus is lined with a soft cushiony layer called the *endometrium,* which thickens and fills with blood in a monthly cycle in preparation for the implantation of a fertilized egg. If fertilization has not taken place, the egg and the unused materials of this uterine lining are discharged in a process called *menstruation.*

Menstruation occurs about every twenty-eight days and lasts approximately five days. Although a twenty-eight day cycle is considered average, there is no definite time for a normal menstrual cycle. A twenty-four day or a thirty-six day cycle can both be considered healthy and normal. A healthy woman's cycle may also vary in length from month to month.

The onset of menstruation occurs in puberty, around age twelve or thirteen, and is called the *menarche.* It usually begins after certain other secondary sexual characteristics, such as the beginning of breast enlargement and the appearance of pubic hair, have occurred.

Menstrual Phases   There are four parts to the menstrual cycle each month: the proliferative phases, ovulation, the secretory phase, and menstruation.

The proliferative phase begins as soon as menstruation has stopped. At this point the endometrial lining of the uterus is quite thin. A new graafian follicle is maturing in the ovary and the follicle is also producing the hormone estrogen. Estrogen causes the endometrium to proliferate—to grow, thicken, and form glands that will secrete substances to nourish an embryo. After about ten days of the proliferative phase, ovulation occurs.

Just before ovulation occurs, the graafian follicle also begins producing progesterone, the other female sex hormone. Progesterone starts the secretory phase by increasing the blood supply to the uterus and causing the newly formed endometrial glands to begin secreting the embryo-nourishing substances. After ovulation, the graafian follicle becomes what is called the *corpus luteum* (yellow body). If the

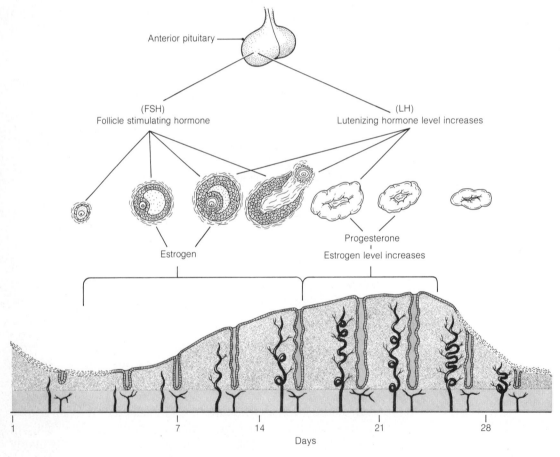

FIGURE 9.3 *A summary of the events occurring simultaneously at the pituitary gland, ovary, and uterine endometrium during the menstrual cycle. Estrogen level inhibits FSH secretion, stimulates LH secretion. Progesterone level inhibits LH secretion.*

egg is fertilized, this egg becomes embedded in the thick endometrium. If the egg is not fertilized, the corpus luteum degenerates after about twelve days into the *corpus albicans* (white body). Hormone production decreases so that the cells and glands of the endometrium begin to die. The lining is then shed in menstruation.

Regardless of the length of the menstrual cycle, menstruation almost always occurs fourteen days after ovulation. The menstrual fluid includes blood and cell fragments, and most of the lining of the uterus is thus shed, but the bottom part is left to form the new lining as the proliferative phase begins again.

Menstrual Discomfort   Some women may experience bloating or swelling of various parts of the body (e.g., the breasts) before the onset of menstruation. This is usually temporary *edema,* which is caused by excess water retention in the body tissues and disappears with the hormonal changes of menstruation. Excess salt may cause the body to retain water at this point in the cycle, so lessening salt intake may provide some relief to many women.

Some women also experience "premenstrual tension," anxieties occurring at about the middle of the cycle and increasing as menstruation approaches. This tension may accompany edema. The exact cause is unknown, though some doctors attribute it to the drop in hormones being secreted at this time.

Dysmenorrhea and Other Problems

About one of every two women experiences varying degrees of *dysmenorrhea,* painful menstruation. Primary dysmenorrhea is associated with an organic disorder; in secondary dysmenorrhea, there is no demonstrable evidence of disease.

Dysmenorrhea varies greatly in its severity from one woman to another. Often it can be relieved with aspirin, other pain killers, heat, or some forms of exercise. In more severe cases, an operation called *dilation* may be required. This consists of widening the cervical canal, the mouth of the uterus. This was used as a method of relief from dysmenorrhea long before there was any good explanation of why it worked. Now it is believed that this procedure destroys some of the nerve fibers that carry pain impulses from the uterus; in extreme cases, certain groups of nerve cells may be entirely removed.

Another method that sometimes is used to reduce or eliminate painful cramps is using oral contraceptives. An anovular cycle (the pill works so that the woman does not ovulate) is often free of cramping, so that the pill may be the answer for a woman who suffers from dysmenorrhea.

A great deal is now known about the physiology of the female reproductive system so that much can be done for the individual who experiences dysmenorrhea, extremely irregular periods, or amenorrhea (lack of periods). A qualified physician can provide information and medical help for these problems.[8]

Menstrual Myths

Various misconceptions about menstruation have existed for years. Among those myths are:

1. A woman should avoid all forms of exercise during her menstrual period. Actually, moderate and regular exercise have been shown to be helpful in alleviating problems of menstruation.
2. A menstruating woman should not swim and she should take showers instead of baths. There is no reason to avoid either swimming or baths.
3. A healthy woman should have a precisely regular cycle. There are many reasons, such as tension, fatigue, travelling, etc., that may make the cycle irregular. Most younger women (ages twelve to twenty-one) tend to have extremely variable cycles. There is usually no reason to be concerned about a variable cycle.
4. Menstruation makes a woman "unclean." This is one of the oldest myths, supported by various cultural and religious beliefs in some societies, but fortunately this idea is disappearing. Odor that has been attributed to the menstrual fluid is actually caused by the oxidation of the blood on the external genitalia or on a sanitary napkin, so it can be prevented by using internal protection. (Since the odor is caused by exposure to air, there is no reason that a perfumed tampon will be any better than an unscented one, and it is, in fact, more sensible to avoid putting unnecessary chemicals into the vagina.)
5. Sexual intercourse should be avoided during menstruation. This myth is associated partly with the myth of impurity or uncleanliness, but there is no reason to refrain from intercourse when it is desired. (A woman who has a diaphragm can insert it to hold the menstrual fluid during the period of heaviest flow. See Chapter 11.)

Menopause

Menopause, the cessation of menstruation, usually occurs sometime between the ages of forty and fifty-five. It is a gradual process, with ovulation becoming less and less frequent due to gradual decline in the ovaries' production of estrogen.

Menopause has often been a time of physical and mental discomfort for many women. We know now that many of the changes during and after menopause are caused by the hormonal changes

[8] Other signs that indicate the need to consult a doctor are: inability to insert a tampon, severe or chronic pelvic pain, vaginal itching or irritation, and bleeding or spotting between periods.

Hysterectomies

In many cases women who suffer from severe uterine cramps or are approaching menopause are advised by their physicians to undergo a hysterectomy. At a time when lowered birth rates and control of fertility and childbirth have vastly reduced uterine disease, hysterectomies are being performed on some 500,000 women a year. It results in death for one out of every 1600 of these women. This procedure for removal of the uterus is the nation's second most frequent major operation. (Only tonsillectomies are performed more frequently.)

The operation, along with the removal of the ovaries and fallopian tubes (a pan-hystero-salpingo-oophorectomy) has been suspected of being unwarranted in a large number of cases. Studies by researchers in California, New York, Maryland, and the Midwest have put the number of questionable hysterectomies in the 15 to 40 percent range.

This is not to imply that the female reproductive organs are always by any means trouble free. There are often good, universally accepted reasons for their removal. These delicate organs and supporting structures are susceptible to cancer, infection, cysts, fibroids, scarring, hemorrhage, and obstruction. Moreover, there are frequent malfunctions: excessive uterine contractions and cramps, uterine tilt (which may lead to infertility or painful intercourse), or prolapse (slippage well out of proper position), which interferes with blood flow and may cause pelvic congestion, back pain, bowel and urinary problems and infections. Fertilized eggs can block the tubes; hormonal imbalances can sabotage the entire system. Incomplete miscarriages can occur and contraceptives carry with them a whole range of potential irritants, infectious organisms, and hormonal upsets.

The best advice to one who finds herself in the position of being advised by her physician to have a hysterectomy is to seek the advice of a second and possibly third qualified physician. Remember, you are the one who will have the operation and you should make the final decision.

occurring—the slowing production of estrogen can produce the symptoms of deficiency. Hot flashes and atrophy of the vagina are the *only* physical signs distinctly characteristic of menopause other than the end of menstrual periods. Other symptoms may be nervousness, tiredness, insomnia, and/or depression. Some women also experience quick mood changes.

Some of the problems of menopause can be alleviated with estrogen therapy. However, there is much controversy over this treatment. Possible side effects include endometrical cancer, vaginal spotting or profuse bleeding, nausea, breast tenderness, fluid retention, and an increase in the size of pre-existing benign tumors of the uterus (fibroids).[9]

[9] See, for example, Francis P. Rhoades, "Minimizing the Menopause," *Sandoz Panorama,* September/October 1969, p. 26. See also "Estrogen Theory: The Dangerous Road to Shangri-La," *Consumer Reports,* November 1976, pp. 642–645.

As mentioned in Chapter 8, menopause need not affect a woman's enjoyment of sexual intercourse and in fact after menopause, sex may be more pleasurable because the threat of unwanted pregnancy is gone. Women have become pregnant during the period of menopause, so contraceptive measures should be continued until ovulation has entirely ceased.

FEMALE SEXUAL RESPONSE

The Sex Drive   The powerful force that motivates our behavior with members of the opposite (and sometimes the same) sex is called the "sex drive" by psychologists and the "libido" by psychoanalysts. In modern industrialized societies, females are said to reach the peak of their sexual drive at about age twenty-five or thirty—at which time this drive may well exceed that of males of a similar age (males usually reach their peak sex drives earlier). Just as different people have different appetites for food and work, so too do individuals have different degrees of sexual drive or need.

It is a recognized fact that one's sexual drive is regulated to a certain degree by one's genetic, instinctive, and environmental situation. Early childhood and upbringing play a major role in determining one's sex drive; attitudes of friends and peers are also important. The stimulus of sexual excitement then is not primarily hormonal in origin. Other factors that play a major role in the female sex drive may include: fear of pregnancy (or diminishing fear), psychological motivations, previous sexual experiences, and general health.

Orgasm   Orgasm in the female can be defined as a sudden peak and release of sexual tension. Yet the feeling of orgasm itself is difficult to describe. It can range from a mild sensual experience to an intense and explosive feeling.

Masters and Johnson describe four phases of sexual response: excitement, plateau, orgasm, and resolution. There are no specific delineations between these four phases, but different responses characterize one phase more than another.

The excitement phases may be the longest phase, when sexual arousal begins. The first reaction to arousal is lubrication of the vagina—the walls become moist—and the inner part begins to expand. The labia minora swell and deepen in color, and the clitoris swells and becomes erect. The clitoris is highly sensitive at this period. The breasts also enlarge and become more sensitive, and the nipples stand erect. The "sex flush" may appear as a rash on various parts of the body. The muscles begin to tighten and the heart rate and blood pressure increase. Breathing becomes faster.

The plateau stage immediately precedes orgasm. At this stage the inner part of the vagina continues to expand while the lower part narrows and becomes more sensitive to pressure. The external genitalia continue to swell and the clitoris retracts under the hood. The breasts continue to swell. The muscles continue to tighten and breathing becomes more rapid.

Orgasm is the release of the sexual tension that has been building up. According to Masters and Johnson, it has three distinct stages. The first stage involves a sensation of "suspension," lasting only an instant, and immediately followed by an "isolated thrust of intense sensual awareness, clitorally oriented but radiating upward into the pelvis."[10] The second stage can be described as a "suffusion of warmth" spreading from the pelvic area to the rest of the body. The third stage involves a feeling of involuntary contraction in the vagina or lower pelvis, described often as "pelvic throbbing."

Unlike men, many women can continue without rest from one orgasm to another. Some women may experience only one orgasm, while others may have three or more in succession (some women experience ten or more).

The last phase of the cycle is resolution. After orgasm has occurred and lovemaking stops, swelling decreases, the muscles relax, and the sexual organs return to their usual states. This period may last half an hour or longer. If the woman reached the plateau stage but did not have an orgasm, the resolution stage might last much longer.[11]

The idea of the vaginal orgasm vs. the clitoral orgasm has been shown to be another myth, especially through the work of Masters and Johnson. They feel that the vagina, tissues, and other organs, and sensitivity are so intricately interconnected that the differentiation does not exist; rather, a woman experiences a *sexual* orgasm.[12]

The Breasts and Sexual Response

The role of the breasts in sexual arousal and orgasm was described above. The sexual responsiveness of women's breasts varies widely. In almost all women, breast stimulation, usually focused on or close to the nipples, can lead to sexual arousal. A Masters and Johnson study found 3 of their study group of 382 women could bring themselves to orgasm simply by manipulating their breasts.[13]

[10] William H. Masters and Virginia E. Johnson, *Human Sexual Response,* Boston: Little, Brown, 1966, p. 135.
[11] Health Collective, *Our Bodies,* p. 47.
[12] Masters and Johnson, *Human Sexual Response.*
[13] Ibid.

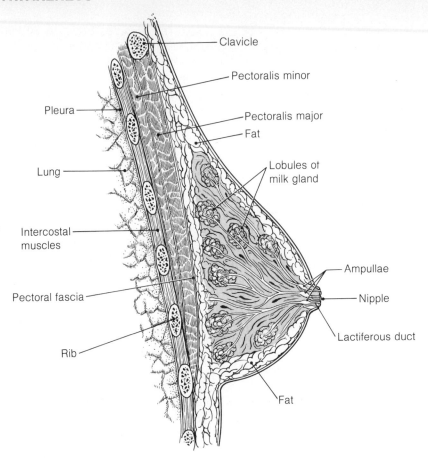

FIGURE 9.4   *The breast.*

Masters and Johnson also found that of 101 women who had just borne children, the 24 who had successfully breastfed their babies had the most intense and rapid return of desire for sexual intercourse after childbirth. They also found that these women sometimes become sexually aroused while breastfeeding their babies, often to the plateau level of sexual response.

Masturbation   Until quite recently, masturbation was considered an unhealthy and unnatural practice. It was believed to cause disease or insanity and was seen as an act of self-abuse. Now we know that masturbation is a normal form of sexual expression and is perfectly healthy. The only "bad" thing about masturbation is the guilt that Is sometimes associated with it because of these old views.

Surveys have found that about 60 percent of high school age females have masturbated compared to 90 percent of males, but this figure may be increasing with the changes in attitudes.

"The Hite Report," a nonscientific study on sexual conduct of females by Shere Hite, says that intercourse alone is a relatively ineffective way for women to achieve orgasm.

Direct clitoral stimulation is the key to female sexual response, it says. Without such stimulation during intercourse, only 30 per cent of the women in the study said they could achieve maximum sexual pleasure.

Of the 82 per cent of women who said they masturbated, 95 per cent could reach orgasm easily and regularly whenever they wanted. "Many women used the term 'masturbation' synonymously with orgasm," Hite notes. "Women assumed masturbation included orgasm."[14]

Women masturbate in many different ways. Some use their fingers or vibrators, others use pillows, streams of water, or other innovations. Most forms of masturbation involve direct or indirect stimulation of the clitoris, but many women also insert something (a finger, a vibrator) into the vagina at the same time.

One woman writer states that masturbation is for her ". . . a form of meditation on self-love," She says, "When I masturbate, I create a space for myself in the very same way I would for a special lover—soft lights, candles, incense, music, colors, textures, sexual fantasies, anything that turns me on."[15]

Whether or not one masturbates, sexual stimulation is for most women both a physical and emotional pleasure, a way of telling herself, "You are loved." Those who have no desire to masturbate are no more or less sexual than those who do; they are simply different in their sexual needs, and such differences are normal. The most important feature of this discussion on masturbation is that *you* should have the final say in what you do with your body.

COMMON SEXUAL PROBLEMS

The word "frigidity" has traditionally been used to cover most female sexual problems. However, this term has degrading and negative connotations. Masters and Johnson use instead the term "female

[14] Shere Hite, *The Hite Report,* New York: Macmillan Publishing Co., Inc., 1976.
[15] Betty Dodson, *Liberating Masturbation: A Meditation on Self Love,* New York: Bodysex Designs.

sexual dysfunction" to describe a range of sexual problems, and the term "female orgasmic dysfunction" for the woman who cannot achieve orgasm as a sexual response.

Female Orgasmic Dysfunction

The term "primary orgasmic dysfunction" can be applied to the woman who has never experienced an orgasm through any means of stimulation. "Situational orgasmic dysfunction" is applied to the woman who has had orgasms but no longer experiences them (or who can achieve an orgasm through masturbation but not through sexual intercourse, for example).

Primary orgasmic dysfunction may be caused by physical problems; the other causes of orgasmic dysfunction are usually psychological. This age of sexual enlightenment has forced a number of people to reexamine their sexual behavior and responses. One drawback is that many people may feel increasing pressure to "perform well;" this type of stress may cause sexual dysfunction in both the male and the female. Fear of pregnancy may also be a causative factor in orgasmic dysfunction. Anxieties, sexual inhibition, or guilt feelings may also lead to orgasmic dysfunction.

A woman experiencing sexual problems can seek help from her physician or a sex counselor. Any physical causes can be treated by her physician; if fear of pregnancy is involved, suitable birth control can be prescribed.

Vaginismus

Vaginismus is an involuntary constriction of the outer third of the vagina that can cause painful intercourse or prevent intercourse altogether. The causes are related to those of orgasmic dysfunction. Therapy, self-understanding and acceptance, a patient partner, and behavior modification are important in the treatment of this condition.

RAPE, THE CRIME AGAINST WOMEN

Rape is on an upward spiral everywhere in the country; there are six rapes an hour in Los Angeles and three a day in Philadelphia. Yet we are only beginning to explore the effects of rape on women and to develop some techniques for dealing with the problems faced by the victim in the aftermath of rape. The woman victimized by a rapist reports the crime, only to be victimized by the system—guilty until she can prove herself innocent.

Rape Prevention   The term "rape" usually conjures up an image of an attack in a dark, deserted alley. Yet 50 percent of all rapes take place in a home (over 50 percent of these rapists break into the house). Thus a woman alone must be conscious of the threat of rape.

The Rape Crisis Center of Washington, D.C. has suggested several precautions against rape:

1. Avoid going alone into dark areas of the city. Most rapes occur in the evening hours.
2. Walk in the middle of the sidewalk rather than close to the curb or buildings where someone might be lurking.
3. Avoid shortcuts that lead through deserted areas, abandoned buildings, or dark alleys.
4. If travelling at night, take a bus instead of the subway. Avoid gypsy cabs; last year in New York alone there were ten complaints concerning molestation of passengers by gypsy cab drivers. While on a bus, stay awake and aware. Sit in the front of the bus near the driver, especially if you are travelling in an unfamiliar area.
5. If a driver pulls over to the curb to ask directions, avoid him. When in your car, avoid giving directions to pedestrians. They can walk over and put a gun to your head.
6. When driving, keep your doors locked and your windows rolled up most of the way.
7. Make sure all doors are locked when your car is parked. Check the back seat before entering your car. Rapists have been known to enter cars and lie in wait for their victim.
8. Buildings: Don't get into an elevator alone with a man. Don't go to the laundry room alone, particularly at night when it may be deserted. Try to go when the room is well populated.
9. Don't let a stranger into your apartment unless you have checked his identification with your superintendent. Better yet, ask your superintendent to accompany him to the apartment.

When a Rapist Attacks   Despite precautions, a woman may find herself confronted with a rapist. She must make a decision to either resist or submit. Some people advise against fighting, for fear that it may cause the rapist to become more violent. Rape is actually a crime of violence, not of passion or sexual desire. However, others urge the woman to fight back in certain ways. If a woman has learned self-defense, she may have a good chance of escaping. New books such as *Against Rape* by Andrea Medea and Kathleen Thompson (New York, Farrar, Straus and Giroux, 1974) contain detailed information on how to fight back.

An article in *Psychology Today* entitled "Don't Take It Lying Down" contains the following suggestions:

·   Yell. Shouting "Fire!" often gets a better response than "Help!" or "Rape!"

- If at all possible, run away, preferably toward a populated area.
- Do not show fear or submissiveness.
- Resist physically. Claw, bite, pull the man's hair, jab him in the neck or solar plexus with an elbow, or give him a fast, short kick in the groin. (A knee in the groin may be a safer defense than a kick, because he may be able to grab your ankle as you kick.) These tactics may give you a chance to escape.

The Washington Rape Crisis Center lists several methods of defense. A woman can strike at the following vulnerable body areas of her attacker.

- *Eyes:* Try to gouge them out. If you put your hands gently along the side of his face, an attacker may think you're going along with him. Wait for the right moment and shove your thumbs into his eyes.
- *Testicles:* Squeeze them as hard as you can. The man's reaction of pain can give you time to get away. If attacked from the rear, reach around and grab the testicles and squeeze hard. This will automatically cause the rapist to loosen his grip on you.
- *Biting, smashing your handbag in an attacker's face, jamming your palm up against his nose, pressing back one of his fingers*—all these may throw your attacker off balance just long enough for you to flee.

Basically, the woman herself must decide whether to resist or submit. The decision may depend on her attacker or the situation.

When Rape Has Occurred

If a woman has been raped, she should get immediate medical attention. Often the first instinct after being raped is for a woman to take a shower or try to remove any traces of the attack from her body (and mind). Instead, she should have a medical exam in case there are any injuries (she may be unaware of internal injuries) and to secure evidence for prosecution of the rapist. She should use her clothes as evidence also, and if the rape occurred in her home, she should not clean up the house until after the police have been there. In addition, the Rape Crisis Center advises the woman to write down, as soon as possible, everything she can remember about the crime.

A woman who has been raped should usually seek out someone —a counselor at a rape crisis center, etc.—to discuss her experience. It is usually a traumatic occurrence and her feelings may be confused. The people at a rape crisis center are trained to deal with these feelings; they can also help the woman if she decides to prosecute, which is usually another difficult experience.

Fortunately, steps are being taken in areas of rape prevention and aid for those who have been raped. Crisis centers are becoming more numerous; more police departments are setting up special units to deal with rape. Following is a list of organizations concerned with preventing rape:

- Center for Women Policy Studies
  2000 P. Street, N.W., Suite 508
  Washington, D.C.   20036
- Chicago Legal Action for Women (CLAW)
  c/o Sharon Moomey-Prokop
  105 Washington
  Oak Park, IL   60302
- Feminist Alliance against Rape
  P.O. Box 21033
  Washington, D.C.   20009
- Men Organized Against Rape
  3417 Spruce Street
  Philadelphia, PA   19174
- Rape Crisis Center
  P.O. Box 21005
  Kalorama Street Station
  Washington, D.C.   20009
- Women Organized against Rape, Inc.
  P.O. Box 17374
  Philadelphia, PA   19105
- Woman's Crisis Center of Ann Arbor
  306 N. Division
  Ann Arbor, MI   48108
- Rape Crisis Center
  46 Pleasant St.
  Cambridge, MA   02139

More attention is being focussed on this terrifying crime by the media. One of the best books on rape is Susan Brownmiller's *Against Our Will: Men, Women, and Rape.* (New York: Simon and Schuster, 1975).

FURTHER READINGS

Bengis, Ingrid. *Combat in the Erogenous Zone.* New York: Bantam Books, 1974.

A frankly independent and individualistic view of love as sexual combat, this book is written by a woman attracted to men yet repelled by the rigidities of sexual roles and role-playing. She examines how sexual relationships grow distorted in contemporary society yet affirms most people's potential for love and tenderness.

Eagan, Andrea Boroff. *Why Am I So Miserable If These Are The Best Years of My Life?* New York: J. B. Lippincott Co., 1976.

A survival guide for the young woman dealing with sexual relationships, romances, and friendships.

Frankfort, Ellen. *Vaginal Politics.* New York: Quadrangle Books, Inc., 1972.

The author hopes to demythologize medicine and its practitioners by making doctors more accountable to the medical, financial, and psychological needs of women. She describes why radical surgery for breast cancer is statistically unwarranted, how menstrual periods can be shortened, and provides a checklist of what should happen during a gynecological examination.

Greer, Germaine. *The Female Eunuch.* New York: Bantam Books, 1970.

A cool, witty, and resourceful portrait of "castrated" women, examining middle class myths of love and marriage, the economic basis for sexual discrimination, and women's capacity for rebellion and revolution against male repression and domination.

Howard, Jane. *A Different Woman.* New York: E. P. Dutton & Co., Inc., 1973.

A Different Woman celebrates life, not ideology. It is at once a brilliant kaleidoscopic portrait of the American woman's coming of age from the 1950s to the 1970s and the tender, witty impassioned autobiography of a girl from the Midwest, now one of the nation's best journalists, coming to terms with her own womanhood.

McBride, Angela Barron. *The Growth and Development of Mothers.* New York: Harper & Row, Publishers, 1973.

A serious attempt to reveal in plain words the complex, sometimes rewarding, always challenging experience of motherhood, told the way it is, not the way it's supposed to be.

Chapter 10

Male
Sexuality

Sexual stereotypes work against all of us, both male and female. Mention male sexuality to the average person and he may respond with images of football players and cowboy heroes. Too few people think of males in terms of sensitivity, caring, or tenderness. Yet the male stereotypes listed in Chapter 10 (aggressiveness, independence, logic, directness, adventuresomeness, self-confidence, ambition, and lack of emotions) can be just as damaging as female stereotypes.[1] Movements for equality of the sexes are helping to destroy some of these stereotypes and allow both men and women to become "liberated." Whatever our sex, we must determine for ourselves how we feel, think, and act. "Don't be just a man (or just a woman)—be a person."

MALE SEXUAL ANATOMY

The male and female sexual/reproductive systems are similar in structure and function. Each system begins as an embryonic cell and differentiates according to genetic determinants. The penis and the clitoris can be compared, for both are sexually responsive and become erect with sexual stimulation. The testicles of the male correspond to the ovaries in the female, for both produce sex hormones. Further, the testicles produce the sperm and the ovaries produce the eggs, which together are the source of new life.

The male reproductive system can best be described by following the course of the sperm from its origin in the testicles to its exit from the penis. The *spermatozoan* is a tiny, one-celled structure

[1] Florence Howe, "Sexual Stereotypes Start Early," *Saturday Review,* October 16, 1971, p. 80.

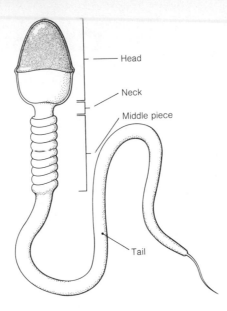

Head

Neck

Middle piece

Tail

FIGURE 10.1   *A spermatozoan. Within the head of the spermatozoan lies the entire genetic code representing the male half of inheritance. The rest of the spermatozoan is concerned only with movement and carries no information whatever.*

with a head and tail. (See Figure 10.1.) The head contains the nucleus of chromosomes and genes, and the tail propels the sperm. The immature sperm cells are called *spermatogonia.* Through a long process (it may take up to seventy-five days), they mature into the spermatozoa.

The *testicles,* like the ovaries in the female, begin their development in the abdomen of the fetus, near the kidneys. While the ovaries normally move very little from their original position, about a month before birth the testicles of the male descend into a pouch of skin called the *scrotum.*

Occasionally, one or both testicles will fail to descend; it is therefore unable to produce sperm. Because the temperature is higher within the pelvis, the sperm cannot become viable, but a lower temperature (2° Centigrade less) in the scrotum makes the production of viable sperm possible. Since each testicle can produce billions of sperm cells, only one testicle is necessary for fertility, but if both testicles fail to descend, the man will be sterile. This condition usually can be corrected by surgery.

The interior of a testicle is filled with *seminiferous tubules,* very narrow tubes in which the male sperm cells are produced. A male sex hormone, testosterone, is also produced here. From the seminiferous

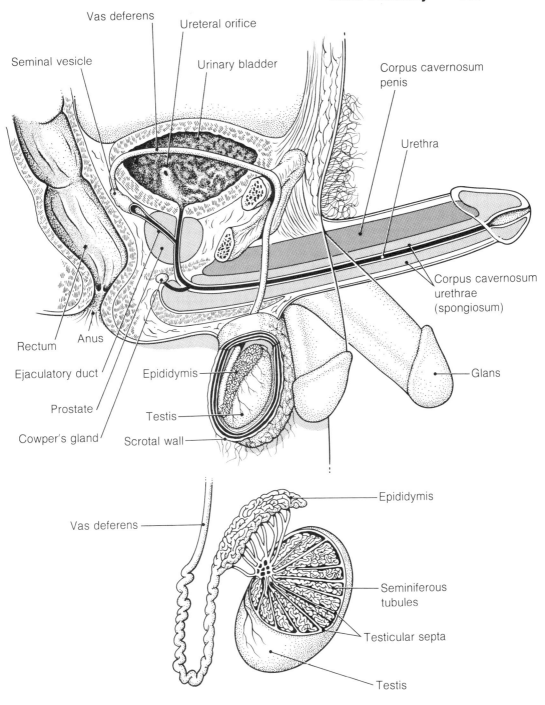

FIGURE 10.2 *The male reproductive system.*

tubules, the maturing sperm cells move into the *epididymis.* This is a long coiled structure resting on the testicle, within the scrotum. If uncoiled, the epididymis would be about twenty feet long. The sperm are stored here, and they mature in a fluid produced by the epididymis, until they are ejaculated or are disintegrated and reabsorbed by the tubules.

Figure 10.2 shows the ejaculatory path of the sperm. From each testicle, an excretory duct called the *vas deferens* carries the sperm cells up into the pelvis, around the bladder, and down toward the urethra.

In erection and ejaculation, secretions from several other glands are added to the liquid containing the sperm to create the seminal fluid. The *seminal vesicles* secrete a substance to make the sperm cells convert into energy for movement; the *prostate gland* secretes an alkaline substance that provides a suitable environment for sperm ejaculated into the vagina, and it also improves the movement of the sperm; and the *Cowper's glands* secrete an alkaline fluid, which in sexual intercourse precedes the sperm to neutralize the acidity in the urethra and lubricate it for their passage. The sperm are finally ejaculated through the erect penis.

The *penis* is composed of spongy erectile tissue called *cavernous tissue.* It contains the urethra, through which urine is excreted and, during ejaculation, the seminal fluid. The end of the penis is called the *glans penis* and is highly sensitive. The glans is separated from the shaft of the penis by an elevated ridge called the *corona.* The penis itself is covered with a thin, loose layer of skin. A fold of this skin, called the *prepuce* or foreskin, extends forward to cover the glans. The skin connecting the glans on the underside of the shaft of the penis is called the *frenulum;* this is also quite sensitive.

When the male is sexually stimulated, the penis becomes engorged with blood. This pressure makes the penis erect and hard. If the man is uncircumcised, the foreskin is retracted from the sensitive glans. Stimulation of the glans eventually brings the man to orgasm and the release of the seminal fluid.

Penis Size   Despite the lack of any evidence to support the idea that "manliness" or virility and sexual adequacy depend on the size of the penis, many men are concerned about penis size. Lack of confidence in his ability to satisfy a woman during intercourse can become very disturbing to the male and possibly even cause secondary impotence. Therefore, it seems worthwhile to devote some space here to a discussion of penis size.

Despite persistent legends of "superpenises," the length of the *average* human penis is three to three-and-a-half inches while flaccid

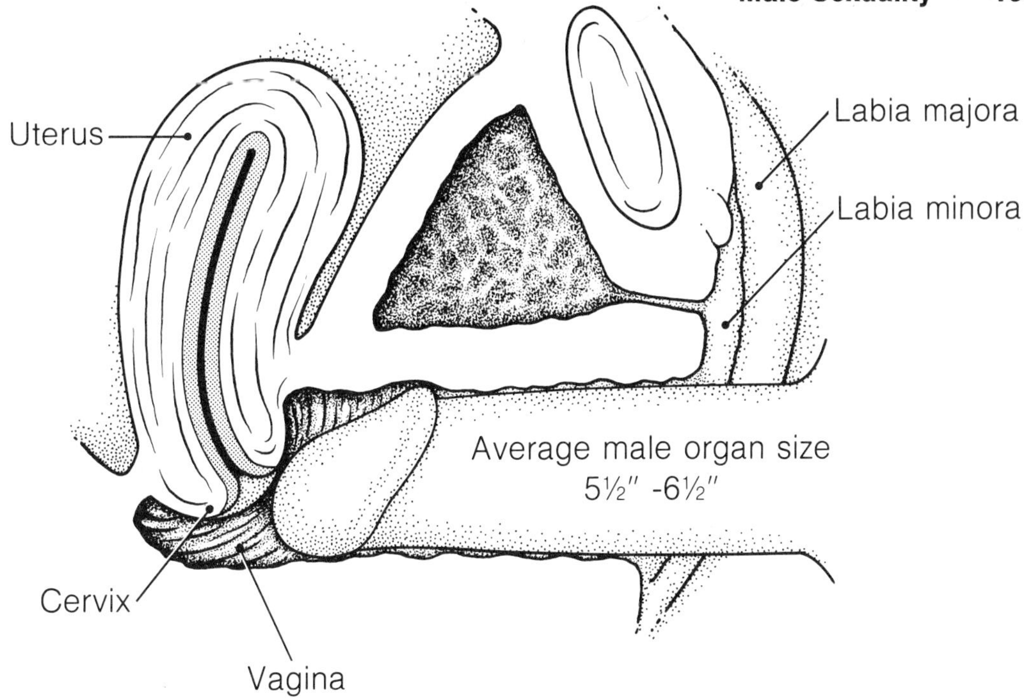

Uterus

Labia majora

Labia minora

Average male organ size
5½" -6½"

Cervix

Vagina

FIGURE 10.3 *The average organ sizes are shown here in comparison.
Because the vagina can adapt easily, the size of the penis need not be a
problem.*

and five to six inches when erect. Although there is a larger variation
from the average in the flaccid state, penises which are small in the
flaccid state increase in size far more than penises that are larger
when flaccid.[2] Small penises may in fact double in size during erection.

Also, the female vagina can adapt to almost any penis. Since
the inner two-thirds of the vagina are distended during sexual arousal,
the length of the penis does not make any difference. Also, the inner
part of the vagina is not a sensitive area; the lower part of the
vagina is more sensitive to pressure, and this is the part that narrows
during intercourse to hold the penis. (See Figure 10.3.) The major
sexual stimulation of the female is caused by friction involving the
clitoris, not from pressure within the vagina. Thus, there is really no
relationship between penis size and the sexual function.

Circumcision   Small glands beneath the prepuce secrete a wax like material
called *smegma*. If this substance accumulates under the foreskin, it
may cause irritation. To simplify hygiene, therefore, the foreskin is

[2] Jan Raboch, "Penis Size," *Sexology*, June 1970, p. 18.

often removed shortly after birth in an operation called *circumcision.* Circumcision originally had religious and cultural connotations, but today it is usually done for health reasons. Despite rumors to the contrary, there is no evidence that circumcision affects sexual response. Therefore, since circumcision neither indicates "normality" nor influences sexual intercourse or responsiveness, the uncircumcised male need not be concerned with being different. He should, however, be particularly careful to retract the foreskin and wash the head of the penis regularly.

MALE SEXUAL RESPONSE

The ability to respond to sexual stimulation is a characteristic of all healthy people. Erection of the penis is basically an automatic response triggered by nervous signals from the spinal cord. Many things can set off these signals. Both sexes may experience sexual stimulation from an erotic book or picture or from a discussion of sex. The major cause of sexual arousal is touch. The starting point of almost all lovemaking and sexual arousal is close bodily contact.[3] For the male, friction of the glans may be caused by sexual intercourse or masturbation.

Sexual Intercourse   The male experiences the same four phases of sexual response as the female: excitement, plateau, orgasm, and resolution.

In the excitement phase, the first reaction to sexual stimulation is the erection of the penis and partial elevation of the testes. Other general effects from a rise in adrenalin (the hormone secreted by the adrenal glands in response to any form of excitement) also occur, such as muscular contraction. Some men experience the sex flush, and in some males the nipples become erect.

During the plateau phase, the testes become fully elevated, and final engorgement causes an increase in the size of the glans and the testicles. Orgasm never occurs without elevated testes, although they may be less elevated in men over fifty years old. Muscle contraction continues in this phase. The heartbeat speeds up and blood pressure may rise. In some men the glans may take on a deeper color.

There are two stages of the orgasmic phase in the male. The first stage involves the muscular contraction and spasm of the vas deferens, the seminal vesicles, and the prostate gland, causing expul-

[3] As to touching, proximity, and so on, see Desmond Morris's brilliant account in *Intimate Behavior,* which catalogues our hangups.

sion of the seminal fluid into the urethra. The inner sphincter muscle closes so that urine will not be mixed with the ejaculate. At this stage of orgasm the male may feel the "inevitability" of ejaculation, and he would be unable to voluntarily stop the rhythmic contractions occurring.

The second stage of orgasm in the male is the ejaculation of the seminal fluid from the penis. Some men may start to perspire immediately after this. As the rhythmic contractions cease, the male experiences the resolution phase.

In the first few seconds after orgasm, the male partially loses his erection. Further loss of the erection occurs more gradually and depends on the age and physical condition of the man, recent sexual activity, etc. Another erection is impossible until the resolution, or recovery, phase is completed.

Masturbation   Males also may satisfy their sex drive through masturbation. As mentioned in Chapter 9, evidence shows that about 90 percent of all males masturbate as compared to 60 percent of all females. The "aura of sin" that clings to the practice of masturbation was also discussed in Chapter 9, but it should again be stressed that it is a healthy and normal outlet for sexual urges.

Generally (at least in the past) males begin to masturbate at a younger age than females: 80 percent of all males have masturbated by age fifteen compared to only 20 percent of all females at this age. Some males masturbate several times a week, others only once or twice a month. Frequency varies widely, and daily masturbation, especially by adolescent boys, is not abnormal or uncommon.

Nocturnal   Many pre-adolescent males may have "dry" ejaculations. One
Emissions   of the first signs of puberty is the wet ejaculation. The other secondary sex characteristics that occur at this time include the deepening of the voice, growth of facial and body hair, enlargement of the penis and the testes, and general body and muscular growth, usually through a growth spurt. Another sign in adolescent boys is the beginning of nocturnal emissions (sometimes called wet dreams), which in fact may be the first appearance of a wet ejaculation.

All males experience nocturnal emissions in varying frequency throughout their lives. Nocturnal emissions are normal releases for sexual tension and cause no physical or psychological harm to those with a healthy acceptance of their own sexuality.

MALE SEXUAL DYSFUNCTION

There are several sexual problems a male may experience. As is true with female sexual dysfunction, most of these problems have some psychological rather than physiological basis. The two most common forms of male sexual dysfunction are impotence and premature ejaculation.

Impotence

Impotence may be defined as failure of the male to achieve or maintain an erection for the purpose of sexual intercourse. The process of erection in the male is a complex response, ordinarily dependent on both psychological and physiological factors. There are two kinds of impotence: organic and functional. Organic impotence stems from physical causes, such an injury, disease (e.g., diabetes or epilepsy), surgery, etc.[4] Less than 10 percent of all cases of impotence are caused by physical factors.

Functional impotence is one of man's most common psychogenic disorders. There are few men who have never experienced temporary functional impotence for one reason or another. Causes may include feelings such as fear, shame, guilt, anxiety, or anger toward sex or toward one's partner. Fatigue or ingestion of alcohol may also cause functional impotence. A male's fear of inadequate performance may make him incapable of achieving an erection. He may worry about bringing his partner to orgasm and the strain may cause temporary impotence.

Any male who finds he is having continuing difficulty in achieving or maintaining an erection for sexual intercourse should consult a physician or someone experienced in sex therapy. The individual may help himself by reviewing past experiences—if, for example, he finds that he usually drinks excessively before intercourse, he may have all or part of the answer. However, one cannot will an erection; in fact, worrying about achieving an erection may make the problem worse.

Premature Ejaculation

Premature ejaculation is the most common male sexual dysfunction, occurring even more frequently than functional impotence. Masters and Johnson define premature ejaculation as an "inability to delay ejaculation long enough for the woman to have an orgasm 50

[4] Bruce G. Belt, "Some Organic Causes of Impotence," *Medical Aspects of Human Sexuality,* January 1973, pp. 152–161.

percent of the time.''[5] This definition thus takes the emphasis away from a specific time period.

Most men experience premature ejaculation at one time or another in their lives. It may occur, for example, when a young man has sex after several weeks of abstinence, but in this situation he will probably achieve another erection shortly thereafter, without premature ejaculation.

The causes for premature ejaculation are often similar to those of impotence, even though at first this seems to be an opposite problem. Fear, guilt, anxiety about performance may again play a part. Masters and Johnson found that most of the men they treated had a history of hurried sexual encounters. Any male who has a consistent problem of premature ejaculation should seek help.

FURTHER READINGS

Duyckaerts, Francois. *The Sexual Bond*. New York: Dell Publishing Co., 1970.

The author explores the hidden feelings and motivations that people bring to their sexual relationships and the inner battles against aggression and anxiety that must be won if the sex act is to be a truly satisfying communication between man and woman.

Henry, George. *Masculinity and Feminity*. New York: Collier Books, 1966.

This book considers the extent to which every man possesses feminine attributes and every woman is, in some respects, masculine.

Man's Body: An Owner's Manual. New York: Paddington Press Ltd., 1976.

Here are clear answers to the questions men ask (or do not ask) concerning his body's functions and possible malfunctions.

Tiger, Lionel. *Men in Groups*. New York: Vintage Book, 1970.

The author suggests that the habit of "male bonding" as he calls it, may be a biological necessary affirmation rather than an escape from apron strings.

Unbecoming Men. New York: Times Change Press, 1971.

A men's consciousness-raising group writes on opposition and themselves.

Vilar, Esther. *The Manipulated Man*. New York: Bantam Books, 1974.

An angry antifeminist account of how women "exploit" men and subject them to countless indignities. Only women, the author maintains, can break the circle of man's manipulation—if they choose to do so.

[5] William H. Masters and Virginia E. Johnson, *Human Sexual Inadequacy*, Boston: Little, Brown, 1970.

Chapter 11

Human Reproduction

The process of conception and birth is sometimes regarded as a miracle. Yet the mystery that once surrounded reproduction no longer exists; most aspects of this complicated sequence are now understood. In view of the concern about overpopulation and unwanted pregnancies, as well as various problems that may arise in childbirth, it is important to be aware of the facts of conception, birth, and birth control.

CONCEPTION

The menstrual cycle and ovulation were discussed in Chapter 9. There it was stated that if viable sperm exists in the fallopian tubes at the time a mature egg is released from the ovary, fertilization can take place.

Fertilization   There are millions of sperm contained in the male ejaculate. This large number is necessary to ensure that conception will be possible, as the process of fertilization is a difficult one.

Most sperm do not even reach the ovum. Upon release into the vagina, the sperm swim in all directions, not necessarily toward the egg. (See Figure 11.1.) Some remain on the penis and are removed from the vagina; others remain in the vagina or the uterus or are discharged from the woman's body; others swim up the fallopian tube that does not contain an egg. The secretions in the vagina or uterus kill off many of the sperm, and others do not have the energy for the long trip up the fallopian tube.

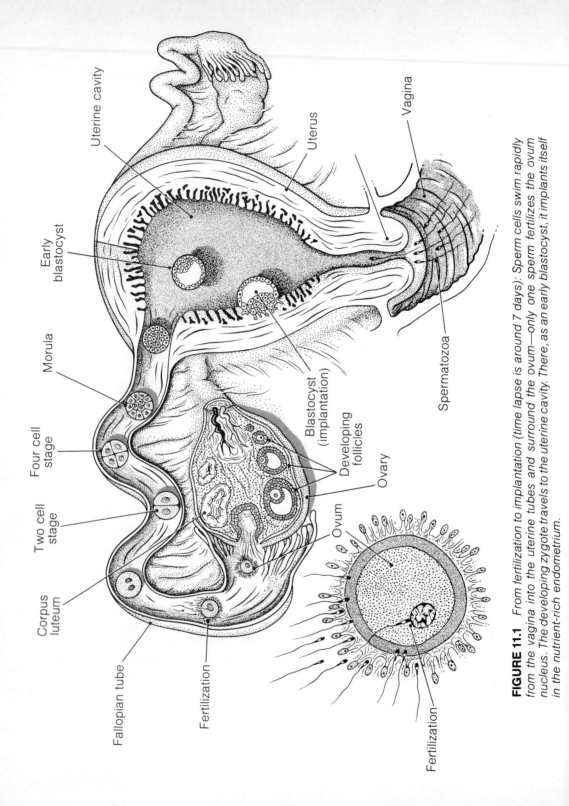

FIGURE 11.1 *From fertilization to implantation (time lapse is around 7 days): Sperm cells swim rapidly from the vagina into the uterine tubes and surround the ovum—only one sperm fertilizes the ovum nucleus. The developing zygote travels to the uterine cavity. There, as an early blastocyst, it implants itself in the nutrient-rich endometrium.*

Uterine cavity

Uterus

Vagina

Early blastocyst

Morula

Blastocyst (implantation)

Developing follicles

Spermatozoa

Four cell stage

Ovary

Two cell stage

Ovum

Corpus luteum

Fallopian tube

Fertilization

Fertilization

The actual penetration of the outer coating of the ovum is a difficult process. All the sperm that have reached the ovum are involved in the process of breaking down the coating, but only one spermatozoan will penetrate the ovum. As soon as it has penetrated the ovum, the coating of the egg thickens so that no other sperm can enter it. When the ovum and the sperm are finally united, they are called a *zygote.*

Most cells in the human body contain forty-six chromosomes. The cells of the sperm and the ovum undergo a division process called *meiosis,* in which the number of chromosomes in each cell is reduced to twenty-three. Then, when the zygote is created, it will contain the normal number of chromosomes, forty-six. The twenty-three chromosomes from the male and the twenty-three from the female determine the genetic characteristics of the embryo; the sex of the embryo is determined by one of the chromosomes from the male.

Once the zygote has been created, this cell undergoes another type of division, called *mitosis.* The cell reproduces itself exactly, providing two new identical cells that then continue the process. After seventy-two hours the zygote has subdivided into thirty-two cells; after four days it has become about ninety cells.

Implantation and Development   The zygote moves slowly down the fallopian tubes while continuing to divide. Once it reaches the uterus, it floats there for about three days. The zygote is becoming what looks like a hollow ball of cells; it is actually filled with fluid. This ball is called the *blastocyst.* (See Figure 11.1.)

Throughout the menstrual cycle, the walls of the uterus have been thickening and otherwise preparing for the implantation of the fertilized egg. About seven days after conception, the blastocyst attaches itself somewhere in the endometrial lining, where it continues to divide and grow.

DETERMINATION OF PREGNANCY

The first sign of pregnancy for most women is the absence of menstruation, but many other factors may cause this, including emotional tension stemming from a fear of pregnancy. Other signs of pregnancy include breast enlargement, nipple secretions, vaginal bleeding or spotting (which sometimes occurs at the time of implantation and is called "implantation bleeding"), frequent urination, and some physical changes in the vagina and labia. Most of these symptoms may also be caused by factors other than pregnancy.

Pregnancy Tests   There are various types of tests used to determine pregnancy. Most are not reliable until at least two or more weeks after the first missed period. One test that has been used most commonly in the past is based on the excretion of gonadotrophins (the follicle-stimulating hormones) in the woman's urine during the early stages of pregnancy. The urine is injected into a lab animal, usually either a frog or a rabbit, and the reaction shows whether or not the woman is pregnant. The results from these tests are known within two or three days.

The "slide test" and the "tube test" also use the female's urine, but they provide results within a few minutes or hours. The reaction of a drop of urine and antibodies against the gonadotropin provides an extremely dependable indication of a pregnancy.

Another test will determine whether a woman's missed period is caused by pregnancy or other factors. The woman is given an injection of large amounts of the female hormones. If she is not pregnant, the hormones should bring on the menstrual flow. There is no menstrual flow if she is pregnant. Most experts believe that this injection will do no harm to an embryo if the woman is pregnant, but recently there has been some controversy about this.

An internal examination by a physician can also determine the positive signs of pregnancy, but this exam is usually not reliable until after about two months or so of pregnancy. One change is called *Hegar's sign.* This is a softening of the area between the cervix and the body of the uterus. This occurs about six weeks after the last menstrual period. Changes in the mucous membranes of the vagina and labia can also be observed.

These tests can be performed by one's personal physician, university health services, or by various reliable clinics or pregnancy counselling services.

PRENATAL DEVELOPMENT

During the first two weeks after conception, the developing cells are called the zygote. After two weeks, the zygote is referred to as the embryo, and after six weeks, it is called the fetus. These differentiations are somewhat arbitrary.

Within a week after fertilization, the cells of the zygote have begun to develop into three distinct layers. The outer layer, or *ectoderm,* will develop into the outer layer of the body, including the skin, the sense organs, and the brain. The middle layer, or *mesoderm,* becomes the bones, muscles, heart, and blood vessels. The innermost layer, or *endoderm,* will develop into the organs of the digestive and respiratory systems.

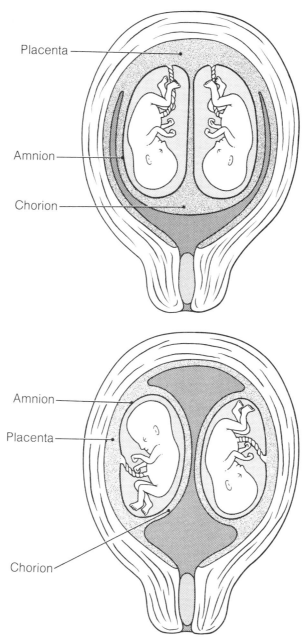

Placenta

Amnion

Chorion

Amnion

Placenta

Chorion

FIGURE 11.2 *Identical and fraternal twins. Identical twins develop from the splitting of a single zygote; they share the same chorion and placenta. Fraternal twins develop when two egg cells are released from the ovaries at the same time and are fertilized by two different sperm; they have separate chorions and placentas.*

During the zygotic and embryonic stages, the development of the umbilical cord occurs and membranes are formed to surround the placenta, as shown in Figure 11.2. This figure also shows the fetal development for twins.

Within a week after conception, the amnion has developed. It is a thin membrane that holds the amniotic fluid, which serves to cushion and insulate the developing embryo.

Surrounding the aminotic sac is the chorion, a thicker membrane that develops about two weeks after fertilization. The chorion extends villi or finger-like projections into the endometrium of the uterus. Although the circulatory systems of the mother and the embryo are separate, the villi provide for the absorption of nutrients, vitamins, antibodies, and hormones by the embryo (from the mother) and for the excretion of its wastes through the mother's system.

Eventually, the placenta develops. This membrane connects the chorion and the endometrium; it is connected with the umbilical cord, the original stalk from the zygote to the endometrium. The umbilical cord replaces the functions of the chorion, in that the nutrients and other substances diffused through the villi are now transferred directly through the blood vessels of the cord. The placenta is the main defensive barrier for the embryo. (See Figure 11.2.)

By the end of the first month of pregnancy, the embryo is still smaller than one-half inch in length, but its heart has begun beating and it has a digestive tract. By the end of the embryonic period, it is about an inch long. Fingers and toes have appeared and the nervous and muscular systems are rapidly developing.

During the fetal period, the other systems and structures continue their development in preparation for birth after nine months of gestation. By the end of the fourth month the fetus is about six inches long and is beginning to expand the uterus. During the fifth month the first fetal movement, or quickening, may be felt by the mother. Prior to the seventh month, the fetus would be unable to survive outside the womb; after this stage, there is an increasing chance of viability, the ability to survive outside the womb.

PRENATAL CARE

When a woman believes she is pregnant, she should have a complete physical exam. This should include a medical history, pelvic exam, and various lab tests.

The medical history should cover the menstrual history to establish a probable date of birth, previous pregnancies, and any abortions, operations, or illnesses. Rubella (German measles) can cause fetal deformities if the mother is exposed early in pregnancy. This therefore should be a concern. Family medical history should also be discussed, to discover tendencies toward multiple births or diseases such as diabetes, heart or kidney problems, or genetic diseases such as sickle-cell anemia or Tay-Sachs.[1]

The pelvic exam will verify the pregnancy and should also include a measurement of the pelvis to see if a normal birth is possible or if a caesarian section (surgical removal of the fetus from the womb) could be necessary.

Certain lab tests should be done. A blood sample will determine type and the presence of the Rh factor. Tests for anemia and for adequate oxygen-carrying capacity of the blood should be done. A urinalysis is important, as is a test for syphilis and a Pap smear (for detection of cancer). A test for rubella immunity will also be done, to confirm the information in the history.

Other topics of concern are diet, weight gain, and drug use. The mother must be sure to receive adequate nutrition so that the fetus can grow and develop in a healthy way. If a woman is planning to nurse her baby, she should be even more aware of her diet, especially in the last weeks of pregnancy. Supplemental vitamins and minerals are important. A large weight gain is neither necessary nor recommended. The average increase is about twenty to twenty-four pounds if the woman is at her proper weight when she becomes pregnant. Only part of this weight will be lost at delivery of the child— most of the remainder will disappear after a few weeks, but the mother may have to exercise and eat sensibly to regain her desired weight.

Studies have shown that women who are heavy smokers have babies of lower birth weights than those of nonsmokers. Moderate amounts of alcohol may in fact be helpful for relaxation to the woman but excess amounts can be harmful to the fetus. The child of a woman addicted to alcohol may experience withdrawal after birth, just as the child of a heroin addict will suffer drug withdrawal. Any sort of drug use should be checked with a physician—even aspirin or excess caffeine (from coffee or tea) is sometimes believed to be harmful.

After the initial visit to the doctor, the woman should return for monthly checkups until the seventh month, when she should go every two weeks. In the last month, weekly visits should be set up until the birth. The visits will be concerned with the position and heartbeat of the fetus, among other factors, and will involve urinalysis and weight and blood pressure checks. The doctor will advise the woman on her diet and weight gain, amount of exercise, sexual activity, and so forth.

[1] Boston Women's Health Book Collective, *Our Bodies, Ourselves,* 2d edition, New York: Simon and Schuster, 1976, p. 258.

What Are a Woman's Odds?

The odds against dying from childbirth in the United States today are about 4,000 to 1, the Health Insurance Institute reports.

But only 25 years ago, a woman's chances were no better than 1,000 to 1.

According to an insurance company study, mortality from disorders associated with pregnancy and childbirth went from 125.8 deaths per 100,000 live births in 1947–48 to 26.2 per 100,000 in 1967–68.

In the decade from 1957–58 to 1967–68, maternal deaths from all causes declined—with the exception of sepsis, which showed no change.

Deaths from toxemia and hemorrhage decreased by over a half, and those from abortion and ectopic pregnancy dropped about a third.

Age and race are still major factors in maternal mortality. Older women are far more likely to die in childbirth than their younger counterparts and the maternal mortality of nonwhite women is still "nearly four times higher" than that of white women.

Source: Medical Times, March 1974.

Problems in Pregnancy

There are certain problems that may arise, affecting the woman and/or the child. There are some indications that may point to the possibility of complications, and women with these symptoms should receive adequate medical care. An older woman, especially one pregnant for the first time, may face difficulties. The dangerous age used to be 40, but many experts now believe that even 35 may be considered "late." A woman who has had a previous child with Downs Syndrome, an open neural tube defect, or any other genetic disease or birth defect should probably consider genetic counseling before becoming pregnant again. Other problems, such as an inborn error of metabolism, can be diagnosed prenatally. Many problems can now be discovered through various tests while the fetus is still in the womb.

Toxemia

Toxemia is a form of poisoning that may occur late in pregnancy and, if untreated, can cause the mother to have convulsions or she may lapse into a coma. The causes of toxemia are not yet understood; many theories have been advanced. Diet seems to have some relation to toxemia; the incidence of its occurrence has been shown in some studies to be much lower among women receiving adequate nutrition. The symptoms include edema (water retention and swelling), high blood pressure, and later, severe headaches, blurring of vision, and abdominal pains. The symptoms must be treated in a hospital in order to avoid harm to the mother and fetus.

Rh Factor

Everyone has either Rh positive or Rh negative blood. When an Rh negative mother is carrying an Rh positive fetus, her blood may develop antibodies that can cross the placenta and destroy some of the red blood cells of the fetus. This can cause mental retardation, anemia, or other disorders in the child. However, the mother will usually not build up damaging antibodies until after one or more pregnancies (or abortions). Problems with these pregnancies can be avoided in several ways, once the condition is known.

When a mother with Rh negative blood gives birth, she should receive an injection of Rhogam within seventy-two hours. This will help prevent dangerous antibody production in future pregnancies. When an Rh negative woman becomes pregnant, the doctor should check the antibody level in her blood throughout her pregnancy. If the level becomes too high, he can give a blood transfusion to the fetus in the womb or to the child immediately after birth.

Miscarriage

About one of every eight or ten pregnancies in the United States ends in miscarriage, or spontaneous abortion. Most of these occur within the first three months of pregnancy; only 25 percent occur later.

Among the causes are: a defective embryo, tumors in the uterus, abnormalities of the cervix, faulty implantation of the embryo, or bleeding between the placenta and endometrium. Certain constitutional diseases, such as tuberculosis, diabetes, syphilis, and malnutrition can induce a spontaneous abortion. Another causative factor can be excessive x-rays or radiation.[2] A miscarriage is rarely caused by factors such as falls or overexertion.

Alan Guttmacher has found three conditions that are associated with a low frequency of spontaneous abortion: youth, the ability to conceive easily, and the absence of any previous abortion.[3]

[2] A pregnant woman should avoid x-rays, as they can cause problems or abnormalities in the child.
[3] Alan F. Guttmacher, *Pregnancy and Birth,* New York: New American Library, Signet Books, 1962.

LABOR AND BIRTH

There are three stages of labor. Most first births in the United States take from thirteen to sixteen hours but may last as much as thirty-six hours. Subsequent births are shorter, usually lasting about six to eight hours. The first stage of labor is usually the longest. This is the preparatory stage. The second stage culminates in the delivery of the baby. In the third stage, the afterbirth is expelled.

The first stage of labor begins with short and mild contractions. They are irregular, occurring about every ten to twenty minutes. Occasionally, the beginning of labor is signalled by the breaking of the amniotic sac so that the fluid within it is released. There also may be some blood-stained mucus discharged from the vagina. During this stage of labor the cervix is dilating (opening) to accommodate the baby. The contractions become more intense and regular, occurring about every three to five minutes until the cervix is dilated to ten centimeters. During this stage, the contractions of the uterus have pushed the baby down into position for birth. The average length of this stage in a first birth is twelve hours.

The second stage of labor begins when the baby's head moves into the birth canal, and ends when the baby is delivered. This stage may take from twenty minutes to an hour and a half. During this part of labor, the woman can "bear down" during contractions to help release the baby (unless she has been heavily anesthetized). Gradually the body of the baby appears, until it is outside the mother, but it is still attached by the umbilical cord. Once all the blood from the placenta has emptied from the cord into the baby's system, the cord is cut. The part attached to the baby eventually shrivels up, leaving the navel. The accumulated fluid and mucus are removed from the baby's nose and mouth, and it usually starts breathing within a minute of delivery. The baby's eyes are treated to avoid possible infection and the infant's heart rate, respiration, muscle tone, reflexes, and coloring are evaluated under what is called the Apgar test.

The third stage of labor lasts about fifteen to twenty minutes. As the uterus begins to contract, the placenta is forced down the vagina and out. The physician checks to make sure all of this material (the afterbirth) has been removed from the uterus.

Types of Childbirth   A woman may choose natural childbirth (without drugs) or she may prefer to rely on various amounts and levels of pain killers and anesthesia. The most commonly practiced type of natural childbirth in the United States is the Lamaze method, developed by Dr. Fernand Lamaze. This method works to relieve pain by having the woman concentrate on special breathing techniques throughout the

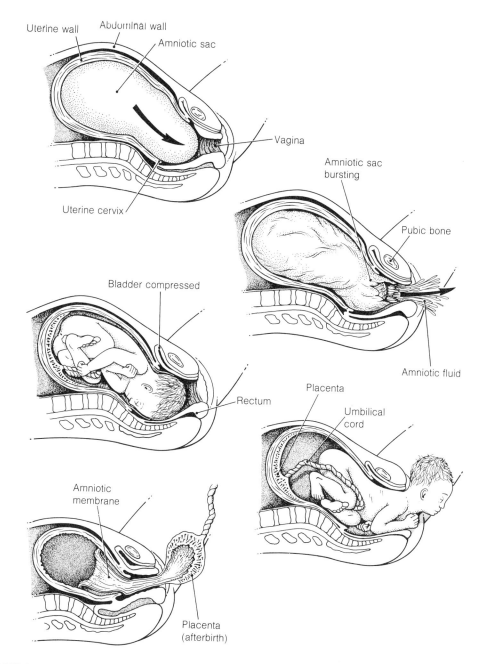

FIGURE 11.3 *The stages of labor: First stage—Uterine contractions intensify, the amniotic sac ruptures, the cervix dilates and the baby moves down the birth canal into birth position. Second stage—The baby's head, and gradually body, move into the birth canal and appear outside the mother; the umbilical cord is cut and tied. Third stage—The uterus begins to contract, and the placenta and amniotic membrane are expelled.*

different stages of labor. She usually prepares for natural childbirth by practicing various exercises and types of breathing. Some advocates of natural childbirth believe no drugs or pain killers should be used; others feel that there is no harm in the mother requesting them at certain points.

Other women may want to be anesthestized for part or all of the birth process. The types of drugs vary in strength and in the areas of the body they affect. These drugs all cross the placenta and are believed to have a depressant effect on the respiration and other reactions of the baby.

The woman may receive general tranquilizers or barbiturates. Anesthesia may be general (the woman is put completely to sleep for the last few minutes of labor), or regional (affecting different parts of the body). The pudendal block anesthetizes only the external genital organs, whereas spinal anesthesia affects the entire birth area. These two types are administered during delivery, whereas other types of regional anesthesia (the caudal and epidural blocks) can be administered throughout the first and second stages of labor. Depending on the amount and type of anesthesia, both the mother and baby can suffer varying reactions and aftereffects. See the box on page 183 for a more detailed explanation of the types of anesthesia.

Induced Labor

Occasionally labor is induced artificially at or near full term. This may be done in cases where the baby's and/or mother's health are endangered—by Rh incompatibilities, toxemia, or diabetes—or for other reasons.

The amniotic sac is first ruptured with a sterile instrument. There is some disagreement over the use of this procedure, and it is not clearly understood why this will bring on labor. If labor does not begin within a certain period of time after the sac is ruptured, the woman is given a synthetic pituitary extract (usually intravenously) to stimulate contractions.

Types of Delivery

The type of birth depends on the position of the fetus within the womb. In almost all births, the head appears first; this is a cephalic presentation. If the baby is positioned so that the feet or buttocks appear first, this is called a breech presentation. In a transverse presentation, the shoulder appears first.

The physician can usually manipulate the baby within the uterus so that the head will be presented first. If this is not possible and there are problems with the delivery a caesarian section may be performed. The mother is given a general anesthetic and the baby is removed surgically through the abdomen. (A woman with a small

Conduction Anesthetics: a cocaine drug such as xylocaine or novocain is injected at a specific location to block nerve impulses to the brain. A skilled anesthetist is essential. The woman remains conscious. She can usually move her legs (unlike with a spinal) but the urge to bear down is inhibited.

Local: eliminates pain by injecting an entire area or single spot to block nerve fibers.

Pudendal block: an injection given through the buttocks toward pelvic bones. The baby is not felt coming out and the mother must be coached to push.

Paracervical block: a needle is placed through vagina to cervix. It sometimes slows the baby's heart after injection. Its use is often in relieving labor pain.

Spinal: this is a dangerous method and mortality is very high when used improperly. Here, the anesthetic is injected into the spinal fluid surrounding the lower spinal cord. Forceps are required in most cases. Low back pain and headaches are side effects.

Saddle block or "low spinal": the injection numbs the part of the body that would touch a saddle. Although less anesthetic is used low back pain can result.

Extradural: the anesthetic is placed in a space lined by ligament and bone external to the dura (tough membrane covering spinal cord and brain), rather than in contact with spinal cord itself.

pelvic bone construction may require a Caesarian delivery.) This operation takes about an hour.

POSTNATAL PERIOD

The mother loses about eleven pounds of weight she has gained during the actual delivery. This is the weight of the baby and the placenta and amniotic fluid. Within a few days the woman will lose more weight as her body excretes much of the excess fluid she has acquired during pregnancy.

As the uterus returns to its normal position and shape, there may be further contractions after birth. There is also a discharge of fluid, which may last for about three weeks, changing from red to yellowish-white.

Unless there are complications, a new mother can be up and around within twelve to twenty-four hours, and she may leave the hospital within three to five days.

Six weeks after the birth, the woman should have a follow-up examination by her doctor. She is advised to wait until after this exam to resume sexual intercourse, but this may vary.

Breast-Feeding   After giving birth, the woman's breasts will become engorged with accumulating fluids. If she has not planned to nurse her baby, she will be given an injection so that milk production will not continue. The fluid that first appears is called colostrum; within a few days this turns to milk.

Masters and Johnson found that the uterus of a nursing mother returns to its normal state much more quickly than that of a woman who does not nurse. The nursing mothers resumed sexual intercourse more quickly than those who did not nurse. In addition, there is some evidence to suggest that women who have nursed children have a lower incidence of breast cancer than those who have never nursed.

BIRTH CONTROL: PREGNANCY BY CHOICE RATHER THAN CHANCE

Birth rates for unmarried teenage girls have more than doubled since 1940. Most of these pregnancies are unplanned and unwanted.

Despite the proliferation of literature on the subject of birth control, many people are still uneducated; they may rely on methods with a high risk of pregnancy or they "forget" to use any birth control at all. Some people are unwilling to consider the consequences of their sexual behavior. Men may not feel concerned with birth control, since it is the woman who gets pregnant. Some women may feel that planning for birth control commits them to a certain sexual philosophy or type of behavior. Other individuals may feel that birth control methods interfere with spontaneity or the enjoyment of intercourse. Religious prohibitions are also a factor.[4]

There are many methods of birth control available, varying in effectiveness, safety, and convenience. Student health services, private physicians, Planned Parenthood, and other local organizations, hospitals, or clinics can provide information and birth control.

[4] See Takey Crist, "Contraceptive Practices among College Women," *Medical Aspects of Human Sexuality,* November 1971, pp. 168–176.

Oral Contraceptives   Oral contraceptives— birth control pills—contain synthetic hormones, estrogen and progestin. The pills are usually taken for twenty-one days of each menstrual cycle, with a break of seven days. To facilitate the proper usage of oral contraceptives, some packages contain twenty-eight pills, seven of which (the last seven) contain no hormones.

There are three kinds of birth control pills. Combination pills include both estrogen and progestin for each day of the cycle. The estrogen inhibits ovulation. The progestin works against pregnancy by increasing the thickness of cervical mucus so that sperm are less likely to reach the fallopian tubes and by retarding the development of the endometrium, so that if an egg is released and fertilized, it is unlikely to become implanted. The pill with only progestin therefore produces these two effects but does not inhibit ovulation. Sequential pills provide only estrogen during the first days of the cycle and then combine estrogen and progestin. The combination pill is the most prescribed today as it is more effective than the other two types and has fewer side effects than the sequential pills, which have higher levels of estrogen.

The pill is the most effective type of birth control today, but there are many possible side effects and risks associated with its use. Side effects may include nausea, weight gain, headache, fluid retention, breast enlargement, depression, decreased sexual desire, vaginal or urinary tract infections, breakthrough bleeding (spotting between periods), and skin problems. These symptoms might occur during the first few months but disappear once the woman's body has adjusted to the different hormonal levels. Other side effects may disappear if the woman switches to a different brand of pill.

There are other more serious risks associated with using the pill. Research has found a definite relationship between birth control pills and increased incidence of blood clots. These may include phlebitis (blood clots in the legs), pulmonary thromboembolism (clots in the lung), and stroke (blood clots or hemorrhage in the brain).[5] A connection between the pill and gall bladder problems has recently been found. The pill does cause some increase in blood pressure,[6] and some studies have indicated a greater risk of heart attack for pill users.[7] Other experts fear a connection between cancer and the pill, but there is no data to support this.

Depending on the medical history, not every woman can take the pill. In general, a decision to take the pill should be carefully considered. Although oral contraception is one of the easiest methods

[5] Women's Collective, *Our Bodies, Ourselves,* p. 190.
[6] It should be noted that the blood pressure usually returns to normal when the pill usage is discontinued.
[7] Women's Collective, *Our Bodies, Ourselves,* p. 190.

> **What the Food and Drug Administration (FDA) Suggests Concerning the "Pill"**
>
> · It is the FDA's present view that estrogen-containing medicines are useful, effective, and safe—when properly used.
> · For birth control pills, FDA now advises that women over 40 should use some other method of contraception.
> · Any woman taking the pill should be examined regularly by her physician.
> · Women with a history of breast cancer or cancer of the uterus or of blood clotting should not take the pill.

of birth control and the most effective one, unfortunately, the research on its effects—especially long-term effects—is still inadequate.

Intrauterine Devices (IUDs)

The IUD is an intrauterine contraceptive device, made of plastic, stainless steel, or copper and inserted into the uterus to prevent pregnancy. Although it has long been known that a foreign object in the uterus will work as a contraceptive device, it is not clear how an IUD works. It is believed that the uterus reacts as to an inflammation, thereby preventing implantation of a fertilized egg. The newer copper IUDs seem to also interfere with enzyme functions within the uterus.

Once the IUD has been inserted by a medical professional, it can remain in place for many years. (The copper devices must be replaced every two to three years.)

There seem to be fewer side effects or complications with an IUD than with the pill. There is usually some initial discomfort or bleeding after insertion. A major drawback is involuntary expulsion, which sometimes occurs, especially in women who have never been pregnant. (This may depend somewhat on the type of IUD used.) Therefore, the woman must be careful, especially at first, to check that the IUD is still in position. (See Figure 11.4.)

One relatively rare possibility is perforation of the uterus by an IUD; this usually occurs only if it has not been inserted properly. Some women have become pregnant while using an IUD; this can cause serious complications.

Diaphragm

The diaphragm is regaining popularity as a means of birth control; although its effectiveness is not as great as that of the pill or the IUD, there are no side effects. The diaphragm is a dome-shaped rubber cup designed to cover the cervix thereby preventing sperm

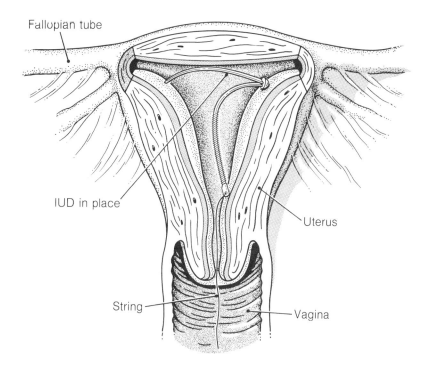

Fallopian tube

IUD in place

Uterus

String

Vagina

FIGURE 11.4   *The Copper 7 IUD in place.*

from entering the uterus. (See Figure 11.5.) It ranges in diameter from two to four inches (50 to 105 mm.).

The diaphragm must always be used with a spermicidal jelly or cream. It must be inserted within two hours (some experts advise half an hour or less) before intercourse—so that the spermicide will still be effective—and must be left in position for at least six to eight hours afterwards, so that all the sperm in the vagina will be killed before it is removed. Each time intercourse is repeated, additional spermicide must be inserted. The diaphragm can safely be left in place for up to twenty-four hours.

The diaphragm must be fitted by a medical professional. It can then be purchased with a prescription at the clinic or a drugstore; the spermicide is available without prescription at drugstores. The diaphragm should be replaced every one to three years, and it must be checked frequently for holes.

Some women may object to the diaphragm, feeling that it is messy or that it interferes with the sex act. Once it is properly in place, neither the woman nor man should be aware of it. Some women (e.g., one with a severely displaced uterus) might not be able to use the diaphragm successfully.

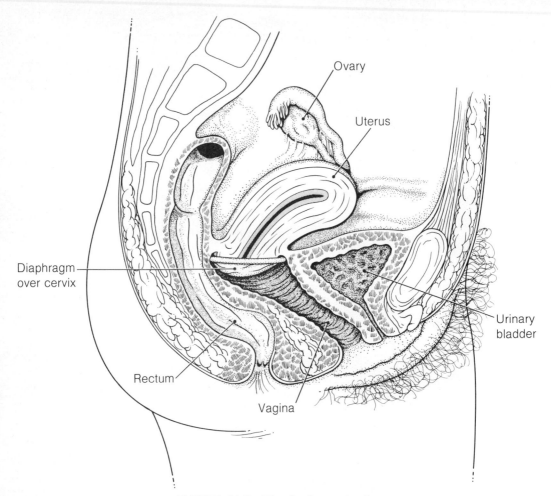

FIGURE 11.5   *The diaphragm in place.*

The pregnancy rate with a diaphragm depends somewhat on the spermicide used, and a great deal on the motivation of the woman using it. Part of the failure rate can be attributed to neglect in using it every time. It is also possible for the diaphragm to become displaced during intercourse (because of the "tenting" effect or expansion of the uterus during intercourse). For this reason, each woman should be fitted with the largest possible size.

Condom   The condom is a sheath made of rubber or animal tissue that fits over the erect penis and prevents the sperm from entering the woman's vagina. Condoms may be purchased at a drug store without prescription, and it has been shown that they cut down on the inci-

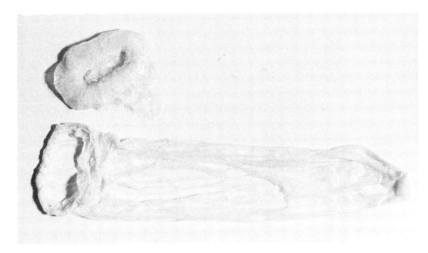

FIGURE 11.6 *The condom, rolled (as packaged) and unrolled.*

dence of venereal disease. The effectiveness of the condom is increased if the woman uses a spermicide.

Some people object to the condom because foreplay must be interrupted. (It is important to put it on before actual intercourse because some pre-ejaculatory fluid that contains sperm might be discharged.) Some men feel that a condom cuts down on sensation. This is less likely with the more expensive condoms—and these are also less likely to tear. Care must be taken when removing the penis from the vagina to avoid leakage around the edges of the condom.

Vaginal Spermicides

Vaginal spermicides may be foam, jelly, cream, or suppositories or tablets, and they are available without prescription. These are inserted into the vagina with a plastic applicator, as close as possible to the act of intercourse. Their effectiveness is much lower than any of the methods previously discussed. Suppositories and tablets are even less effective because they are not spread throughout the vagina. It is much safer to use the spermicides in combination with a condom or diaphragm.

The inconvenience of inserting the spermicide before intercourse may restrict the spontaneity of the sex act. In addition, certain of the stronger preparations may irritate the vagina or penis.

Rhythm Method

The rhythm method is based on determining the days on which the woman is fertile. A woman usually ovulates fourteen days before the beginning of menstruation. Sperm can live within the woman's body for up to seventy-two hours; the ovum will survive only about

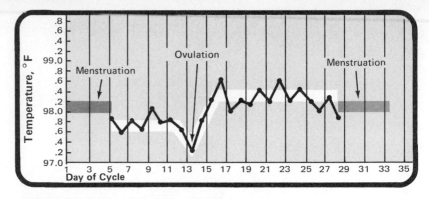

FIGURE 11.7 *Body temperature during the menstrual cycle: predicting ovulation by use of a temperature chart.*

twenty-four hours if it is not fertilized. Thus, theoretically there are only a few days each month during which a woman can conceive.

It is difficult to predict the exact date of ovulation. Most women using the rhythm method are advised to take their temperatures daily, because the body temperature rises slightly the day or two after ovulation and can thus be an indication of a woman's cycle. (See Figure 11.7.) A woman with an irregular cycle will find it impossible to rely on the rhythm method; in general, it is not effective. Both partners must feel highly motivated to avoid pregnancy, as they must practice abstinence for a week or so of unsafe days.

Coitus Interruptus   Coitus interruptus, or withdrawal, is not an effective means of birth control. Its effectiveness depends upon the withdrawal of the penis from the vagina before ejaculation, theoretically preventing the deposit of sperm. However, the pre-ejaculatory release experienced by many men contains a high concentration of sperm. In addition, the man may not withdraw in time.

For most couples, withdrawal destroys the spontaneity and much of the enjoyment of sex because the man must be constantly prepared to withdraw, and the woman must be concerned with whether or not he will act in time.

Douching   Douching (flushing out the vagina) immediately after intercourse should not be considered a method of birth control. Sperm can be deposited directly at the cervix so that many will have entered the uterus before douching. It is possible that douching may push *more* sperm into the uterus.

Sterilization

Two million Americans of childbearing age have found complete freedom from both contraceptive methods and unwanted pregnancy by undergoing sterilization, and more and more people are considering this alternative. Each year an additional 100,000 persons request sterilization as a permanent method of contraception. Five years ago most sterilization procedures involved women, whereas today, 70 percent of the candidates are men.[8]

Sterilization is legal in all states, but many doctors are unwilling to perform the operations on young unmarried people. At present, these operations should be considered permanent—the effects are usually not reversible. A woman may be sterilized through either a tubal ligation or the endoscopic techniques. The operation for men is a vasectomy.

Tubal Ligation

A tubal ligation is the more traditional method of female sterilization, and it is usually done immediately following childbirth. An abdominal incision is made, a small part of each fallopian tube is cut out, and the ends are tied off. This procedure is shown in Figure 11.8.

This method does not affect the menstrual cycle and ovulation at all. The ova are still produced, but can go only part way down the tube. They are absorbed into the body. Thus, sterilization does not change the hormonal balance of the woman or have any effect on sexual activity or female characteristics.

Endoscopic Techniques

There are three more recent methods of sterilization for a woman— the endoscopic techniques. The doctor uses a needle-like tube that contains a light and mirrors for locating the fallopian tubes, a cutting instrument, and an instrument to cauterize and seal off the cut ends.

In the *laparoscopy,* a small incision is made in the woman's naval; in the *culdoscopy* and the *hysteroscopy* the instrument enters through the vagina. Only local anesthesia is needed for endoscopies, they take a short time, and they involve fewer complications than tubal ligations. They are often performed on an out-patient basis so that the woman is able to walk out within a short time.

Vasectomy

A vasectomy takes only about half an hour and can be performed under local anesthesia in a clinic or doctor's office. It involves making

[8] Association for Voluntary Sterilization, *Questions and Answers on Sterilization,* New York, 1970, p. 1.

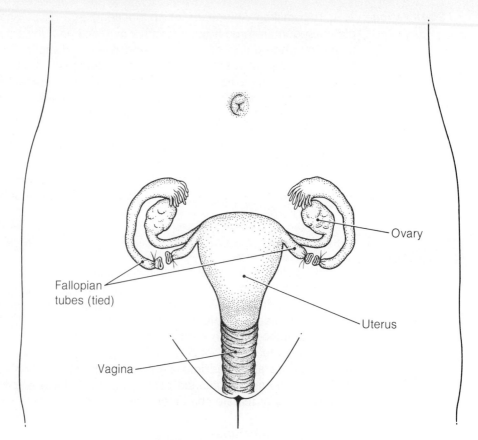

FIGURE 11.8   *A tubal ligation.*

a small incision on either side of the scrotum, then cutting and tying off the vas deferens, so that sperm will be blocked. See Figure 11.9.

The operation in no way affects a man's sexuality. His body still produces sperm, but they are absorbed into his system. The operation does not interfere with his ability to have an erection or ejaculation.

ABORTION

In 1973 the U.S. Supreme Court made abortion legal in all states. Every woman in the United States now has the same right to an abortion during the first six months of pregnancy as she has to any other type of surgery.

During the first trimester (three months) of pregnancy a woman has the right to an abortion without qualification. The decision is hers and her physician's. During the second trimester, the decision is

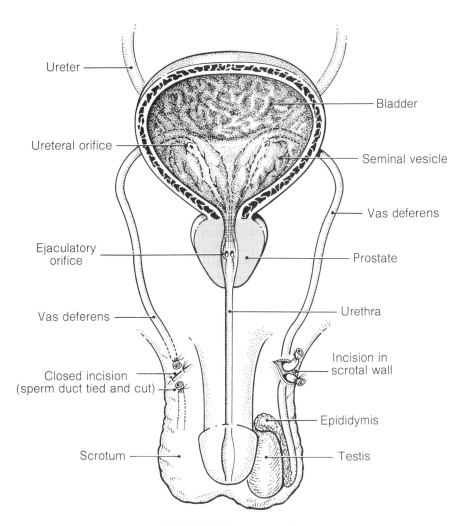

Ureter

Ureteral orifice

Ejaculatory
orifice

Vas deferens

Closed incision
(sperm duct tied and cut)

Scrotum

Bladder

Seminal vesicle

Vas deferens

Prostate

Urethra

Incision in
scrotal wall

Epididymis

Testis

FIGURE 11.9 *A vasectomy.*

still the woman's, but the state can impose conditions to safeguard her health. Once the fetus has reached a point of possible viability (from twenty-four to twenty-eight weeks) the state may prohibit an abortion except in cases where the woman's health is endangered by the pregnancy.

Abortion Counseling   An abortion is a physical and emotional experience. There are many qualified abortion counselors and services to deal with these effects. Pre-abortion counseling can help to prepare the woman by providing an understanding of abortion and the procedures involved.

It can make her aware of alternatives to abortion and provide contraceptive education. It can also help her to cope with any emotional aftereffects.

Methods of Abortion   There are three basic techniques for abortion: dilation and curettage, vacuum suction, and saline injection. Either a dilation and curettage procedure or a vacuum suction is used early in the pregnancy; a saline injection must be used in the later weeks.

Dilation and Curettage

Dilation and curettage (D and C) is the more traditional method for abortion during the eighth to twelfth week after a woman's last menstrual period; some doctors will perform a D and C through the fifteenth week, but there is controversy about the desired procedure for a later abortion.

A D and C is a surgical procedure that is also used for problems with infertility, menstrual periods, etc. The woman is given general anesthesia, so a D and C abortion must usually be performed in a hospital. The doctor uses dilators to gradually stretch the cervical opening until he can insert a curette. This is a metal loop that has a blunt, sharp, or serrated edge, mounted on a long thin handle. The doctor uses the curette to loosen the fetus and placenta from the uterine walls. The woman may then receive an injection of Ergotamine, a drug similar to the hormone that induces labor, to contract the uterus and aid in the expulsion of the fetal matter. The doctor usually also uses ovum forceps to remove all the material from the uterus.

Possible complications include perforation of the uterus, hemorrhage, or infection. There is also the possibility of incomplete abortion, in which case an infection would set in and another D and C would be necessary. There is a bloody discharge for a few days following the abortion.

Vacuum Suction

A vacuum suction abortion (also called dilation and evacuation, or D and E) is a newer and safer method than the D and C. It is the most widely used method in the United States during the seventh to twelfth week after the last menstrual period, while the D and C is still used for twelfth- to fifteenth-week abortions.[9]

A vacuum suction abortion requires only local anesthesia. The cervix is dilated until a vacurette can be inserted into the uterus. This

[9] Women's Collective, *Our Bodies, Ourselves,* p. 225.

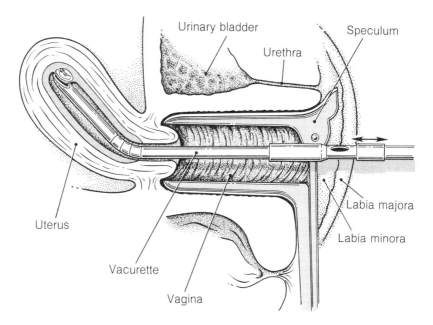

FIGURE 11.10 *A vacurette.*

is a hollow metal tube (shown in Figure 11.10) connected to a suction pump. The fetal tissue is gently sucked out of the uterus by controlled pressure. Both a D and C and a vacuum suction abortion take only about fifteen minutes.

The possible complications of a vacuum suction abortion are the same as those of a D and C, but they are less likely to occur. There is usually less bleeding.

Saline Injection

An abortion performed sixteen to twenty-four weeks after the last menstrual period must be done using a saline (or prostaglandin) injection. This method is more traumatic physically and emotionally than those used in earlier weeks of pregnancy.

A local anesthetic is injected into the skin of the woman's abdomen. A long thin needle is then inserted into the amniotic sac and an abortion-causing solution injected. This is usually a concentrated salt solution, but recently prostaglandins have sometimes been used. These are contraction-causing hormones.[10] Usually within several hours the woman goes into labor, and the fetus and placenta are delivered. If a saline solution is used, the fetus will be dead, but with prostaglandins, it may survive for several hours.

[10] Ibid., p. 225.

There are more risks and complications with this type of abortion than with the other methods. There is the possibility of saline shock, hemorrhage, or infection.

INFERTILITY

Although many people are concerned with methods of birth control and the prevention of pregnancy, there are others who are concerned because they cannot conceive. Ten percent of the couples in the United States are unable to have any children and another 15 percent are unable to have as many as they would like. Some of these couples have problems that can be cleared up, but others will never be able to reproduce. A temporary inability to conceive is called infertility, and a permanent inability to reproduce is called sterility.

In 35 percent of the couples who cannot reproduce, the female is infertile; in another 35 percent it is the male. The other 30 percent face infertility because of combined problems.[11]

Female Infertility

A number of things can cause infertility or sterility in the female. Various infections or diseases of the reproductive system can be factors. Tumors or other growths may be responsible for preventing the sperm from reaching the egg. The fallopian tubes may be blocked because of a congenital defect or earlier infections (such as gonorrhea).

It is also possible that the egg will not mature, because of a hormonal imbalance. There may be factors preventing the egg from being fertilized or penetrated by the sperm. An egg may become fertilized but fail to become implanted in the uterus.

Some of these medical problems can be corrected surgically or with hormone treatment. Other factors such as malnutrition or emotional stress can play a part in infertility; when these problems are alleviated, conception may occur.

Male Infertility

There are three major causes of male infertility or sterility. These are blockage of the sperm ducts, low sperm production, and low motility (movement of the sperm).

The passageways through which the sperm travel may be blocked because of infections or disease. There are numerous factors related to sperm production and motility. Among these are injury, congenital defects, overexposure to x-rays, diseases such as mumps, poor health or nutrition, and psychological problems.

[11] Ibid., p. 318.

Again, some of these problems can be treated surgically or with hormones. Temporary infertility may result from high temperatures in the testicles, where the sperm are produced—temperatures too high for sperm production may be caused by saunas, hot baths, etc. Sperm production decreases if a man has intercourse very frequently; thus a man with a low sperm count may be able to impregnate his partner if they have intercourse only at certain times close to ovulation.

Infertility of the Couple   Some couples may have combined problems. For example, a woman may have an allergic response to her partner's sperm, creating destructive antibodies. There are certain positions and times for intercourse that can make fertilization more likely. Many of these combined problems can be solved.

ALTERNATIVES TO NATURAL CONCEPTION

If a couple finds that they cannot conceive naturally and they still want to have children, there are two alternatives—artificial insemination and adoption.

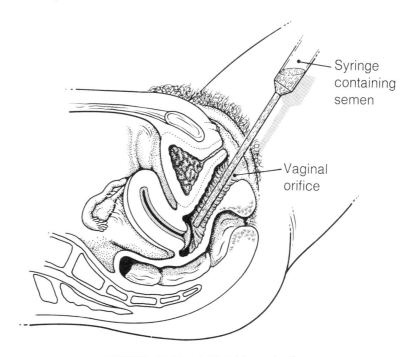

FIGURE 11.11 *Artificial insemination.*

Artificial Insemination: Difficult Questions

When an obstetrics patient chooses artificial insemination, the physician may get some hard-to-answer questions from her or her spouse. Answers that may help can be equally hard to come by, states the Institute for Business Planning, a publisher of financial information. "There are few court decisions and even fewer statutory guides." Here are some of the "best answers" the firm's attorney-editors were able to muster for questions asked by patients and physicians.

· What are the physician's legal liabilities? There are no reported cases on the doctor's legal posture, the institute says. "His situation may depend on whether the insemination is to be viewed as adulterous or not" and liability may also conceivably turn on the "legitimacy or illegitimacy of the resulting child."

· Can the wife be considered guilty of adultery? The California Supreme Court says the wife is not guilty, but in Illinois there are unreported lower court decisions "facing both ways on this issue."

· Will the child be considered legitimate? One state supreme court (Calif.) has decided the child is legitimate. Oklahoma has a law that provides for adoption and legitimizing of the child, but, again, New York and Illinois have lower court rulings "going off in opposite directions."

· Must the husband support the child? Where he consents to the insemination, he does have support obligation "even where the child may be viewed as illegitimate."

· Does the child inherit through the husband or through the semen donor? It is not clear whether the child will inherit through the donor, but he will through the husband if he is considered legitimate and the husband is considered "the father." (There are no court cases on this question.)

Source: Medical World News, December 21, 1973.

Artificial Insemination

Artificial insemination involves many questions but it may be a good solution for some infertile couples. In this procedure, sperm are deposited near the female's cervix at the time she should be ovulating. The sperm may be from her husband or an anonymous donor. Conception may then occur and pregnancy and birth proceed naturally.

Adoption

A second alternative for the infertile couple is adoption. The process of adoption is usually long and involved. There are fewer and fewer infants available for adoption because of increasingly effective use of birth control and the availability of abortions. Also, more unmarried women decide to keep their children. Agencies must take care to protect the adopted child and make sure the adopting parents are making a well-considered decision. The number of children available varies in different locations, and some couples may find this an attractive possibility.

FURTHER READINGS

Arms, Suzanne. *Immaculate Deception*. Boston: Houghton Mifflin Co., 1975.

Provides a new look at women and childbirth in America.

Bing, Elisabeth. *The Adventure of Birth*. New York: Ace Books, 1970.

Experiences in the Lamaze method of prepared childbirth are explored.

Callahan, Daniel. *Abortion*. New York: Macmillan Co., 1970.

A comprehensive and sensitive study of abortion in all its medical, legal, social, and ethical implications.

Fraser, Dean. *The People Problem*. Bloomington, Ind.: Indiana University Press, 1971.

What you should know about growing population and vanishing resources.

Ingelman-Sundburg, Axel. *A Child Is Born*. New York: Dell Publishing Co., 1974.

A very practical guide for the expectant mother.

Leboyer, Frederick. *Birth Without Violence*. New York: Alfred A. Knopf, 1976.

The author presents his radical yet supremely simple techniques for easing the birth trauma.

Milinaire, Caterine. *Birth*. New York: Harmony Books, 1971.

The development of the embryo from conception to birth described in relation to woman's mind/body.

Rorvik, David. *Woman's Medical Guide*. New York: Avon Books, 1976.

Authoritative, sensitive, up-to-date guide with a special section containing one hundred health questions most women ask.

Sarvis, Betty and Rodman, Hyman. *The Abortion Controversy*. New York: Columbia University Press, 1974.

A comprehensive account of the moral, social, legal, and medical issues involved in abortion.

Trussell, James and Chandler, Steve. *The Loving Book*. New York: World Publishing, 1972.

Offers a comprehensive understanding of birth control and human sexuality.

5

PEOPLE AND DRUGS

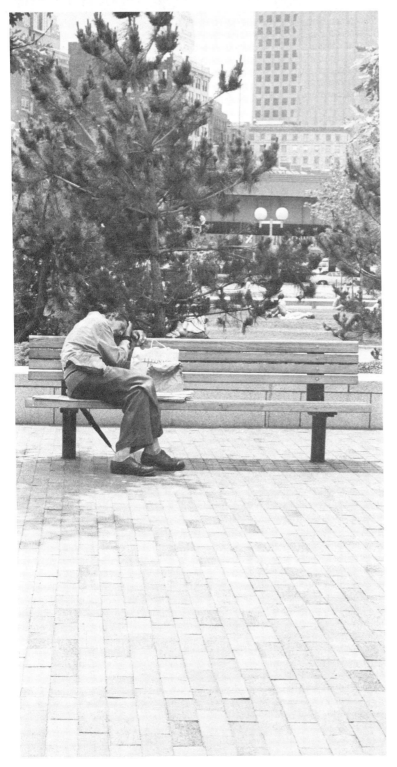

What a curious feeling. I
must be shutting up like
a telescope.

. . . First, however, she
waited for a few minutes
to see if she was going to
shrink any further: she felt
a little nervous about this:
"for it might end, you
know," said Alice to
herself," in my going
out altogether . . ."

Lewis Carroll
Alice in Wonderland

Chapter 12

Tobacco
and Health

Americans smoke about 500 billion cigarettes a year, or about 3,000 per person. This means they spend about $15 billion each year on cigarettes alone (not including pipe tobacco, etc.). Not only is smoking an expensive habit, it is costly to the health of both the smoker and the nonsmoker. Cigarette smokers die at earlier ages than non-smokers and they experience more days of disability than non-smokers.[1] Figure 12.1 shows the percentages for both sexes.

WHY DO PEOPLE SMOKE?

In view of all the negative publicity about smoking and tobacco, why do people continue to smoke? The answers to this question have both social and psychological roots.

People use smoking cigarettes as a means of relaxation. They feel smoking relieves their tensions. When tension is especially great, as during periods of war, consumption of tobacco rises dramatically. During both world wars there was a 50 percent increase in demand for cigarettes in the United States. Yet the nicotine in a cigarette is actually a stimulant; physiologically, it does not act as a tranquilizer.

Some authorities suggest that a cigarette represents a reward, one that the smoker can treat himself to whenever he wants. Some people just enjoy smoking.

Young people often see smoking cigarettes as a form of self-assertion or a sign of adulthood. They begin smoking in imitation of adults around them, in expression of an unconscious desire to be

[1] See Edward M. Brecher, *Licit and Illicit Drugs,* New York: Consumers Union, 1972, and *The Report of the Surgeon General's Advisory Committee on Smoking and Health,* Washington, D.C.: U.S. Government Printing Office, 1964.

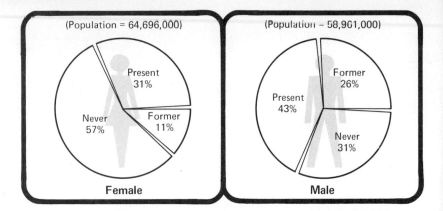

FIGURE 12.1 *Percentage of male and female smokers and nonsmokers, age 17 and over. Source: U.S. Department of Health, Education and Welfare, Chart Book on Smoking, Tobacco & Health, p. 4.*

adult. There is often the feeling that with smoking comes the power and privileges of adulthood. The act of smoking is viewed as a symbolic break with childhood. Teenagers are especially concerned with being accepted by their peers, so they may smoke in an attempt to conform to popular standards of behavior—because of peer pressure.

Recent studies have shown that youngsters whose parents smoke are more likely themselves to smoke. If older brothers and sisters have begun to smoke, there is increased likelihood that younger children will also smoke. Smoking, after all, is learned behavior.

A great deal of research must be done before we fully understand the factors that lead people to find smoking an enjoyable (or unbreakable) habit. Extensive research has already been done on the negative effects of smoking to health.

EFFECTS OF SMOKING

Tobacco smoke, a product of combustion, is a mixture of gases, vaporized chemicals, and millions of minute particles of ash and other solids. The minute particles, or particulate matter, are called *tar.* It contains nicotine, a toxic substance that is part of tobacco, and other products from the partial burning and distillation of the tobacco. The tar contains at least seven compounds that are proven to be cancer-producing (*carcinogenic*) agents and others that have been found to be cancer promoting.

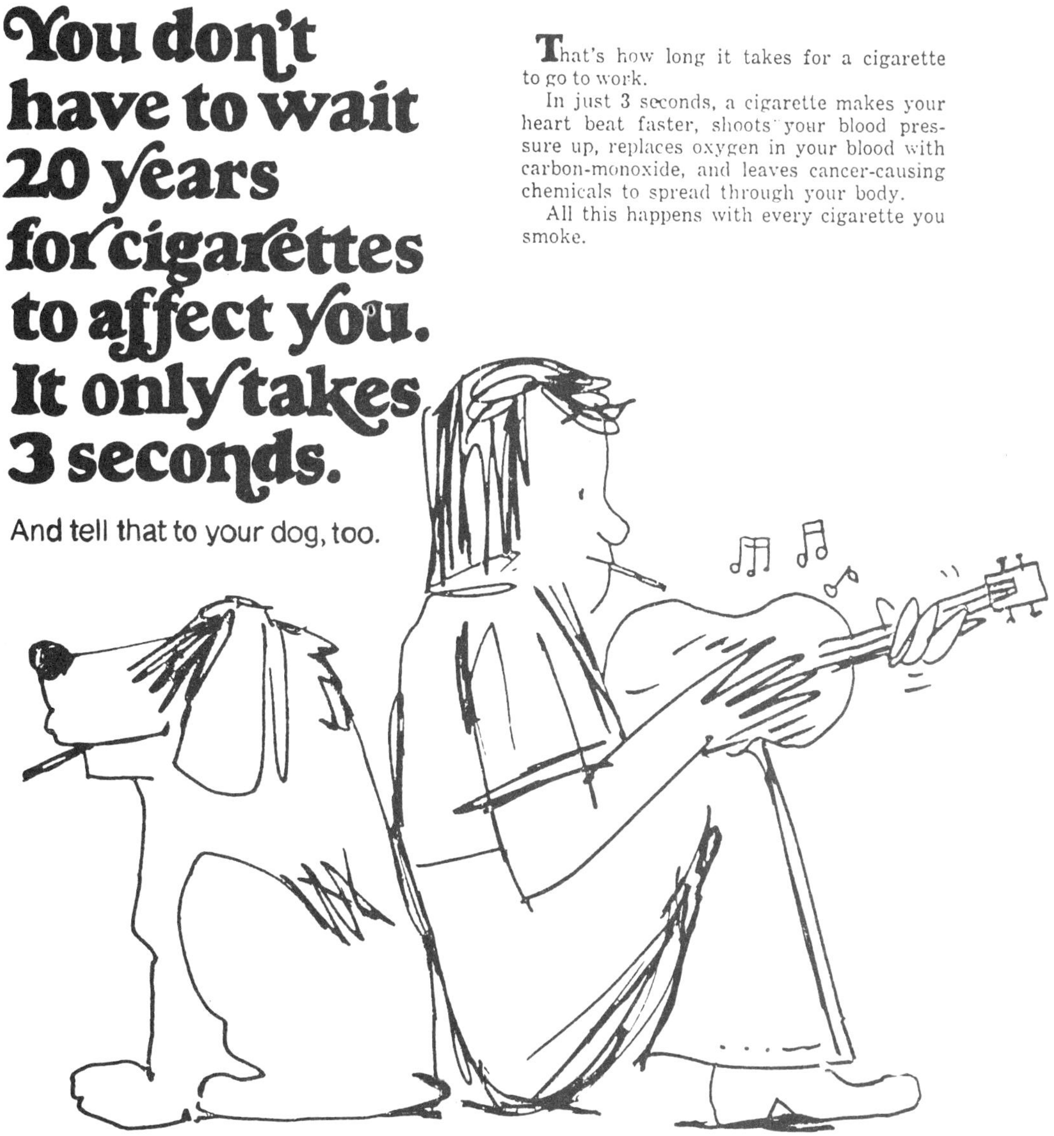

You don't have to wait 20 years for cigarettes to affect you. It only takes 3 seconds.

And tell that to your dog, too.

That's how long it takes for a cigarette to go to work.

In just 3 seconds, a cigarette makes your heart beat faster, shoots your blood pressure up, replaces oxygen in your blood with carbon-monoxide, and leaves cancer-causing chemicals to spread through your body.

All this happens with every cigarette you smoke.

FIGURE 12.2 (*Source:* National Clearinghouse for Smoking and Health, 5401 Westbard Avenue, Bethesda, Md. 20016.)

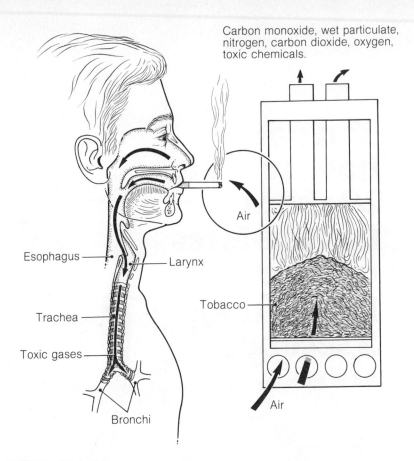

Carbon monoxide, wet particulate, nitrogen, carbon dioxide, oxygen, toxic chemicals.

Air

Esophagus

Larynx

Trachea

Tobacco

Toxic gases

Bronchi

Air

FIGURE 12.3   *Chemical composition of smoke. Tobacco smoke contains many chemical compounds, some of which are known carcinogens, or cancer-causing agents.*

Figure 12.3 shows the composition of tobacco smoke. Over 90 percent of the smoke is various gases; the rest is particulate matter (8 percent). Nitrogen makes up the greater part of the smoke (59 percent), with carbon dioxide (13.6 percent), oxygen (13.4 percent), carbon monoxide (3.2 percent), and small amounts of numerous other chemicals.

When smokers inhale, the smoke with all its toxic substances is drawn in through the mouth and throat and down into the lungs. Of the many effects on the smoker's health, cancer (especially lung cancer), chronic bronchitis, emphysema, heart disease, and circulatory impairment are among the major ones. Figure 12.4 shows comparative mortality rates from these diseases for smokers and nonsmokers.

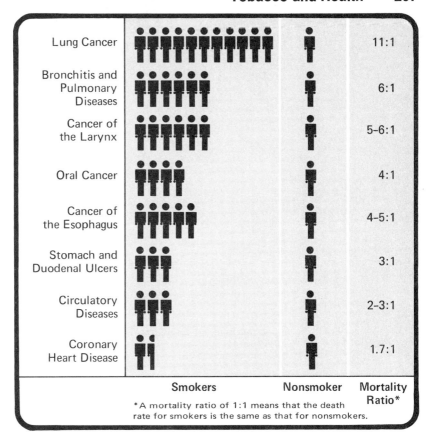

	Smokers	Nonsmoker	Mortality Ratio*
Lung Cancer			11:1
Bronchitis and Pulmonary Diseases			6:1
Cancer of the Larynx			5–6:1
Oral Cancer			4:1
Cancer of the Esophagus			4–5:1
Stomach and Duodenal Ulcers			3:1
Circulatory Diseases			2–3:1
Coronary Heart Disease			1.7:1

*A mortality ratio of 1:1 means that the death rate for smokers is the same as that for nonsmokers.

FIGURE 12.4 *Mortality ratio of smokers to nonsmokers for several diseases. Source: Adapted from U.S. Department of Health, Education and Welfare,* Progress Against Cancer, *1970, p. 41.*

Lung Cancer   As smoke is drawn into the breathing passages and air sacs of the lungs, the gases and particulate matter settle into the surrounding membranes. One point of great concentration is at the division of the large breathing tube (bronchus) into two smaller tubes, the bronchi. At this point, the smoke slows its movement, causing the particulate matter to be deposited along the bronchial lining. This area is where most lung cancers begin.

As the cells and tissue of the lining begin to react to the continued irritation of tobacco smoke, the cilia (fine hairlike growths) along the surface of the lining begin to slow and stop their natural cleansing function. The cilia work to remove irritating substances from the lungs through mucus. Eventually, however, the cilia may actually disappear, so that the carcinogens remain in contact with the sensitive cells in the lining. It is this contact over long periods of time that is believed to cause cancer.

This initial change in the reaction of the lungs to tobacco smoke is called *hyperplasia.* The smoker may develop a cough—the response of the lungs to try to remove the toxic substances from their lining—during this period. As the cells of the lining change further, *carcinoma in situ* develops, a condition that is the precursor to cancer. Many of the symptoms of both hyperplasia and carcinoma, such as the smoker's cough, hoarseness, etc., are accepted as a normal part of smoking, so that cancer is not diagnosed until a later and more serious stage.

Other Types of Cancer

A strong association has been established between tobacco smoking and cancer of the esophagus, larynx, pharynx, mouth, and cheeks, so that a cause-and-effect relationship seems likely. Pipe and cigar smokers also are more prone to cancers of the tongue and lips than nonsmokers.

Research has also revealed a connection between cigarette smoking and cancer of the bladder in the male. Thus far, the data is not sufficient to prove a causative relationship, but in 1967 two large

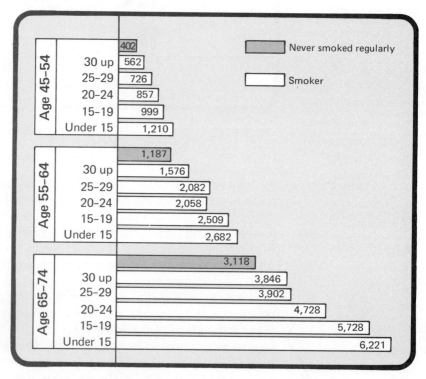

FIGURE 12.5   *Death rates of smokers by age smoking began, per 100,000 population. Source: U.S. Department of Health, Education and Welfare,* Chart Book on Smoking, Tobacco & Health, *p. 13.*

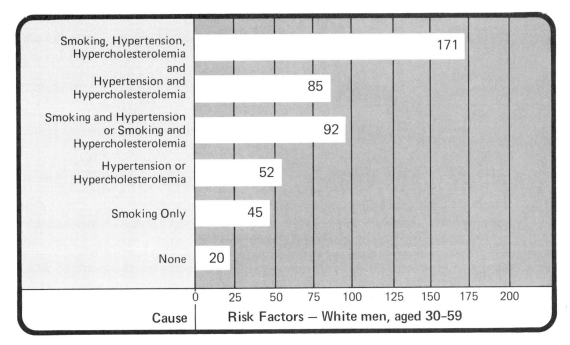

FIGURE 12.6 *First major coronary event: Smoking, hypertension, and high blood cholesterol levels (hypercholesterolemia) are all major risk factors for heart attack and sudden death from coro-* *nary heart disease. When any two or all three of these factors are present, the risk is much greater. Source: Facts: Smoking and Health, National Clearinghouse for Smoking and Health, 1971.*

population studies (covering 1.3 million people) showed that those who smoked more than one pack a day had a death rate from bladder cancer twice that of nonsmokers. In 1968 additional research data emphasized this relationship and also linked smoking with cancer of the pancreas.

Respiratory Disease   Cigarette smoking is the major cause of chronic bronchitis in the United States and greatly increases the risk of dying from bronchitis or emphysema. Deaths from chronic bronchitis and emphysema had risen from 2,300 in 1945 to 23,000 by 1965.

Chronic bronchitis is an inflammation of the bronchial tubes. The first symptom is a cough, which signifies the reaction of the irritated area against an accumulation of mucus. The cough becomes established and other symptoms such as wheezing and shortness of breath appear. Research has shown that these symptoms are more prevalent in women who smoke heavily than in men. In the later stages of the disease, the persistent coughing and irritation may damage the delicate walls of the alveoli (air pockets in the lungs), causing the elastic tissue of the lungs to degenerate, leading to emphysema.

Warning for Pipe, Cigar Smokers

Cigaret smoking is an established risk factor in heart disease. But a new study suggests pipe and cigar smokers run a risk as great as many cigaret smokers. Dr. Oscar Auerbach of the Veterans Administration Hospital in East Orange, N.J., and Dr. Harry W. Carter of St. Barnabas Medical Center in Livingston, N.J., studied the hearts of 1,056 deceased men and compared their stages of heart disease and their smoking habits. "The proportion of cigar and pipe smokers who had moderate and advanced atherosclerosis [fatty deposits on an artery's inner walls] was about the same as those smoking one or two packs of cigarets per day," they report with two American Cancer Society epidemiologists in the journal Chest.

Source: The National Observer, March 5, 1977.

Pulmonary emphysema is defined as a loss of functioning lung tissue accompanied by overinflation of the remaining tissue. It results from obstruction of the bronchioles (small bronchial tubes) so that the ability to exhale is affected. When the smoker exhales, the bronchial tubes contract and air is trapped by the mucus accumulated

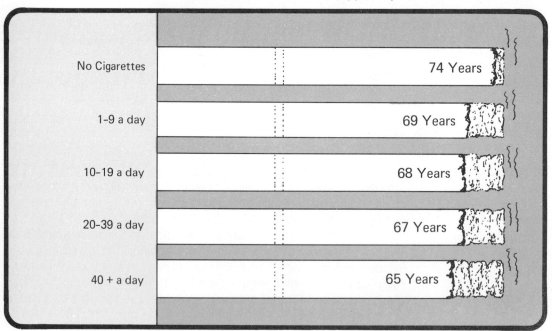

FIGURE 12.7 *According to the American Cancer Society, a 25-year-old man can expect to live to 74—if he doesn't smoke. If he does, the illustration above shows what happens to his life expectancy.*

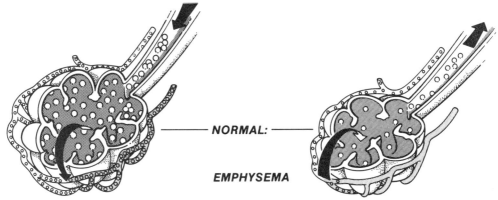

NORMAL:

EMPHYSEMA

(1) Healthy: The alveoli expand for intake - snap back for exhalation.
(2) Diseased: Air enters a diseased alveolus but is poorly expelled owing to a saggy-balloon effect and tube collapse.

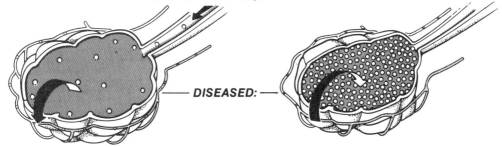

DISEASED:

FIGURE 12.8 *Emphysema.*

from smoking. Eventually the tissue and cells are damaged and stop functioning. Coughing and shortness of breath or wheezing are also symptoms of emphysema. In the later stages, bloating of the chest cavity may occur because of the trapped air and inflated tissue in the lungs.

Heart Disease and Circulatory Impairment

Nicotine from cigarettes stimulates the part of the nervous system that controls the heart and blood vessels. The combination of the nicotine and carbon monoxide in tobacco smoke exerts a strain on the heart, making smokers far more susceptible to heart disease than nonsmokers. As lung function becomes impaired by smoking, the heart must work harder in using the remaining air sacs. More smokers also die from coronary artery disease than do nonsmokers.

The stimulus of nicotine may cause high blood pressure. Buerger's disease is another ailment of the circulatory system related to

---

Cigarettes Safer If Kept Out of Mouth

A smoker who keeps his cigarette in his mouth between puffs (a "drooping" smoker) is more likely to have chronic bronchitis than one who smokes in the usual fashion.

The excess of chronic bronchitis among drooping smokers presumably is a result of greater exposure of their bronchi to the damaging substances in tobacco smoke than that occurring in persons who smoke comparable amounts in the normal manner. The actual volume or concentration of smoke may not be greater for the drooping smoker, but perhaps he inhales a greater proportion of "sidestream" smoke. This smoke, which arises from the mouthpiece and burning cone during puff inter-missions, may contain more tar than the "mainstream" smoke that emerges from the mouthpiece during puffing. In any event, the observed variations in the rates of chronic bronchitis cannot be explained on the basis of differences in age, rate of cigarette consumption, type of cigarettes, or social class of the two types of smokers.

Among 5,438 men age 40 years or older, the incidence of chronic bronchitis was about 42 percent in the 460 drooping smokers and about 34 percent in the 4,978 who smoked in the usual manner.

J. Rimington, M.D., St. Thomas' Hospital, Stockport, England. Chronic bronchitis: method of cigarette smoking. *Br Med J I:776–778, 1973.*

---

smoking. The smoke causes a constriction of the small arteries in the hands and feet; in extreme cases it can lead to gangrene (tissue decay caused by oxygen starvation when the blood supply is obstructed), necessitating amputation.

Other Problems

There has long been evidence that cigarette smoking aggravates sinusitis (inflammation of the sinus tissues). Meaningful relief from this condition can be obtained when the person stops smoking. Persons with ulcers are especially advised not to smoke, since tobacco smoke aggravates both peptic and gastric ulcers.

Clinical studies have also linked smoking to oral diseases other than cancer. Both gingivitis (inflammation of the gums) and bone deterioration occur more often in smokers than in nonsmokers. Some of these problems are related to the buildup of tartar or plaque caused by nicotine.

Smoking and Pregnant Women

There is now a substantial body of evidence to show that smoking during pregnancy can have a retarding influence on fetal growth. Women who smoke have babies with significantly lower birth weights than those of nonsmokers. In addition, spontaneous abortions and stillbirths are more common in women who smoke. The U.S. Public Health Service reports that there are 4,600 stillbirths each year that can be attributed to smoking. Neonatal (newborn) deaths and illness

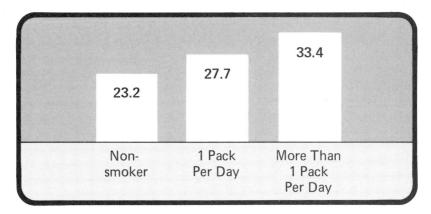

FIGURE 12.9 *Smoking and pregnancy: Fetal and infant deaths per 1,000 total births, in smoking and non-smoking women. Source: Ontario Department of Health.*

are also higher among infants whose mothers smoke. (See Figure 12.9.) The woman who smokes may not only harm the fetus but also handicap her child in early infancy.

Smoking and Teenagers   Despite the evidence against smoking, teenagers continue to take it up and, in fact, are beginning to develop the habit earlier and earlier. Some are confirmed smokers by the age of thirteen or fourteen.

Recent research into the effects of smoking on teenagers emphasizes the dangers for all. Evidence shows that high school students with from one to five years of smoking experience suffer from excessive coughing, increased sputum production, and shortness of breath. These young smokers also show lower lung volumes, probably reflecting small airway obstructions. An additional fact to consider is that the earlier age for taking up smoking means that by the time the females become mothers, they have suffered the effects of smoking for many years, thereby increasing the risk of problems in pregnancy.

NONSMOKERS' RIGHTS

Another deterrent to smoking should be that even nonsmokers suffer the consequences. The *U.S. Surgeon General's Report of 1972* accumulated much evidence of the ill effects tobacco pollution exerts on those who do not smoke:

> An idling cigarette contaminates the air for approximately twelve minutes. Smoke from an idling cigarette contains

almost twice the tar and nicotine of an inhaled cigarette and thus may be twice as toxic as smoke inhaled by the smoker. One test made in Germany showed that the smoking of several cigarettes in a closed room makes the concentration of nicotine and dust particles so high that the nonsmoker inhales as much harmful tobacco as the normal smoker inhales from four or five cigarettes.[2]

Researchers have also found that a room full of smokers can raise the carbon monoxide content of the air to between 20 and 80 parts per million. The acceptable maximum in most industrial situations is 50 ppm. If inhaled carbon monoxide enters the blood stream in sufficient quantities, it can cause headache, dizziness, lassitude, and heart and lung damage. In a closed automobile, where the smoke from ten cigarettes can produce carbon monoxide levels of up to 90 ppm, the concentration can interfere with the ability of the driver to judge time intervals, thereby increasing the possibility of accidents.

Nonsmokers suffering from allergies or heart or lung disease may experience stronger and immediate adverse reactions to tobacco smoke. Individuals wearing contact lenses (and even those who are not) experience tearing and discomfort in smoke filled rooms.

The National Interagency Council on Smoking and Health states that nonsmokers have a right to breathe clean air, free from harmful and irritating tobacco smoke. This right supersedes the right to smoke when the two conflict. Nonsmokers have the right to express—firmly but politely—their discomfort and adverse reactions to tobacco smoke. They have as well the right to voice their objections when a smoker lights a cigarette without first asking permission.

QUITTING

Like anything else involving the human personality, the decision to quit smoking is complex. Because each individual may have a different reason for smoking, no one method for quitting or cutting down will be successful for every smoker. Quitting smoking can probably be achieved most effectively by the person who is honestly and positively motivated to stop. If the person really wants to quit, his will power is more likely to overcome his habit.

For those who are determined to quit, there are some practical steps to consider:

[2] U.S., Department of Health, Education and Welfare, *The Health Consequences of Smoking: A Report of the Surgeon General,* Washington, D.C.: U.S. Government Printing Office, 1971.

Smoking and Type A

Why are some people able to quit smoking while others are not? Results from a new University of Michigan study provide at least a partial answer to this question.

In a study of 200 administrators, engineers, and scientists at the National Aeronautics and Space Administration, the University of Michigan researchers found that personality, job stress, and the social nature of the person's occupation—that is, whether or not it involves working with people—are the key factors in governing a person's ability to quit smoking.

Those smokers with Type A personalities—hard driving, competitive, and with heavy work loads—have the least success in quitting, and Type B smokers are the most successful in quiting.

The research team noted that the quitters also tend to have fewer job responsibilities and pressures and to work in object-oriented occupations. Engineers, for example, had a higher quit rate than did administrators.

The investigators say that they do not have enough information to determine whether personality or work load constitutes the major stumbling block to giving up cigarettes. However, they strongly suspect that the major culprit is Type A personality. And, indeed, a number of other studies have shown that those with this type of personality actively seek out high-pressure, people-oriented professions.

Robert D. Caplan, Sidney Cobb, and John R. French, Jr.: Relationships of cessation of smoking with job stress, personality, and social support. J. App. Psychol., 60: 211, 1975. For reprints: Robert D. Caplan, Institute for Social Research, University of Michigan, Ann Arbor, MI 48106.

1. *Smoke one less cigarette each day.* For some, the gradual method is the easiest. They may smoke one less cigarette each week, or they may cut down by one each day. One less cigarette a day means twenty-eight fewer a month!
2. *Try switching to another brand.* Some people find that they do not enjoy smoking any other brand than their favorite so that it is easier to quit entirely.
3. *Anticipate those times that tempt you and try not to smoke during these "prime times."* If you anticipate the times—after meals, when you are tense, etc.—when you most want to smoke, you will be more conscious of your desire to quit at these times. Keeping a list of the times you smoke may help you see your reasons for smoking.
4. *Pick a "Q" day.* Pick a certain date as a special time when you are really going to quit. Some people find motivation from their friends who are aware of this firm decision.

5. *Outside help.* Some medical authorities view heavy smoking as a psychological problem that can be helped by some form of group therapy. Hypnosis is helpful in some cases. Use of drugs to quit smoking is more likely to be harmful or simply ineffective.

Table 12.1 *Tar and nicotine content of cigarettes. Source:* National Clearinghouse for Smoking and Health, Rockville, Md., 1971.

Brand	Type	Tar (mg/cig)	Nicotine (mg/cig)	Brand	Type	Tar (mg/cig)	Nicotine (mg/cig)
Alpine	King, M	18	1.2	Galaxy	King	20	1.4
American Brand	King (HP)	19	1.3	Half & Half	King	24	1.7
	King	21	1.4	Herbert Tareyton	King, NF	29	1.9
Belair	King, M	17	1.3	Home Run	Reg., NF	19	1.4
	100 mm, M	18	1.4	Kent	Reg.	9	0.6
Benson & Hedges	Reg. (HP)	17	1.2		King (HP)	16	1.0
	King (HP)	18	1.3		King	17	1.1
	100 mm	19	1.4		King, M	18	1.1
	100 mm, M	20	1.4		100 mm	20	1.3
Bull Durham	King	30	2.0		100 mm, M	18	1.2
Camel	Reg., NF	25	1.5	King Sano	King	7	0.3
	King	19	1.3		King, M	6	0.3
Camel Talls	100 mm	20	1.4	Kool	Reg., NF, M	21	1.5
Carlton	Reg.	1	0.1		King, M	18	1.4
	King	3	0.3		100 mm, M	19	1.4
Chesterfield	Reg., NF	25	1.5	L&M	King (HP)	18	1.2
	King, NF	29	1.8		King	19	1.3
	King	19	1.3		100 mm	19	1.4
	King, M	18	1.2		100 mm, M	19	1.3
	101 mm	19	1.4	L.T.C.	King	10	0.7
Domino	King, NF	27	1.4	Lark	King	17	1.2
	King	21	1.3		100 mm	18	1.2
Doral	King	14	1.0	Life	100 mm	10	0.6
	King, M	14	1.1	Lucky Strike	Reg., NF	28	1.8
DuMaurier	King (HP)	17	1.2	Lucky Filters	King	21	1.6
Edgeworth	King (HP)	18	1.3		100 mm	22	1.6
Export	100 mm	19	1.5	Mapleton	Reg., NF	29	1.3
English Ovals	Reg., NF (HP)	24	1.8		King	23	1.2
	King, NF (HP)	30	2.4	Marlboro	King (HP)	18	1.3
Eve	100 mm	17	1.3		King	19	1.3
	100 mm, M	18	1.2		King, M	18	1.2
Fatima	King, NF	31	1.9		100 mm (HP)	19	1.5
Frappe	King, M	10	0.4		100 mm	20	1.5

NF = Nonfilter (all other brands possess filters)   PB = Plastic box   M = Menthol   HP = Hard pack

---

Lower Tar—Lower Risk

A report from the American Cancer Society has found that though the safest course by far is not to smoke at all, the low-tar and low-nicotine cigarette brands really are safer than the stronger ones.

Low tar and nicotine cigarettes were defined as those containing less than 17.6 milligrams of tar and 1.2 mg of nicotine; the high-tar brands contained more than 25.8 mg of tar and 2 mg of nicotine. Since the survey was concluded in 1972, results do not take into account the many brands introduced recently that are even lower in tar and nicotine.

According to the survey, the mortality rate from lung cancer was 26 per cent lower among the low tar and nicotine smokers than among those who smoked stronger brands. For heart disease, the mortality rate was 14 percent lower.

However, the number of cigarettes smoked remains a major factor in determining the health risks. People who smoked more than one pack of the lower tar cigarettes a day had a greater lung cancer mortality than did those who smoked less than a pack of the high tar variety. And nonsmokers fared best of all, with a lung cancer mortality 85 percent lower than low tar smokers.

For those who want to control their smoking but feel they do not want to quit, there are some more healthful tips:

1. *Cut down.* The more you smoke, the worse it is for your health. Even a few cigarettes less can make some difference.
2. *Smoke your cigarettes only part-way down.* The last few puffs of a cigarette are the most toxic and dangerous. The risks from smoking still exist but are somewhat less if you only smoke part (even half) of the cigarette.
3. *Switch to another brand.* Filter cigarettes and brands with less tar and nicotine have been proven to be less harmful.
4. *Try not to inhale.* The risk to the lungs is lessened somewhat if you inhale less and not as deeply.
5. *Get a regular physical checkup (including a chest x-ray).* If you must continue to endanger your health, learn to be aware of changes and warning signals in your body.

The ultimate solution rests with the individual. One can ignore the overwhelmingly negative evidence on smoking and continue this habit, or one can decide to stop.

Remember the Ingredients of Success:

1. Find a motive or reason for stopping.
2. Change your behavior.
3. Change your attitude.

A positive attitude—a feeling that you are giving yourself a gift will be most helpful. Consider the benefits of withdrawal—getting a habit under control, a renewed feeling of self-confidence, the reduced risk of being stricken and crippled at mid-life by one of the chronic diseases associated with smoking: emphysema, bronchitis, cancer, heart disease.

Source: U.S. Dept. of Health, Education and Welfare.

FURTHER READINGS

Allen, William A., Angermann, Gerhard; and Fackler, William A. *Learning to Live Without Cigarettes.* Garden City, N.Y.: Doubleday & Company, Inc., 1968.

This book is divided into three sections. The first section offers the smoker insights into the mental and physical aspects of smoking and provides the most recent findings and techniques available for breaking the cigarette habit. The second section offers the professional a fund of resource materials for use in developing smoking-control programs for youth and adult groups. And the third part of the book provides an easy-to-read question-and-answer section on the principal health hazards of cigarette smoking.

Eysenck, H. J. *Smoking, Health and Personality.* New York: Basic Books, 1965.

The author is concerned with the relationship between smoking, personality, and such diseases as lung cancer and coronary thrombosis.

Chapter 13

Alcohol Use and Abuse

Alcoholism is the nation's number one drug problem. Although there can be no accurate count of all alcoholics in the United States, estimates range from 4 to 9 million and up, and authorities are convinced that the rate is rising steadily. One sign of this is the increasing evidence of juvenile alcohol abuse. The drug of choice for teenagers has become alcohol. Ironically, many parents are relieved to discover their children are having trouble with alcohol rather than with less familiar (and sometimes less harmful) drugs.

WHY PEOPLE DRINK

People drink for a variety of social, cultural, psychological, and/or medical reasons. They drink at parties or celebrations with friends and relatives. They drink in religious ceremonies. They drink at meals to complement their food. Some people drink to relax. Others drink because it is a habit.

Most people's drinking is *integrative drinking.* Alcohol is used as an adjunct to other activities. Among groups such as orthodox Jews or native Italians in which alcohol is part of religious or social traditions, there is a low incidence of problem drinking despite almost universal use of alcoholic beverages.

Most Americans drink moderately and safely, for some of the above reasons. Yet other people drink alcohol for the anesthetizing effect it produces. These people may drink for courage, to forget their worries, to escape. They can not enjoy themselves without liquor. They use alcohol as a drug and often drink for the definite purpose of getting drunk. Eventually, these people cannot do without alcohol.

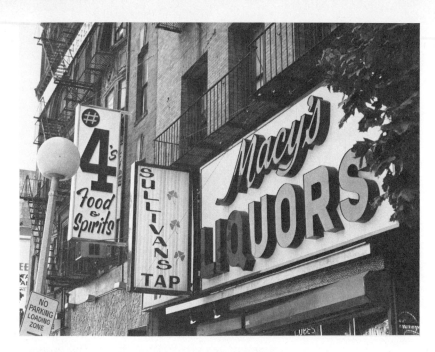

FIGURE 13.1 *We live in a society where it is customary to drink. It is the abstainer who strikes us as the more abnormal. With alcohol we offer hospitality and display our sociability. Though we frown on drunkards we are suspicious of teetotallers. (Neil Kessel and Henry Walton,* Alcoholism, *Baltimore, Md.: Penguin Books, 1965.)*

HOW ALCOHOL AFFECTS THE BODY

When a person drinks an alcoholic beverage, 20 percent of the alcohol is absorbed almost immediately into the bloodstream through the stomach. Unlike most other foods, alcohol does not go through a lengthy digestive process. The other 80 percent of the alcohol is processed only slightly more slowly through the gastrointestinal tract into the bloodstream. The blood then carries it to all parts of the body, including the brain. Only moments after ingestion, alcohol can be found in all the tissues, organs, and secretions of the body.

Alcohol was long regarded as a stimulant; actually, it is a depressant. The "stimulus" effect occurs because of the depressive action on certain parts of the brain, which causes the person to lose his inhibitions (and, gradually, his control).

Moderate quantities of alcohol affect various parts of the body. The heart rate increases, the blood vessels of the arms, legs, and skin

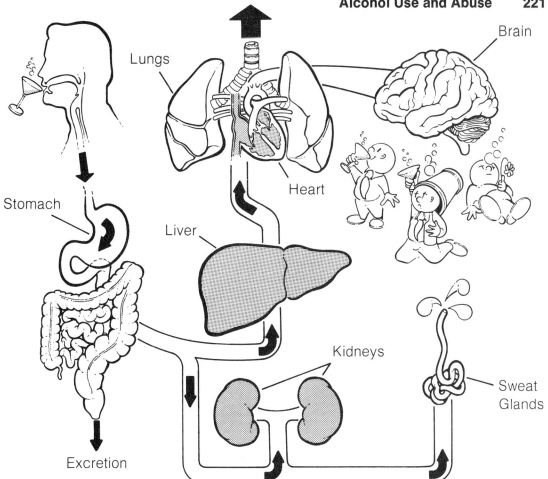

FIGURE 13.2 *Alcohol flow chart. Once the alcohol enters the bloodstream, it is carried to all parts of the body. Some of the alcohol is lost through expiration, sweat, and excretion. The amount that finds its way to the brain depends on a number of factors, but if the level gets too high it can cause unconsciousness or even death.*

dilate slightly, and blood pressure decreases somewhat. The production of gastric secretions increases, and the appetite is stimulated. Urine output is also markedly stimulated, though alcohol will not damage the kidneys.

It is believed that alcohol first affects the parts of the brain that control "learned behavior." This is what causes people to talk more freely, become more aggressive, and so on when intoxicated. Higher levels of alcohol in the blood depress brain activity further, to the point that memory and muscular coordination and balance are affected. Higher blood alcohol levels produce a state of lessened control in which judgment and sensory perceptions are impaired or dulled. If steady heavy drinking continues, the alcohol can anesthetize certain parts of the brain, causing coma or death.[1]

Thus, it is the level of alcohol in the bloodstream that determines intoxication and drunkenness. The rapidity with which alcohol enters the bloodstream and affects the brain depends on several factors:

- *How fast one drinks.* The half ounce of alcohol in an average mixed drink, a can of beer, or a glass of wine can be burned up (oxidized) by the body in about one hour. If you sip your drink slowly and do not have more than one drink an hour, the alcohol will not have a chance to build up in your blood, and you will feel little effect. Gulping your drink, on the other hand, produces immediate intoxicating effects and depression of various brain centers.
- *Whether your stomach is empty or full.* Eating, especially before you drink, will slow down the absorption rate of alcohol into your bloodstream and you will have a less marked response to it.
- *What you drink.* Wine and beer are absorbed less rapidly than hard liquors because they contain small amounts of nonalcoholic substances that slow down the absorption process. These substances are removed from hard liquor in the distillation process. Diluting liquor with most other liquids, such as water, also helps slow down the absorption rate, but mixing liquor with carbonated beverages can increase the rate of absorption.
- *How much you weigh.* Any given amount of alcohol has a greater effect on a 120-pound person than on a 180-pound person. Because of additional body weight, the heavier person will experience smaller blood-alcohol concentrations. See Figure 13.3.
- *What sex you are.* Research has shown that women get drunk more easily than men. Studies have found that even when a woman and man are matched in terms of weight, food intake, and so forth, the woman reaches a higher blood-alcohol level and a state of drunkenness faster than the man. The effects of alcohol have also been found to vary at different stages in the menstrual cycle.

HARMFUL EFFECTS OF ALCOHOL

All substances that exert an effect on the brain are potentially dangerous. Heavy use of alcohol can cause irreversible damage to one's health; however, responsible prolonged use of alcohol has been widely practiced throughout history without negative effects or consequences.

There is no evidence that moderate use of alcohol is harmful. In fact, statistics indicate that moderate drinkers live longer than those

[1] Recent studies have evolved a theory that alcohol affects the reticular formation of the brain, the major regulatory structure of behavior and perceptions. (See National Institute of Mental Health, Public Information Branch, *Alcohol and Alcoholism,* Washington, D.C.: U.S. Government Printing Office, 1967.

Drinks (1 ounce of liquor or a can of beer)	Body weight in pounds								Influenced
	100	120	140	160	180	200	220	240	
	% Blood alcohol								
1	.04%	.03%	.03%	.02%	.02%	.02%	.02%	.02%	
2	.08	.06	.05	.05	.04	.04	.03	.03	rarely
3	.11	.09	.08	.07	.06	.06	.05	.05	
4	.15	.12	.11	.09	.08	.08	.07	.06	
5	.19	.16	.13	.12	.11	.09	.09	.08	possibly
6	.23	.19	.16	.14	.13	.11	.10	.09	
7	.26	.22	.19	.16	.15	.13	.12	.11	
8	.30	.25	.21	.19	.17	.15	.14	.13	definitely
9	.34	.28	.24	.21	.19	.17	.15	.14	
10	.38	.31	.27	.23	.21	.19	.17	.16	

Laboratory studies show that intoxicating effects of alcohol will begin to impair simulated driving tasks when blood alcohol levels are about 50mg/100ml (expressed in the above chart as 0.05 percent). Most people reach this level when 2–3 one-ounce drinks or 3–4 beers are consumed within a 40-minute period. To determine the effect of time on blood-alcohol levels subtract 0.01 percent for each 40 minutes of drinking. For example, a 180-pound man who takes eight drinks in four hours will probably reach a level of 0.11 percent (0.17 percent of the above chart less 0.06 percent for the six 40-minute time periods).

FIGURE 13.3 *A quick guide to one's ability to "hold his liquor." Source: Adapted from Julian A. Waller, MD, "Guide for the identification, evaluation, and regulation of persons with medical handicaps to driving," The American Association of Motor Vehicle Administrators, 1967.*

who do not drink at all.[2] A lower rate of heart attacks has been found among moderate drinkers than among abstainers, ex-drinkers, or heavy drinkers.

Most of the people in the United States who choose to drink do so without harm to themselves or others. Whether alcohol usage is responsible or dangerous depends on many variables, most of which are as yet unknown. Moderate drinking is defined as consumption of not more than two mixed drinks, four glasses of beer, or half a bottle of wine a day. Habitual consumption of more than these amounts is considered heavy drinking.

Excess intake of alcohol can produce a fairly immediate result in the form of a hangover. The long-range physical effects of alcohol in excess amounts can include cirrhosis of the liver, oral cancer, and brain damage.

[2] U.S., Department of Health, Education and Welfare, *Second Special Report to the Congress on Alcohol and Health,* Washington, D.C.: U.S. Government Printing Office.

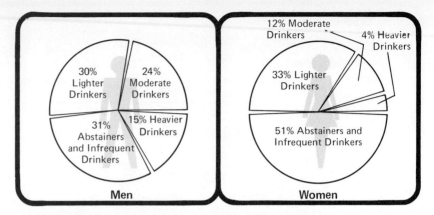

FIGURE 13.4 *Percentage of types of drinkers by sex (USA). Source: U.S. Department of Health, Education and Welfare,* Second Special Report to the Congress on Alcohol and Health, *p. 13.*

Hangover   A hangover is the body's reaction to irresponsible drinking, such as consuming too much alcohol at any time or drinking when tired, hungry, or under stress. The chemistry of hangovers is not entirely understood, but it is known to be related to the chemicals other than alcohol in the liquor. Therefore, a hangover from bourbon or wine may be worse than one from vodka, which is almost pure alcohol.

The symptoms of a hangover include nausea, dry mouth, gastritis (inflammation of the stomach lining), diarrhea, chills or sweating, headache, anxiety and shakiness, and extreme fatigue. There is no scientific evidence to support the curative claims for coffee, raw eggs, oysters, steak sauce, vitamins, etc. The most efficient treatment is rest, aspirin, light nourishment, and plenty of water.

Liver Damage   The connection between alcohol abuse and liver damage, including eventual cirrhosis of the liver, is well known. Cirrhosis can be defined as a contraction and hardening of the liver. It occurs eight times more frequently in alcoholics than in nondrinkers.

Although researchers are not yet certain of the exact causes of this type of liver damage, they believe it is related to the combination of the toxic effects of alcohol and a nutritionally poor diet (as alcoholics drink more, they eat less). Alcohol plays a major role in producing fat deposits in the liver. Alcoholic hepatitis is another common result. Both of these effects cause the sclerosis (hardening) that precedes alcoholic cirrhosis.

Excessive alcohol ingestion affects all parts of the liver's functioning and associated systems, and it can also damage other tissues, such as the stomach lining.

Oral Cancer   It has been shown that a heavy drinker faces approximately the same risk of developing cancer of the mouth and throat as a person who smokes more than two packs of cigarettes a day. If the individual is both a heavy drinker and a heavy smoker, the risk he faces is fifteen times greater than that of a nondrinker and nonsmoker.

Effects on the Brain   Scientists have demonstrated that degeneration of the brain can accompany heavy alcohol consumption. Heavy drinking over many years can produce serious nervous or mental disorders.

The chronic alcoholic is both psychologically and physiologically addicted to alcohol. When alcohol intake ceases, withdrawal symptoms occur. These include delirium tremens (the D.T.s), characterized by hallucinations and uncontrollable shaking, and other physical reactions.

SOCIAL AND PSYCHOLOGICAL IMPLICATIONS

Some of the more destructive effects of excessive drinking are auto accidents, unhappy marriages, broken homes (from divorce and desertion), lost jobs and impoverished families, and deprived or displaced children. Drinking as a social crutch and auto accidents caused by drunkenness are two problems of concern especially to teenagers or college students.

Drinking To Relate   Using alcohol as a means of relating to others in some way has special significance to young people. Drinking seems to provide an instant and easy way of relating to others in a "seemingly real, close, and positive way." It is also used to increase sexual feelings by relaxing inhibitions or hiding fears. Many people find that alcohol can help them relax, feel less inhibited, respond more freely, and feel more sexual.

The problem is that these results are usually only temporary. Alcohol is not a cure for inadequate or inhibited feelings, but only an escape from them. The individual is not learning to deal with these responses or to overcome them—he is only hiding them. Alcohol may thus become a crutch necessary to face any social situation.

A person who uses alcohol to alleviate feelings of sexual inadequacy is compounding his problems. Since alcohol is a sedative, it tends to depress bodily functions. A woman may therefore not respond fully in sexual experiences and be unable to achieve orgasm.

A recent study by the National Institute of Alcohol Abuse and Alcoholism (NIAAA) shows teenage drinking is reaching epidemic proportions.

The study disclosed:

· There are now about 1–3 million teenage males and females nationwide who drink daily or on weekends.
· Of these, about 700,000 ranging in age from 12 to 17, have serious drinking problems, with more than half considered alcoholics.
· Sixty percent of those killed in driving accidents involving drinking throughout the country in the past few years were teenagers, according to the National Highway Traffic Safety Administration (NHTSA).

As mentioned in Chapter 10, excessive drinking can lead to functional impotence. The male drinks because he is afraid he will be inadequate, but the alcohol makes him inadequate. A vicious cycle of drinking in sexual situations to overcome fears or inadequacy can be established quickly.

Auto Accidents   Tests have shown that the impairment of the ability to drive safely begins with the first drink and progresses steadily with continued

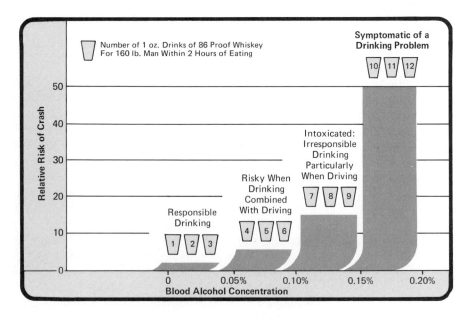

FIGURE 13.5 *Drinking and highway safety.*

drinking. Figure 13.5 shows the relative risk of crashing with each additional drink. Unfortunately, as one drinks more, there is also less awareness of the increasing loss of faculties and judgment. The drinker may be unaware of his condition and feel that he is capable of driving; in addition, he may become belligerent and insist on driving. Not only is he endangering his own life—his car makes the highway unsafe for others.

Statistics have shown the drinking driver to be a factor in 50 to 60 percent of all automobile fatalities. The drinking pedestrian is a factor in the same percentage of adult pedestrian fatalities. Of these drinking drivers and pedestrians, approximately half are alcoholics and half are "merely social drinkers."

Of importance especially to young people is the recent finding by the Insurance Institute for Highway Safety that state laws reducing the legal drinking age to eighteen represent a "social policy that carries a price in increased fatal motor vehicle collisions."

The Institute compared figures for drivers under twenty-one in Michigan, Ontario, and Wisconsin—where the drinking age was recently dropped from twenty-one to eighteen—with those for young drivers in Indiana, Illinois, and Minnesota, where the age is twenty-one. Data indicated that in the first year after the legal drinking age was lowered, fifteen- to twenty-year-olds were involved in 2.6 to 3.3 more fatal crashes than would have been expected.

THE NEED FOR CONTROL

Many individuals use alcohol without abusing it. In the United States, nine out of ten adults who drink do so without evident damage to themselves or society. They have established sensible patterns in their use of alcohol:

- They drink at appropriate times and under appropriate conditions.
- They limit their intake.
- They look upon moderate drinking as a pleasant means of relaxing, adding to the enjoyment of meals, as a long-accepted part of family or religious ceremonies, and even as an aid to their health —but they avoid intoxication or drunkenness.

Yet the other one person out of every ten is a problem drinker. He faces the probability of severe harm to himself and others because of this dependency.

There is no commonly accepted definition of alcoholism. Some people believe that even an individual who has two or three drinks every day is an alcoholic. Most authorities agree on some variation of

---

Production Loss Tops 89 Billion

The cost of alcohol abuse and alcoholism to the occupational sector can be gauged in part by an estimate cited in the *Second Special Report to the U. S. Congress on Alcohol and Health from the Secretary of Health, Education, and Welfare.* The report estimated that the production loss by male workers alone as a result of alcohol problems totaled $9.35 billion a year.

Source: National Clearinghouse for Alcohol Information of the National Institute on Alcohol Abuse and Alcoholism, December 23, 1974.

---

the view that a person is an alcoholic if his drinking interferes with his functioning in society or affects his health. Some experts differentiate between a "heavy drinker," a "problem drinker," and an alcoholic. The heavy and problem drinkers are psychologically dependent on liquor to varying degrees, and the alcoholic is the individual who is both psychologically and physiologically dependent. However, the lines between the three categories are not distinct.

Alcohol Education

Andrew Weil discusses the use and abuse of alcohol in his book *The Natural Mind.* He believes that "the Americans who get into trouble with alcohol are those who begin to use it without ritualistic rules and forms; uncontained by ritual, their drug use becomes unstable and begins to disrupt their lives."[3]

Just as we educate people in the principles of driving before we let them loose on the highway, we should educate them in the healthy uses (or rituals) of alcohol before allowing them to drink. The idea of educating individuals to drink moderately and safely is not new; it is inherent in the habits and attitudes of those cultural groups and people who have demonstrated over centuries an ability to use alcohol with a minimum of harm. Yet, with the increasing problem of alcoholism in the United States, a more comprehensive program of education is needed.

The time to begin such education is as early in childhood as possible, especially in view of rising teenage alcoholism. Studies have indicated that the lowest incidence of alcoholism occurs in groups where the children are exposed to alcohol and sensible drinking practices early in life.[4] Among the most important principles that should be expressed in any form of alcohol education are these:

[3] Andrew Weil, *The Natural Mind,* Boston: Houghton Mifflin, 1972, p. 108.
[4] *Alcohol and Alcoholism,* p. 28.

> ## 450,000 Child Drunks
>
> DETROIT—An estimated 450,000 American children are drunks, according to an expert on alcoholism, and many are taught by their parents.
>
>   "It is sad but true that we live in a drinking society and that drinking often is taught as a social grace to children," said John Melner, executive director for the Detroit area of the National Council on Alcohol.

- *It is not essential to drink.* Abstinence should be socially acceptable. Any individual—youth or adult—who decides to abstain from alcohol for moral, medical, economic, religious, or other reasons should not be pressured to drink by other members of the society. If any such pressuring does occur, the individual should feel no need to give in to it.
- *Excessive drinking does not indicate adult behavior or virility.* In an adult society, a man can no more establish his masculinity nor a woman her sophistication by an ability to drink large amounts of alcohol than with an ability to drink large amounts of milk. Intoxication should not be socially acceptable. Excessive drinking indicates a lack of maturity or a poor self-concept.
- *Safe drinking depends on specific physiological and psychological boundaries.* An educated person can drink moderately and safely, avoiding dangerous blood-alcohol levels. He further realizes that drinking is not the answer to emotional problems—rather, it can be the cause of new problems.

Alcohol education should not mean, nor be restricted to, "alcoholism education" for those already facing such a problem. Instead, it should be considered part of any instruction on the use of potentially dangerous drugs and should be included in all such health education programs.

Seeking Help   Our society has long preserved many wrong ideas and attitudes about problem drinking and alcoholism, labeling these as moral weaknesses to be hidden or endured in silence. Fortunately, alcoholism is now recognized by most people as a disease or form of sickness, so that the alcoholic is seen to need and deserve help. Assistance programs are now available in most communities for the troubled drinker.

In 1935, two alcoholic men discovered that although each had been unable to maintain sobriety alone, they were able to achieve it together by helping each other. This led them to a desire to help other alcoholics who wanted to stop drinking. This was the origin of Alcoholics Anonymous, a world wide self-help organization that has helped many thousands of alcoholic persons to recover.

A.A. charges no dues or fees, keeps no lists, and gives out no membership cards. It works totally on a person-to-person level. It presents a program for sober living in the form of twelve suggested steps. Regular attendance at meetings helps members maintain motivation, identify with other sober alcoholics, form new interpersonal relationships, and help one another. Members are prepared to help other alcoholics who are in need at any time of the day or night.

A.A. is listed in almost all telephone directories. If there is no such listing in your phone book, the national office of A.A. will provide the information you need. Write: Secretary, Alcoholics Anonymous, P.O. Box 459, Grand Central Station, New York, N.Y. 10017 (Telephone: 212–686–1100).

Many other organizations exist to help treat alcoholism, to provide education on alcohol-related problems, or to perform research. Following is a partial list; the Appendix contains a fuller list of alcoholism treatment resources.

· **Al-Anon.** This organization, which works very closely with AA, is composed of the wives, husbands, and other relatives of alcoholics. They meet regularly to discuss problems related to alcoholism and to try to find better ways to help their family members to recover. The basic purpose of Al-Anon is to give people support and strength in facing and overcoming the problem in their own families. To find the nearest Al-Anon group near you, write or phone the AA national office listed above.

· **Al-Ateens.** This is another voluntary group similar to but separate from Al-Anon. The children of alcoholics belong to this group and meet regularly to learn about the disease, how to cope with its damaging manifestations in their own lives, and to discuss ways to help their parents. For further information, write or phone the AA national office listed above.

· **National Institute on Alcohol Abuse and Alcoholism (NIAAA).** Established in 1970 as a part of the National Institute of Mental Health, the NIAAA serves as a focal point for all public health services in the field of alcoholism. It includes four divisions: Prevention, State and Community Assistance Programs, Special Treatment and Rehabilitation Programs, and Research. For further information, write to:

  National Institute on Alcohol Abuse and Alcoholism,
  5600 Fishers Lane
  Rockville, Md 20852

· **National Council on Alcoholism (NCA).** This is the only voluntary health organization devoted to alcoholism. The NCA publishes many articles, pamphlets, and books on alcoholism, which may be obtained either free or for a small charge from any of the 160 affiliated councils across the country. These local affiliated Councils on Alcoholism are also referral centers and are often particularly useful for patients who initially resist the idea of attending AA meetings or even talking with an AA member. Trained consultants are available for your patients. There is no fee involved. There is absolute confidentiality between patient and consultant and sessions are on a one-to-one basis. For many people this helps to remove the first stumbling block to recovery. The NCA also has research grants, predoctoral and postdoctoral fellowships, and supplementary grants available for biomedical research in alcoholism.

- **North American Association of Alcoholism Programs (NAAAP).** This organization is composed of directors or administrators of government-supported alcoholism programs for treatment, education and research. Both individuals and agencies hold membership. For further information on seminars, meetings, and other activities of this group, write:

  North American Association of Alcoholism Programs
  1130 17th Street N. W.
  Washington, D. C. 20036

- **Rutgers Center of Alcohol Studies.** Rutgers has one of the best known schools for alcoholism studies. The school is both a research center and a place where health professionals can take technical courses on the treatment and control of alcoholism during a summer school session. The Rutgers school also publishes technical information on alcoholism, especially directed to the health professional. A catalogue of their publications and an announcement of their courses may be obtained by writing to:

  Center of Alcohol Studies
  Rutgers University
  New Brunswick, N. J. 08903

- **Utah School of Alcohol Studies.** The University of Utah also has an excellent school of alcohol studies, which provides training not only for health professionals but for community leaders as well. For further information, write:

  Director
  University of Utah School of Alcohol Studies,
  Salt Lake City, Utah 84112

- **State Commissions on Alcoholism.** Many, but not all, states have an agency dealing with alcoholism and related problems. In some states, this may be a part of the State Department of Health or Welfare, or—as in New York State—the Department of Mental Health. In others, the agency may be an independent one established by the governor or the legislature. There are two fast ways of locating such a state-wide agency: one is through the state government's telephone information service in the capital city. Probably faster, however, is by phoning your nearest affiliated NCA council—often listed under Alcoholism Information and Referral Center.

Helping Others   The person close to someone who drinks too much also suffers a great deal. Problem drinkers can hurt their families, friends, fellow workers, employers, and others around them. Many of the programs listed above (especially Al-Anon and Al-Ateens) can help the person involved with an alcoholic to learn to deal with the drinker and with his own problems and feelings that stem from such a relationship.

Usually, unless the alcoholic himself has a sincere desire to overcome his problem and is willing to seek treatment, the concerned individual will not be able to do much for him. However, there are things he can do to alleviate the burdens. With compassion, patience, and understanding, someone close to a problem drinker can play a key role in his desire to seek treatment and his eventual recovery. Three stages of help can be to:

- Learn about the illness and become familiar with sources of treatment
- Guide the problem drinker to help when he is ready to seek it
- Support the person during and after treatment

The National Clearinghouse for Alcohol Information has suggested some steps to follow (and others to avoid) while waiting for the "right time" to suggest or find treatment for the alcoholic.

Do:
- try to remain calm, unemotional and factually honest in speaking with the problem drinker about his behavior and its day-to-day consequences
- Let the problem drinker know that you are reading and learning about alcoholism, attending Al-Anon or Alateen, and the like
- Discuss the situation with someone you trust—a clergyman, social worker, a friend, or some individual who has experienced alcoholism either personally or as a family member
- Establish and maintain a healthy atmosphere in the home, and try to include the alcoholic member in family life
- Explain the nature of alcoholism as an illness to the children in the family
- Encourage new interests and participate in leisure-time activities that the problem drinker enjoys. Encourage him or her to see old friends
- Be patient and live one day at a time. Alcoholism generally takes a long time to develop, and recovery does not occur overnight. Try to accept setbacks and relapses with calm and understanding
- Refuse to ride with the alcoholic person if he insists on drinking and driving.[5]

Do not:
- attempt to punish, threaten, bribe, preach, or try to be a martyr. Avoid emotional appeals which may only increase feelings of guilt and the compulsion to drink
- Allow yourself to cover-up or make excuses for the alcoholic person or shield him from the realistic consequences of his behavior
- Take over his responsibilities, leaving him with no sense of importance or dignity

[5] National Clearinghouse for Alcohol Information, "Someone Close," Box 2345, Rockville, Maryland 20852.

- Hide or dump bottles, or shelter the problem drinker from situations where alcohol is present
- Argue with the alcoholic person when he is drunk
- Try to drink along with the problem drinker
- Above all, do not accept guilt for another's behavior.[6]

FURTHER READINGS

Cooperative Commission on the Study of Alcoholism *Alcohol Problems.* New York: Oxford University Press, 1967.

This report deals with the history of alcohol use and of alcohol drinking in America. It discusses means of preventing problem drinking, reviews recent advances in research and personnel training, and describes treatment services available. It also outlines plans for a coordinated approach to alcohol problems on a national level.

Goshen, Charles E. *Drinks, Drugs and Do-gooders.* New York: Free Press, 1973.

The author takes a look at the entire emotional debate concerning drug use, and how the nation has reacted to laws attempting to curb "pleasure seeking" through chemical means in the past.

Kessel, Neil and Walton, Henry. *Alcoholism.* Baltimore, Md.: Penguin Books, 1965.

This book begins by considering what distinguishes the excessive from the social drinker, what alcoholics are like, and what their chances are of recovery.

[6] Ibid.

Chapter 14

The Mood Modifiers

THE DRUG CRISIS

The 1937 edition of the *United States Dispensatory* (the standard American reference book on drugs) contained some 3,090 entries. Thirty years later 2,470 of these preparations were no longer listed because they had been proven ineffective; new drugs had brought the total to 1,508. These figures symbolize the pharmacological revolution which brought the science of drugs from a position of a rather humble collaborator with medicine to a position as its most intimate associate.

Today the "drug problem" stems from the sheer multiplicity of drugs, their availability, and their acceptance by society. For example, there are some forty-four different antibiotics now being sold in the United States, including fifteen varieties of penicillin alone. Between 800 and 900 different drugs are used fairly extensively nationwide, and new ones appear at the rate of about thirty to forty each year. Some of the older drugs disappear as more effective ones take their place. Generally, the newer drugs are more powerful and much more effective than those used in the past. However, they have many more side effects, and must be used with greater caution.

Prescription Drugs Can Be Deadly   Since the first studies were undertaken more than a dozen years ago, the estimated number of deaths due to adverse drug reactions has been continually rising. These are deaths due to legal drugs, legally obtained—mostly by prescription—and used only for bona fide medical reasons.

Some of the major complications of prescription drugs can be attributed to: doctors prescribing a dangerous drug when a safer one is available; using the wrong drug or using the right drug in the wrong way; using a drug of no known therapeutic value, or any number of other mistakes (i.e., wrong drug, wrong dosage, wrong method of administration, wrong patient, or failure to give the prescribed drug).

Studies of prescription patterns as long ago as twenty years show that doctors prescribed for everything including the common cold, for which there is no cure. Thus, it is important first of all to use prescription drugs exactly as the doctor directs. An overdose or underdose, or failure to take the medicine at the proper intervals can lessen its effectiveness in restoring a person to good health; it can also be dangerous. Secondly, one should always tell his doctor if he is taking other drugs. The potential for dangerous drug interactions is always present. Finally, one always should ask a doctor what he is prescribing. Remember, you are paying for this service and you have a right to know exactly what is being done.

It is important to remember that a physician writes a prescription for a definite purpose in the treatment of a specific person. It follows that when a prescription is no longer of use to the patient for whom it was prescribed, it should be discarded. This is true for several reasons: (1) the active ingredients may lose their therapeutic value; (2) any new condition, even if it appears to be similar, may require a different medication; and (3) keeping old drugs beyond their period of usefulness creates the possibility for accidents and poisoning through misuse by children.

Over-the-Counter Drugs

Although over-the-counter drugs are not as likely to be fatal as those dispensed by prescription, any drug can be dangerous if it is not used properly. Even aspirin or products such as stomach aids may cause problems when taken in combination with other drugs.

Some of these nonprescription drugs have been used in excess for "turning on." Other medicines such as certain cough syrups and stay-awake and go-to-sleep preparations which are sold without prescription may cause psychological dependence. Many of these contain ingredients designed to relieve pain; unfortunately, very often these drugs only mask more serious symptoms of illness, delaying proper medical diagnosis.

Aspirin—A Dangerous Drug?

Aspirin was introduced in powder form in Germany before the turn of the century, and the tablet form came into use in the United States in 1915. In this country alone, about 15,000 tons of aspirin are produced (and presumably consumed) each year.

Because the incidence of serious adverse reactions to aspirin is low, it must rank as one of the safest of drugs; however, it may be responsible for gastrointestinal hemorrhage or bronchial asthma in susceptible individuals. More serious is the fact that aspirin poisoning is one of the leading drug killers of young children.

Beware the Message

Another way in which nonprescription medicines and drugs contribute to the drug abuse problem is by the implication of their advertising. When children and adolescents repeatedly see and hear that they should take substances for minor physical and emotional difficulties, they become conditioned to believe in the concept that a pill a day will keep the doctor away. Perhaps this message is part of the reason so many people turn to what are called the "mood modifying" drugs. The widespread use of tobacco and alcohol was discussed in the last two chapters, so here the discussion will concentrate on other drugs. Marijuana, hallucinogens, stimulants, barbiturates, and narcotics—these are the most commonly used (and misunderstood) drugs today.

MARIJUANA

Marijuana is used by many groups in our society, from high school kids to middle-aged businessmen, and it is probably associated with more controversy or misinformation than any other drug. Although it has frequently been considered an hallucinogen, it is actually in a class by itself. It may share some characteristics with the other classes of drugs, but pharmacologically it really is none of these. What we do know is that marijuana is an active intoxicant.

Marijuana is a combination of the crushed leaves, flowering tops, and sometimes stems of the hemp plant, *cannabis sativa.* (The term "marijuana" comes from a Mexican or Spanish word meaning "intoxicant.") The flowering tops of the female plant (which is usually more bushy) secrete a sticky resin, tetrahydrocannabinol (THC), that is the major psychoactive (mind-affecting) ingredient of the plant. The THC content of various parts of the plant varies; the small stems and leaves contain the greatest concentration, with the roots, larger stems, and seeds containing very little. The percentage of THC in a plant varies according to conditions of growth, harvesting, and curing, as well as climate. Marijuana grows wild in many countries, including the United States, but the plants in this country are very low in psychoactive material. (See Table 14.2.)

Hashish is the crude resin of the plant, which is usually collected by scraping the leaves. As it is this resin that contains the

TABLE 14.1   CONTROLLED SUBSTANCES: USES AND EFFECTS

	Drugs	Schedule*	Often Prescribed Brand Names	Medical Uses	Dependence Potential: Physical
Narcotics	Opium	II	Dover's Powder, Paregoric	Analgesic, antidiarrheal	High
	Morphine	II	Morphine	Analgesic	High
	Codeine	II III V	Codeine	Analgesic, antitussive	Moderate
	Heroin	I	None	None	High
	Meperidine (Pethidine)	II	Demerol, Pethadol	Analgesic	High
	Methadone	II	Dolophine, Methadone, Methadose	Analgesic, heroin substitute	High
	Other Narcotics	I II III V	Dilaudid, Leritine, Numorphan, Percodan	Analgesic, antidiarrheal, antitussive	High
Depressants	Chloral Hydrate	IV	Noctec, Somnos	Hypnotic	Moderate
	Barbiturates	II III IV	Amytal, Butisol, Nembutal, Phenobarbital, Seconal, Tuinal	Anesthetic, anti-convulsant, sedation, sleep	High
	Glutethimide	III	Doriden	Sedation, sleep	High
	Methaqualone	II	Optimil, Parest, Quaalude, Somnafac, Sopor	Sedation, sleep	High
	Tranquilizers	IV	Equanil, Librium, Miltown Serax, Tranxene, Valium	Anti-anxiety, muscle relaxant, sedation	Moderate
	Other Depressants	III IV	Clonopin, Dalmane, Dormate, Noludar, Placydil, Valmid	Anti-anxiety, sedation, sleep	Possible
Stimulants	Cocaine†	II	Cocaine	Local anesthetic	Possible
	Amphetamines	II III	Benzedrine, Biphetamine, Desoxyn, Dexedrine	Hyperkinesis, narco-lepsy, weight control	Possible
	Phenmetrazine	II	Preludin	Weight control	Possible
	Methylphenidate	II	Ritalin	Hyperkinesis	Possible
	Other Stimulants	III IV	Bacarate, Cylert, Didrex, Ionamin, Plegine, Pondimin, Pre-Sate, Sanorex, Voranil	Weight control	Possible
Hallucinogens	LSD	I	None	None	None
	Mescaline	I	None	None	None
	Psilocybin-Psilocyn	I	None	None	None
	MDA	I	None	None	None
	PCP‡	III	Sernylan	Veterinary anesthetic	None
	Other Hallucinogens	I	None	None	None
Cannabis	Marihuana Hashish Hashish Oil	I	None	None Potential use in prevention of glaucoma	Degree unknown

*Scheduling classifications vary for individual drugs since controlled substances are often marketed in combination with other medicinal ingredients.
†Designated a narcotic under the Controlled Substances Act.
‡Designated a depressant under the Controlled Substances Act.

Dependence Potential: Psychological	Tolerance	Duration of Effects (in hours)	Usual Methods of Administration	Possible Effects	Effects of Overdose	Withdrawal Syndrome
High	Yes	3 to 6	Oral, smoked			
High	Yes	3 to 6	Injected, smoked	Euphoria, drowsiness, respiratory depression, constricted pupils, nausea	Slow and shallow breathing, clammy skin, convulsions, coma, possible death	Watery eyes, runny nose, yawning, loss of appetite, irritability, tremors, panic, chills and sweating, cramps, nausea
Moderate	Yes	3 to 6	Oral, injected			
High	Yes	3 to 6	Injected, sniffed			
High	Yes	3 to 6	Oral, injected			
High	Yes	12 to 24	Oral, injected			
High	Yes	3 to 6	Oral, injected			
Moderate	Probable	5 to 8	Oral			
High	Yes	1 to 16	Oral, injected	Slurred speech, disorientation, drunken behavior without odor of alcohol	Shallow respiration, cold and clammy skin, dilated pupils, weak and rapid pulse, coma, possible death	Anxiety, insomnia, tremors, delirium, convulsions, possible death
High	Yes	4 to 8	Oral			
High	Yes	4 to 8	Oral			
Moderate	Yes	4 to 8	Oral			
Possible	Yes	4 to 8	Oral			
High	Yes	2	Injected, sniffed	Increased alertness, excitation, euphoria, dilated pupils, increased pulse rate and blood pressure, insomnia, loss of appetite	Agitation, increase in body temperature, hallucinations, convulsions, possible death	Apathy, long periods of sleep, irritability, depression, disorientation
High	Yes	2 to 4	Oral, injected			
High	Yes	2 to 4	Oral			
High	Yes	2 to 4	Oral			
Possible	Yes	2 to 4	Oral			
Degree unknown	Yes	Variable	Oral	Illusions and hallucinations (with exception of MDA); poor perception of time and distance	Longer, more intense "trip" episodes, psychosis, possible death	Withdrawal syndrome not reported
Degree unknown	Yes	Variable	Oral, injected			
Degree unknown	Yes	Variable	Oral			
Degree unknown	Yes	Variable	Oral, injected, sniffed			
Degree unknown	Yes	Variable	Oral, injected, smoked			
Degree unknown	Yes	Variable	Oral, injected, sniffed			
Moderate	Yes	2 to 4	Oral, smoked	Euphoria, relaxed inhibitions, increased appetite, disoriented behavior	Fatigue, paranoia, possible psychosis	Insomnia, hyperactivity, and decreased appetite reported in a limited number of individuals

Source: Drug Enforcement Administration, U.S. Department of Justice.

Table 14.2 *Varieties of Cannabis*

Potency	How Prepared and Consumed
MILD: MARIJUANA (European and American name) DAGGA (South Africa) KIF (North Africa) BHANG (Indian name, usually involves only leaves, is drunk and is usually somewhat richer in THC than American marijuana)	The leaves and sometimes the stems and even seeds or entire plants are ground up and smoked or baked into cookies. The potency varies with THC content.
INTERMEDIATE: GANJA (India)	Leaves close to the flowering tops of well-cultivated plants are harvested. Smoked, drunk, or baked into sweets. Not used outside India.
HIGH: CHARAS (India) HASHISH	The resin which contains almost all the THC in the plant is scraped from the leaves near the flowering tops, pressed into blocks, and usually smoked.

THC, hashish can be up to ten times more potent than marijuana. Hash oil can be extracted from the hashish. Its potency varies with the sophistication of the procedures used for extraction, but it is about two to three times as strong as crude hashish, and twenty to thirty times more powerful than the common grade of marijuana.

Effects   The effects of marijuana or hash depend on the personality and tolerance of each individual, the amount, how it is used (smoked or eaten), quality of the drug, and the circumstances or "setting" in which it is used. Marijuana may induce either stimulation or depression. THC is often considered an hallucinogen with some sedative properties.

Marijuana usually induces a feeling of relaxation or introspection. When introduced into the system it stimulates various brain centers, so that perception of sights, especially colors and sounds may be enhanced. High concentrations of THC in hash sometimes produce hallucinations, but these never occur with marijuana or lower concentrations. The sense of time may be altered or expanded, so that ten minutes seems like half an hour. There may be other pleasant sensations and changes in the senses of touch and taste.

A person who is high on marijuana can usually return to his normal state if desired—a reversal of effect that is not possible with alcohol. Any aftereffects are mild; there is no hangover. Marijuana is nonaddictive, and there is no evidence that its use leads to harder

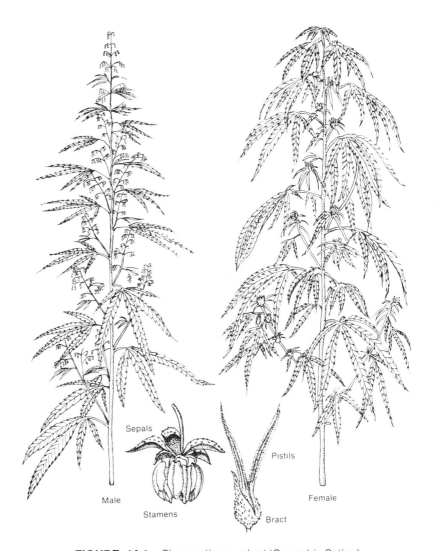

Male

Sepals

Stamens

Pistils

Bract

Female

FIGURE 14.1 *The marijuana plant* (Cannabis Sativa).

drugs.[1] Furthermore, there has been no research that has shown that it causes either genetic or chromosomal damage.

The user's tolerance to marijuana does not increase, so greater amounts do not become necessary to produce the same stimulating effects. In fact, research has found that tolerance actually diminishes. This is apparently because THC remains in the body for a long time

[1] Norman E. Zinberg, "The War Over Marijuana," *Psychology Today,* December, 1976.

(about 48 hours) and is available to enhance the effects when marijuana is next used.

Marijuana and Sexuality

Two studies regarding the influence of marijuana use on sexual performance or sexuality have recently come up with some interesting results.

A study conducted by the Reproductive Biology Research Foundation indicates that marijuana may cause temporary sterility in males. Researchers found that 35 percent of the marijuana users surveyed had reduced sperm counts; however, this effect seemed to be reversible. When the men stopped using marijuana, the sperm counts gradually returned to normal.

An additional finding was that the male marijuana smokers had testosterone (the male hormone) levels 44 percent lower than nonsmokers. This could possibly cause temporary impotence. Again, the effect was reversible—the testosterone levels returned to normal when marijuana use was discontinued. This finding could be related to the claim by other experts that males who are habitual marijuana users experience some growth of their breasts. This idea is the center of much controversy, but would seem to be connected with changing hormone levels.

A British report entitled *The Cannabis Experience: An Interpretive Study of the Effects of Marijuana and Hashish* concluded that cannabis has significant aphrodisiac properties. This claim was based on study of cannabis as a stimulus to sensory perceptions and other experiences. The vast majority of men and women surveyed made statements such as: "Sex is much nicer when you're high," "It always seems to go on longer," "Everything about it is improved," and "To turn on and go to bed with a member of the opposite sex is an incredible experience."

This conclusion—that cannabis is an aphrodisiac—is controversial. One also has to consider the environment or setting and personalities involved in the influence of marijuana on sex. If one is in a situation where sex is anticipated while smoking marijuana, the results are often positive, but to label marijuana as a sexual stimulant is probably misleading. Thus far, most evidence suggests that it does nothing more than lower sexual inhibitions, thereby increasing sexual pleasure.

Marijuana and Motivation

Some studies link marijuana use with loss of motivation and reduction in capacity to think straight. Norman E. Zinberg, one of the country's foremost authorities on the use and effects of marijuana, has concluded that these studies are totally unfounded. He cites a very important Jamaica study on long-term users and nonusers, revealing that ". . . no differences in motivation between users and nonusers . . ." was found.[2]

The belief that marijuana causes irreversible brain damage goes back to the 1930s, but Zinberg found no evidence to support that contention. "Lung damage due to marijuana smoking is mentioned now and again, but this particular fear, which is probably realistic, has been partially negated by the fact that marijuana, unlike nicotine, causes vasodilatation (enlargement) and expansion of lung bronchioles."[3]

Dr. Zinberg does suggest some caution. He states:

> Obviously there are areas of concern. Drawing any hot substance into the lungs cannot be good for anyone, but we should remember that no marijuana smoker in this country uses as many cigarettes a day as tobacco smokers do. Also, marijuana is an intoxicant; and despite the research showing that someone high on marijuana does better on a driving simulator than someone high on alcohol, driving under the influence of any intoxicant must be considered a real danger. Finally, it is my absolute conviction that adolescents below the age of 18 should not use intoxicants of any kind, whether nicotine, alcohol, or marijuana. The 14-, 15-, or 16-year-old struggling to develop in this complex society needs as clear a head as possible. One argument made some years ago for the legalization of illicit substances was based on the possibility that parents and other authorities could more readily control above-ground use of licit substances than they could control the underground use of illicit substances.[4]

Marijuana and the Law   There is great and continuing debate over the legalization of marijuana. Many people are against decriminalizing its use until further research has been conducted, especially on the long-term effects of the drug. On the other hand, many feel that marijuana has already been shown to be far less harmful than either tobacco or alcohol. In addition, use of marijuana in our society today is so widespread it seems counterproductive to classify so much of the population as criminal.

[2] Ibid.
[3] Ibid.
[4] Ibid.

It is useful to recognize that the removal of criminal sanctions does not condone marijuana use. As in other aspects of medicine, the dictum "First do no harm" is worth remembering. Many have come to feel that the costly effects of marijuana laws on the criminal justice system far outweigh the deterrent value of these criminal penalties. The retention of a noncriminal fine (as in Oregon and California) lets everyone know that marijuana use is not being encouraged. In any event, it is essential that we separate the health issues surrounding marijuana use from the legal issues. Health research alone will not solve this social problem of drug abuse legislation. The social policy decisions must involve other issues as well.

THE HALLUCINOGENS

The hallucinogens have been variously described as psychedelic, mind-altering, consciousness-expanding, or mind-blowing. The most common of these drugs are LSD, mescaline (or peyote), STP (DOM), and psilocybin.

Lysergic Acid Diethylamide (LSD)   Almost half a century ago, a Swiss chemist, Albert Hofmann, accidentally discovered the psychoactive properties of lysergic acid diethylamide, or LSD. This is a very potent, odorless, colorless, and tasteless drug. Little research was conducted on this substance after Hofmann's discovery until the 1960s, when it became the subject of considerable controversy, first at Harvard and then throughout the country.

Effects

LSD is either a white powder, a tablet, or a clear liquid. The effects usually begin to occur within twenty to forty-five minutes after taking the drug. This latency period may vary from fifteen minutes to three hours, depending on the way it is taken and other factors. The duration of an average "trip" varies from five to twelve hours.

LSD is absorbed into the blood very quickly and is rapidly distributed throughout the body. It significantly affects the nervous system, producing both physical and psychological reactions. The physical reactions include a wide range of motor and sensory phenomena. The most common motor phenomena are increased muscular tension, tremors or twitches and jerks, and complex twisting movements. Other effects include an acceleration of the pulse rate, a rise in blood pressure, dilation of the pupils and blurring of vision, sweating and chills, and increased salivation. Some of these effects, such as the change in pulse rate, may vary according to the trip.

Perceptual changes are the most frequent and constant part of an LSD trip. Hallucinations, increased visual imagery, and illusions are common. These visions may involve colors, geometric patterns, and architectural perceptions, but they are usually more complex, centering on human faces and figures. Prolonged after-images (visual images that remain fixed on the retina) may occur. In some individuals the thought processes are accelerated; in others, they are retarded. There is usually difficulty in concentrating, and often confusion.

Some individuals may experience euphoria, but others feel extreme anxiety. Sexual feelings may be inhibited, or they may become a dominant aspect of portions of the trip. Much depends on the personality of the individual, his thoughts before taking LSD, and the environment during his trip.

A short period of tolerance may develop. If an individual takes LSD within three days of an earlier trip, he may need an increase in dosage for the same effects. But beyond this period, tolerance drops back to normal. Physical dependence does not occur, though psychological dependence may develop.

Bad Trips and Flashbacks.   For various reasons, an individual may experience a bad trip. His state of mind (set), the purity of the drug, where he is when taking the drug, and the amount of LSD can all be factors in causing a bad trip. A person feeling anxious or one who is emotionally upset is more likely to have this reaction. The experience may change from a state of euphoria to one of panic. The psychedelic reactions and hallucinations become so confused and involved that the person has trouble in removing himself from the experience. The psychological perceptions and distortions affect him more deeply.

In some cases a bad trip can cause psychotic reactions. Even if the person has been able to come out of the experience, it may become a traumatic part of his life that he can't reject or forget. If he has had trouble relating to his experiences during the trip, he may have problems integrating the perceptions of the trip afterwards.

One related result is the flashback. This is best defined as a spontaneous recurrence of some aspect of a trip, usually long after the drug itself has worn off. Flashbacks occur most often after bad trips.

There are two likely explanations of the causes of flashbacks. One is that the person has "learned" new ways of perceiving his environment, so that this learning stays with him to recur occasionally or even frequently. This explanation applies more to flashbacks that involve visual distortion. Another explanation is that the individual may find himself in a situation similar to the situation or perceptions of the trip, and this repeated occurrence may trigger a flashback. Flashbacks may also be set off by other drugs.

Research on LSD

Much of the research on LSD has centered on its chromosomal or genetic effects. Currently, it is believed that pure LSD is not damaging to chromosomes but "street" LSD is so often mixed with other substances that one cannot be certain of its effects.

Other studies have focused on the positive potential of LSD. It has been used as an experimental treatment for depression or alcoholism and in psychotherapy. It has also been used in programs involving patients with terminal cancer.

Some of the most interesting of this type of research is being conducted by Dr. Stanislav Grof at the Maryland State Psychiatric Center. He believes that LSD research conducted under carefully controlled clinical settings is important in answering some of the questions about the dimensions of human personality. He found a typical pattern in the patients he treated of gradual improvement followed by a period of rapid deterioration, and a final reawakening establishing high levels of adjustment and stability.[5]

Clearly, more research is necessary to answer the questions about the positive and negative effects of LSD and its possible value to man.

Mescaline (Peyote)   Peyote is a small cactus that grows in the southwestern United States and in Mexico. The rounded tops of the cactus (peyote buttons) may themselves be chewed for the hallucinogenic effect, but a usual reaction is violent nausea. Therefore, mescaline, the most active of the various alkaloids in the cactus, is usually extracted. It can also be created synthetically. It usually appears as a white powder.

Effects

A typical mescaline trip lasts from four to twelve hours, depending on the amount. Mescaline is chemically related to amphetamine, so it produces a stimulating effect. The most pronounced effects are on the vision, so that colors and visual images seem brighter and more profuse. This overstimulation also produces wavering outlines and

[5] Robert W. Ferguson, *Drug Abuse Control* (Boston: Holbrook Press, Inc., 1975), p. 143.

other distortions similar to those induced by LSD. The visual hallucinations caused by mescaline usually seem to follow a pattern—geometric figures, then familiar scenes and faces, and finally unfamiliar visions.[6] It is these visions that have made peyote part of various religious rituals. The Native American Church has a special governmental exemption allowing it to use peyote in religious sacraments.

The major difference between mescaline and LSD is that mescaline does not seem to provoke the rapid emotional changes often experienced with LSD. A feeling of contentment and peace is a common reaction.

Some tolerance may develop to mescaline as with LSD, but it occurs more slowly. Psychological dependence can develop, but physical dependence does not occur. Prolonged use of mescaline can cause behavioral changes; as with LSD, this is most likely in individuals with some previous disturbances or subliminal psychosis.

Psilocybin and STP   Psilocybin and STP are two other common hallucinogenic drugs. Psilocybin and psilocin are derived from the *psilocybe mexicana* mushroom, which grows mainly in Mexico. Its effects are similar to those of mescaline. Again, there is no evidence of physical dependence, but psychological dependence will develop.

STP is a derivative of mescaline. A drug developed by Dow Chemical, DOM, has the same chemical formula. The reactions to STP are similar to those of LSD. The experience may last up to twenty-four hours, depending on the dose. Flashbacks have also been reported.[7]

STIMULANTS

There are a variety of substances that act as stimulants, elevating mood, preventing fatigue, or causing short-term improvements in performance. Coffee, tea, and cigarettes are all stimulants. The major stimulating drugs that are abused in the United States are the amphetamines and cocaine.

Amphetamines   The pharmaceutical industry manufactures annually an enormous amount of amphetamines. Eight million pills are lawfully produced, packaged, and consumed each year. Most amphetamines

[6] Ibid., p. 153.
[7] Ibid., pp. 144–145.

are used by housewives, students, businessmen, physicians, truck drivers, or athletes. Students use them to prevent fatigue while studying, truck drivers use them when traveling long distances, athletes use them for a burst of energy. They are used by many people to lose weight. They are sometimes prescribed for hyperactive children (in whom they act as a depressant rather than a stimulant). These people are the majority of amphetamine users; those who inject high doses intravenously are only a tiny fraction of the total number of users or abusers.

Effects

Two of the most common forms of amphetamines are Dexedrine and Benzedrine. Among the physical effects of these drugs are increased heart rate, rise in blood pressure, increased muscle tension, and stimulation of the adrenal glands. These effects produce hyperalertness and wakefulness. In fact, since the adrenal gland is stimulated, the body is in a sense reacting (as to stress) with the fight-or-flight syndrome.[8] Amphetamines appear to affect the "pleasure center" of the brain, so that users may experience a sense of euphoria or well-being and a feeling of self-confidence or increased mental and physical powers.

Some of these symptoms alone make amphetamines dangerous. The habitual user is over-ruling the fatigue his body is experiencing. He may become confused or disoriented. Loss of appetite is an additional effect, so that harmful weight loss may occur. Although amphetamines are not physically addictive, tolerance builds up quickly and psychological dependence does occur. Symptoms of dependence include restlessness or irritability, talkativeness, tension and anxiety, decrease in muscular coordination, and/or extreme cheerfulness. Long-term use affects the heart and liver. Chronic use of heavy doses can result therefore in heart irregularities and hepatitis, as well as brain damage and death. Excessive doses can lead to psychosis.

A third form of amphetamines is methamphetamine (Methedrine, or "speed"). Speed is usually injected into the body, producing a "rush" (euphoric flash or intense high). The speed user experiences the same reactions as the chronic heavy user of other amphetamines, though usually at a more intense level. The user experiences marked euphoria, along with a sense of extreme physical strength and mental capacity. Sexual feelings and pleasures are often intensified.

As a speed user develops tolerance to the drug, he requires stronger doses with more dangerous results. Symptoms of toxicity

[8] Ibid., p. 122.

begin to appear—these include vivid visual, auditory, and even tactile hallucinations. Other effects may be severe chest pain, unconsciousness, psychosis, and other symptoms described above.

Cocaine   Cocaine is the alkaloid contained in the leaves of the coca plant, which grows mainly in the Andes. It acts as a depressant to produce a numbing effect when used locally (as an anesthetic), but its general effect in the body is pronounced stimulation of the central nervous system. In fact, it is one of the strongest stimulants known to man.

Pure cocaine is a white crystalline powder. In the United States its purity varies with the number of dealers who have handled it. It may be diluted (cut) with milk sugar, quinine, or similar substances.

Effects

The reactions to cocaine vary with the physical and emotional state of the person, the quality and quantity, and how the drug is taken. The most popular method in the U.S. today seems to be inhaling (snorting) the powder through the nostrils. Heavy users may inject it as a liquid into the bloodstream.[9]

Small doses of cocaine, when snorted, produce a cold or numb sensation in the nose and palate. The user feels powerful and elated. In general, it increases the heartbeat, speeds up breathing, raises body temperature and blood-sugar levels. It also causes dilation of the pupils of the eyes and dryness of the throat. Injection of cocaine produces much more severe reactions.

Chronic use consequently produces increasingly unpleasant hyperstimulation, nausea and digestive disorders leading to weight loss, chronic insomnia and even death. Snorting cocaine over a long period of time will gradually cause erosion and perforation of the nasal membranes. When large doses are used, the euphoria is mixed with anxiety and suspicion. Paranoid delusions accompanied by visual and auditory hallucinations may occur. The syndrome of toxicity is similar to that resulting from amphetamines, but less severe.

Addiction and Withdrawal

According to Lester Grinspoon and James B. Bakalar, "cocaine can be considered habit forming only in the sense that people who try

[9] Some drug addicts may mix cocaine and heroin together for injection, a combination called a "speedball." This prolongs the effects of cocaine, though lessening the stimulant effect. Heroin addicts rarely get high from heroin, so they use this combination to supply their heroin craving and produce a high or rush.

it are likely to continue using it if they can obtain it easily.'"[10] Simply put, if it is available and affordable, people will want to use it.

Grinspoon and Bakalar also state that,

> cocaine produces no clearly defined withdrawal syndrome, since it is not a depressant. It may, however, cause the same kind of uncomfortable but physiologically unspecific feeling of need associated with nicotine, caffeine, and amphetamines.
>
> Even in its severe forms, coming down from stimulants does not cause a desire for more. Unlike the heroin addict, the amphetamine or cocaine abuser feeling the effects of overindulgence does not seek more of the drug to relieve his misery. On the contrary, he may have to wait out and sleep off the effects of his body's reaction to the overstimulation before he can take an interest in the drug's euphoriant powers again.[11]

BARBITURATES

The barbiturates are general depressants. The consumption of barbiturates in the United States is close to one million pounds a year, or about 4.5 billion doses. They are most commonly prescribed as sleeping pills. They are also used clinically to relieve mental stress, as a pre-anesthetic medication, as diagnostic and therapeutic aids in psychiatry, and to control convulsions.

Effects   The depressant effect of barbiturates is nonspecific, so that they are capable of producing a sedative effect on a wide range of functions, including those of the neurons throughout the brain and the skeletal and cardiac muscles. The effect on the central nervous system varies from mild sedation to unconsciousness and coma, depending on the dosage. Moderate dosages may create an initial effect of euphoria by lowering inhibitions, followed by the depressant effect. There is no one clear-cut response; it depends upon the individual using the drug. Some people may experience no effects at all from a moderate dose, while others may become dizzy or nauseated. In rare cases, a high fever or delirium may result.

Excessive dosage levels (which may vary according to the individual and the situation) can cause barbiturate poisoning, involv-

[10] Lester Grinspoon and James B. Bakalar, *Cocaine: A Drug and Its Social Evolution.* New York: Basic Books, 1977.
[11] Ibid.

Barbiturates and Booze

The barbiturates have become the most commonly misused legal drug, second only to alcohol. The person who has become a frequent user of barbiturates, and then makes the mistake of combining this drug with alcohol puts himself in even more serious jeopardy. These two categories of drugs have an additive effect in causing respiratory depression, coma, and death. Barbiturates or tranquilizers should never be prescribed for a person who is a known alcoholic, and a person who uses alcohol should never concomitantly take a legally prescribed barbiturate. The withdrawal phenomenon upon abruptly stopping barbiturates, which have been used for 30 days or longer in milligram quantities of 600 milligrams or above, frequently produce symptoms of restlessness, agitation, loss of appetite, headache, nausea, vomiting, and sometimes convulsions, coma, and death.

Barbiturate withdrawal certainly presents itself as a medical emergency. Unlike the person who uses narcotics, the barbiturate dependent individual should never be treated for withdrawal symptoms outside of a hospital setting. The heroin addict will have an uncomfortable time, should he stop his drug of abuse abruptly; but he will not die. Narcotic withdrawal is uncomfortable, it is undesirable, but it is not fatal.

Source: From a Report by Ronald J. Dougherty, M.D., Chairman, Committee on Drug Abuse, New York Academy of Family Practice.

ing convulsions, coma, and/or death. Prolonged use of excessive amounts may cause anemia or even degenerative changes in the liver. Toxic psychosis and delirium may also result. These dangers are even more likely if barbiturates are taken intravenously.

An additional danger of barbiturates is accidental death. A person using them as sleeping pills may take an overdose by taking a second dosage after becoming groggy and forgetful from an earlier dose. Barbiturates are the cause of death in many suicides, both accidental and intended. Furthermore, the combination of alcohol and barbiturates is extremely risky, since both are depressants. Alcohol lowers the lethal dosage of barbiturates for an individual; if he takes these pills and drinks, coma or death may result.

Increasing tolerance and both psychological and physical dependence occur with all barbiturates. These may occur rapidly and from only small or moderate dosages. Withdrawal symptoms are very serious and extremely dangerous.

Withdrawal should always be done under hospital supervision. Otherwise convulsions and toxic psychosis may occur. The central nervous system is deeply depressed in barbiturate addiction, and recovery is difficult. Without medical supervision, death may occur.

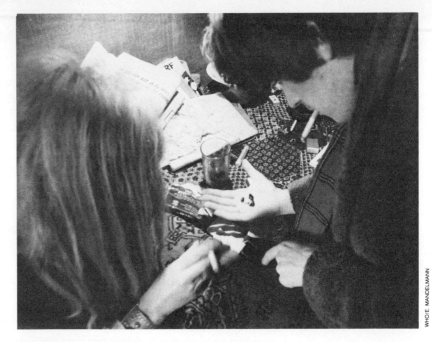

FIGURE 14.2   *For some, drugs and alcohol are nothing more than a lonely trip to nowhere.*

NARCOTICS

Narcotics include the opiates—opium and its derivatives—and synthetic drugs similar to opium. Narcotics usually have a depressant effect upon the central nervous system. All these drugs are addictive. Morphine is used medically to relieve pain and sometimes by addicts, but the drug most often abused in the United States is heroin.

Heroin   Heroin is an indirect opium derivative created from morphine. It is found as a white or off-white odorless crystalline powder. The color depends on how it has been cut or adulterated. The heroin user usually progresses from snorting to skin popping (injecting the liquified drug just beneath the skin) to mainlining (injecting the drug directly into the bloodstream).

Effects

Heroin acts as both a spinal and cerebral depressant. The user will have pin-point pupils that react slowly, if at all, to light, slower breathing, and retardation of the functions of the nervous system, glands, and organs.[12] A person's size and metabolic rate, the other drugs he is using or has used, and his emotional state will all affect his reaction to heroin. Usually, however, the most pronounced result is a rush, or euphoric spasm, which may last for several hours. At this time the user is lethargic, drowsy, and withdrawn. These effects are caused by the fact that heroin has its heaviest effect (and concentration) in the corpus striatum portion of the brain, which seems to be important in integrating motor activity and perceptual information.

Heroin use can cause other severe physical problems. Hepatitis occurs frequently, usually from unsterile needles. Other diseases may be transmitted this way. Bacterial infections causing inflammation of the lining of the heart and surrounding tissues account for about 9 percent of all deaths of heroin addicts.

Another danger stems from the way the drug is cut. Usually substances such as quinine or milk sugar are used, but heroin may also contain poisons such as strychnine, crystallized battery acid, and other drugs such as LSD or amphetamines.

Inadvertent overdose is a constant possibility. Again, this is usually a result of the adulteration of the drug. The user has no way of telling the strength of the drug he has purchased. While at some times it may be too weak to produce a rush, at other times the percentage of pure heroin may be high enough to produce overdose and death. An overdose severely depresses respiration and also causes pulmonary edema (filling of the lungs with fluid).

Tolerance and dependence occur very rapidly with heroin. The effects of each injection usually last only five to eight hours, so that the addict must have another injection or he will experience withdrawal symptoms. These symptoms last for a period of about three days, increasing in intensity. The first results are chills and sweating, yawning, watery eyes, running nose, and sneezing. Loss of appetite, severe cramps, and dilated pupils are part of the second stage. In the final stage, vomiting and diarrhea are added to the list of symptoms.

CAUSES OF DRUG ABUSE

Drug use and abuse is becoming epidemic in the United States. Experts are only now beginning to make progress in understanding why individuals, especially young people, use and abuse drugs.

As mentioned earlier, ours is a very drug-conscious society. Many parents routinely give vitamins, aspirin, and other drugs to

[12] Ferguson, op cit., p. 64.

their children (some of which are "candy coated" to taste better). Many adults rely on alcohol, tobacco, amphetamines, and/or barbiturates. This widespread emphasis and dependence can be a determining factor in a teenager's interest in marijuana or other more dangerous drugs.

Peer pressure was mentioned as a cause for teenage cigarette smoking, and it is equally important in drug use. Marijuana smoking has spread from the colleges down to even the elementary schools. Drug use of some sort is considered the "in" thing by many young people, a way to demonstrate maturity. If one of a group of friends is exposed to drugs, it is likely that all the members will experiment. (Studies have also shown that young people who experiment with drugs at an early age, also experiment with sex at an early age.)

There are two basic classes of drug users or abusers. The first group consists of the less heavy users. They may use drugs because of curiosity, for experimentation, because of peer pressure, or from a desire for sociability. Some people may experiment initially with drugs because of emotional problems—these are more likely to become part of the second group.

The second group is made up of the heavy drug users and the addicts. They use drugs as an escape. Many of these abusers are suffering from underlying mental disturbances; some of these people are psychoneurotics or psychotics. These individuals would rather resort to drugs than face their problems, so a cure for them is difficult.

DRUG COUNSELING AND TREATMENT

There are many unanswered questions and problems in our methods of drug treatment. One of the most controversial programs is the use of methadone to treat heroin addiction. Methadone is a synthetic narcotic, so that many people view its use as the substitution of one addiction for another. Yet, a methadone maintenance program can allow the addict to live a normal life. Other problems center around the many widely held drug misconceptions in our society. Teenagers realize that many of the so-called facts about marijuana are actually untrue "scare tactics"; consequently, they don't believe the dangers of other more serious drugs.

Perhaps one of the best answers to the problem of drug abuse is an extensive program of education. Most drug treatment centers today realize that drug use is not limited to any one type of person or any particular part of society. Therefore, our youth should be made aware of the problems and dangers of all drugs. Many high schools (and some elementary schools) have set up drug counseling centers. Mental health centers and hot lines have been established to deal with drug questions and problems, and there are other individual counselors available.

Students themselves can set up support groups of those who are concerned about drug use and abuse. These students therefore can both educate themselves and help others who are concerned or involved with drugs. The Drug Enforcement Administration of the U.S. Government can provide information. (A listing of the thirteen Regional Offices is included in the Appendix on page 379.) Drug counseling centers and libraries can also supply literature and answers.

FURTHER READINGS

Blum, Richard H. and Associates. *Society and Drugs* and *Students and Drugs*. San Francisco: Jossey-Bass Publishers, 1969.

These two volumes provide the reader with a comprehensive coverage of the psychoactive drugs including LSD, heroin, alcohol, marijuana.

Bloomquist, E. R. *Marijuana*. Beverly Hills, Calif.: Glencoe Press, 1968.

A thorough and factual look at the drug marijuana.

Braden, William. *The Private Sea: LSD and the Search for God*. New York: A Bantam Book, 1967.

This book examines the death of God, Zen, pantheism, and the psychic revolt through the eyes of those who have used psychedelic drugs.

Brecher, Edward M. *Licit and Illicit Drugs*. Boston: Little, Brown & Co., 1972.

From the Consumers Union, the complete drug book—everything from cocaine to caffeine—with recommendations for workable drug laws.

Evans, Wayne O. and Kline, Nathan S. (eds.) *Psychotropic Drugs in the Year 2000.*

A succinct review and integration of present knowledge and likely future discoveries enable one to gain an overview of the actual and the possible impact of drugs on the world.

Grinspoon, Lester. *Marijuana Reconsidered.* Cambridge, Mass.: Harvard University Press, 1971.

A psychiatrist's analysis of marijuana in America—its psychological, physiological, and social effects—and the implications of its continuing presence.

Gustaitis, Rasa. *Turning On*. New York: The Macmillan Co., 1969.

The story of a woman who turns, first with LSD and then with the human potential movement.

Kaplan, John. *Marijuana: The New Prohibition*. New York: Pocket Books, 1971.

This book explores some of the crucial questions, including the law, relating to marijuana. The author's conclusion is that marijuana should be legalized.

Lingeman, Richard R. *Drugs From A to Z: A Dictionary.* New York: McGraw-Hill Co., 1969.

This book combines scientific data with the history and lore surrounding narcotic, stimulant, depressant, and hallucinogenic drugs.

Margolis, Jack S. and Clorfene, Richard. *A Child's Garden of Grass.* New York: Pocket Books, 1970.

This unpretentious little book has something to say to those who have, to those who haven't but want to, and even to those who don't want to but would like to stay informed about marijuana.

Masters, R.E. and Houston, Jean. *The Varieties of Psychedelic Experience.* New York: Dell Publishing Co., Inc., 1966.

An extremely thorough and comprehensive book on the effects of LSD on human personality.

Pope, Harrison. *Voices from the Drug Culture.* Boston: Beacon Press, 1971.

Gives sound ideas on why middle and upper class youth have turned to drugs and what the drug subculture is like.

Smoking and Health. Princeton, N.J.: D. Van Nostrand Co., Inc., 1970.

The complete report of the advisory committee to the Surgeon General of the Public Health Service on tobacco and health.

Tart, Charles T. *On Being Stoned: A Psychological Study of Marijuana Intoxication.* Palo Alto, Calif.: Science and Behavior Books, 1971.

A study of marijuana in relation to touch, taste, smell, pleasure, and enhanced sexual enjoyment. A must book for those who are interested in marijuana research.

Wallgren, Henrik and Barry, H. *Actions of Alcohol.* Vol. 1 & 2. New York: Elsevier Pub. Co., 1970.

A quite comprehensive review of experimental work on the effects of alcohol on the living organism.

Weil, Andrew. *The Natural Mind.* Boston: Houghton Mifflin, 1972.

Deals with altered states of consciousness—with and without drugs—and the inadequacies of conventional ways of thinking about drugs, current drug laws, and drug control programs.

6

HEALTH
IMPAIRMENTS

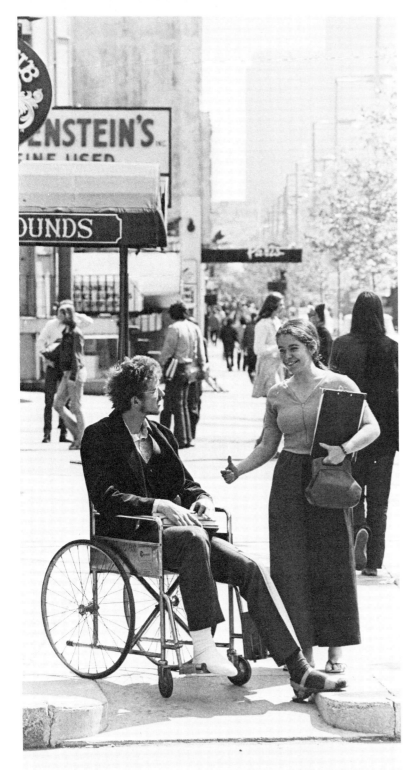

All interest in disease
and death is only another
expression of interest
in life . . . .

Thomas Mann
The Magic Mountain

Chapter 15

The Communicable Diseases

René Dubos' conception of health as a quality of life that is determined by ecological and evolutionary principles provides a foundation for an understanding of diseases and the disease process. Dubos suggests that life involves the continual interplay between individuals and their environments so that health is controlled by the nature of these interactions. Thus, health is a state of social, mental, and biological fitness resulting from the responses and adaptations of individuals to their external world.[1]

Since these relationships are continually in flux, the characteristics of health vary from place to place and from one time to another. The manner in which disease affects populations, then, will change with different individual and environmental factors. The past demonstrates this, as the relative effects of various diseases in terms of morbidity, mortality, and disability have fluctuated from one historical period to another.[2]

THEORIES OF DISEASE CAUSATION

The differential occurrence and distribution of diseases have supplied the foundation for theories of disease causation throughout history. Early civilizations connected the seemingly random outbreaks of disease with moral and religious behaviors, so that primitive forms

[1] René Dubos, *The Mirage of Health,* New York: Anchor Books, 1959.
[2] René Dubos, *Man, Medicine, and Environment,* New York, Mentor Books, 1968, pp. 87–113.

of disease prevention were marked with periods of fasting and human sacrifices or other offerings to placate the gods.[2]

Subsequent theories moved away from disease as a consequence of man's behavior and moved toward environmental causes. Man began to associate the incidence of disease with conditions of blood and bile as well as with general aspects of his external environment. During this period people believed, for example, that swamp vapors were responsible for diseases (e.g., *malaria*). Some of the prevention measures arising from these beliefs—such as efforts at sanitation—actually did contribute to a reduction in disease.

The development of the microscope marked a turning point in conquering the spread of communicable disease. Micro-organisms were discovered to be the causes of disease, and led to the understanding of the germ theory.

With the development of the germ theory, new possibilities for disease control appeared. Efforts were concentrated on the elimination of infectious agents and the isolation of infected persons. New discoveries in chemotherapy (drug treatment) of disease and immunizations made disease control more possible.[4]

Today the germ theory is only part of the explanation for the spread and incidence of disease. The multifactorial theory of disease causation, like Dubos' conception of health, views the occurrence of disease as dependent upon the interaction of many individual and environmental factors. Individual factors such as genetic susceptibility, age, sex, race, behavior, and natural resistance may determine whether or not one becomes host to a certain group of pathogens (disease-causing germs). Environmental determinants of disease might include climate, weather, the presence of infectious agents, socioeconomic conditions (housing, nutrition, occupation, etc.), and the availability of health services.

THE DISEASE PROCESS

All communicable diseases have certain components in common. These include infectious agents, a reservoir of infection, a mode of transmission, and a host who is susceptible to infection. All communicable diseases are caused by specific microorganisms, which are referred to as pathogens, infectious agents, causative agents, or

[3] Gaylord Anderson, "Landmarks of Communicable Disease Control—Past and Future," *Canadian Journal of Public Health,* 61, no. 5, September/October 1970, p. 374.
[4] Ibid., p. 377.

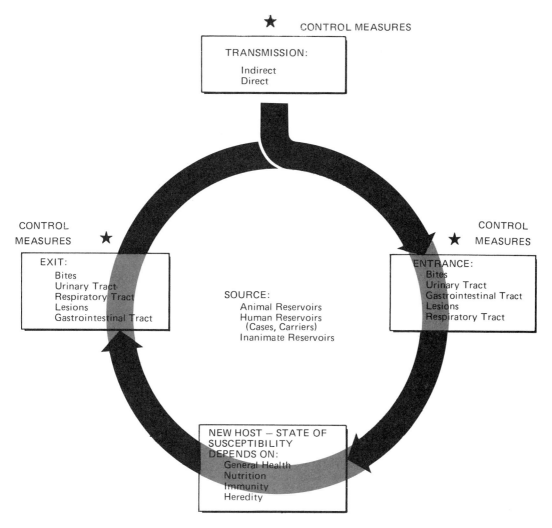

FIGURE 15.1 *The disease process. (Adapted from John Hanlon, Principles of Public Health Administration (St. Louis: C. V. Mosby Company, 1969), p. 338.*

etiologic agents. Most of the micro-organisms in our environment are harmless; relatively few are pathogens. There are six types of disease causing agents: bacteria, viruses, rickettsia, fungi, protozoa, and worms.

The disease process whereby a pathogen affects an individual is a definite cycle of events. Control measures can be aimed at different stages of this cycle.

Stages of Communicable Diseases

The four basic stages in the progress of a communicable disease are transmission and infection, incubation, the clinical period, and recovery or convalescence. The pathogen must be transmitted from a reservoir—another human being, an animal, or an inanimate object—to a susceptible host. A disease may be passed from an infected person to another by direct or indirect contact, or it may be transmitted by a vector. Vectors are insects or animals that can carry pathogens from one individual to others. Some people may also be carriers, meaning that they are not suffering symptoms of illness themselves, but can infect others. Infection occurs when the pathogen gets into the host's body through a point of entry such as a wound, a body opening, or a vector bite.

The time interval between the establishment of the pathogen within the body and the appearance of clinical symptoms is called the incubation period. The incubation period varies in duration with each specific disease but is usually a few days to a few weeks. It may be as short as two or three hours or as long as several months. During the incubation period, the pathogen multiplies until it is abundant enough to overcome the body's natural defenses against disease. Communicable diseases are usually contagious during the incubation period, especially in its later stages.

During the clinical period, symptoms of illness appear. The first symptoms may be general (nonspecific) and are similar for many diseases. Soon after these symptoms, specific symptoms occur according to the disease.

The last stage in the disease process is convalescence, or the recovery period. In this stage, the body's natural defenses work to overpower the infectious agents, which may have been weakened by some form of treatment. As the natural defenses function more and more effectively, the symptoms gradually disappear. The infectious agents are still present in the body at this point, however, and

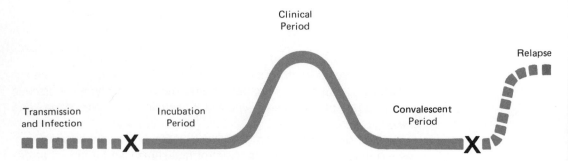

FIGURE 15.2   *The stages of communicable diseases.*

may regain their influence if a convalescing person weakens his defenses by resuming full activity too soon—bringing on a relapse.

PREVENTION AND CONTROL OF COMMUNICABLE DISEASES

The human body has various natural defenses against disease; another protection against infection is immunity of different types. In addition, there are certain steps the individual can take to help avoid disease.

The Body's Natural Defenses

The human body has both outer and inner sets of defenses against disease-causing organisms. The skin and mucous membranes are an important part of the first-line barrier against disease. The tiny hairs, or cilia, in the nostrils and the other parts of the respiratory system work to prevent pathogens from penetrating the body. Tears, saliva, and other body secretions all contain the enzyme *lysozyme,* which destroys many infectious agents.

If any pathogens do succeed in breaking through the first-line barrier, they are met by a complex internal system of defense. The white blood cells, or *leukocytes,* perform a dual role in protection. They are capable of breaking down and destroying infectious agents and they also can contain the pathogens, restricting the infection to a certain area and impeding its spread to the rest of the body. Another bodily reaction to infection is the production of interferon. This is an antivirus chemical that works to protect surrounding cells from invasion by the viruses.

A fever is a symptom of infection that can be regarded as a defense against serious illness. Most pathogenic microbes will not survive at temperatures more than a few degrees above the normal body temperature, so the fever temperatures work to destroy the infection. A rise in body temperature also stimulates the production of the white blood cells to destroy pathogens. However, a high temperature can be harmful to the normal body functions.

Immunity

Antibodies are substances in the human body that work to destroy disease-causing organisms (antigens). By fighting these organisms, antibodies can make the individual immune to various communicable diseases. There are two types of immunity that protect the human body—active and passive.

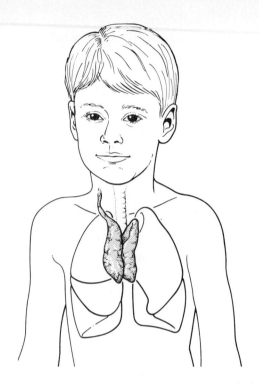

FIGURE 15.3   *The Thymus Gland. Recent research has helped define the role of the butterfly-shaped thymus in protecting the individual from disease. This gland seems to manufacture specialized cells which are sent out to such organs as the lymph nodes, bone marrow, and spleen, where they become lymphocytes able to recognize foreign substances (antigens) introduced into the body. The thymus is most active and at its largest in childhood; in an adult it is only a fraction of its early size, but continues to influence the functioning of the body's protective immunity system.*

In active immunity the individual produces his own antibodies. This may be caused by infection from a specific disease or injection of specific antigens. An individual who has become infected by a disease may build up enough specific antibodies against this disease to remain immune for long periods of time. With an injection of certain antigens—called artificial immunization—the body will also be stimulated to produce its own antibodies. It may take days or weeks for active immunity to develop, but it can persist for years. Booster injections may be required to keep the antibody level high.

In passive immunity, the individual receives protective antibodies but does not produce any himself. Passive immunity can be transferred through the placenta to the fetus so that a child will have some protection in the first few weeks of life. Breast feeding can also transfer immunity from the mother to the child. Passive immunity can

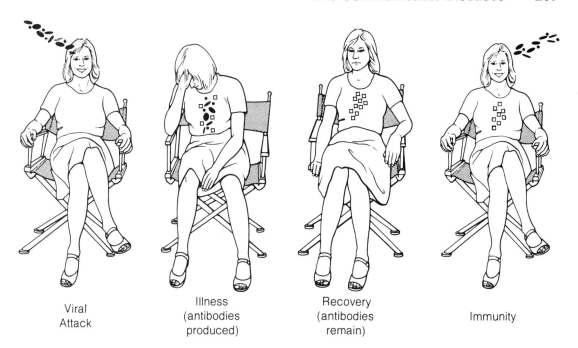

| Viral Attack | Illness (antibodies produced) | Recovery (antibodies remain) | Immunity |

FIGURE 15.4   *Active Immunity. Immunity to a virus may be achieved by an individual who has recovered from an episode of illness caused by that virus. An understanding of this phenomenon, as illustrated above, has enabled scientists to perfect methods of protecting populations against some of the more serious viral diseases. Vaccines are prepared that stimulate the formation of protective antibodies without causing illness.*

be acquired through an injection of antibodies or antitoxins. It provides only temporary protection, but does provide immunity quickly and therefore is used as an emergency measure when a person has been exposed to a contagious disease.

Chemotherapy   In addition to injections for immunity, drugs of various sorts are effectively used in treating many communicable diseases. The sulfa drugs, discovered in the 1930s, were the first antimicrobial drugs; since then numerous others have been developed. These drugs may either kill the invading pathogens or suppress their growth or multiplication. Chemotherapy has been least successful against virus-caused communicable diseases, but some new drugs seem more effective.

Prevention through Action   An individual can take some important steps to help prevent serious complications from arising from some of the more common communicable diseases. These preventive measures include good

Table 15.1 *Immunizations Commonly Used in the United States*

Type of Immunization	Who Should Be Immunized	Effectiveness of Immunization and Frequency of Booster Doses
Cholera	Foreign travelers	Only partial immunity; renew every 6 months for duration of exposure
Diphtheria	All adults in good health with no previous immunization; travelers	Highly effective; renew every 10 years
Influenza	All adults of any age, especially those with chronic disease of the heart, respiratory tract, or endocrine system	Renew every year (because viral strains change easily)
Mumps	Most helpful to children and young adults who have not had mumps	Believed to confer lifetime immunity
Polio	All adults, particularly travelers, those exposed to children, and those in health and sanitation industries	Long-lasting immunity; with oral immunization virulent booster every 10 years. With Salk vaccine should boost every year
Rabies	Only those bitten by rabid animal	A vaccination each day for 14 to 21 days beginning soon after the bite
German measles	Mainly for children	Highly effective; need for boosters not established
Measles	Mainly for children	Highly effective; usually produces lifelong immunity
Tetanus	Everyone	Very effective; renew every 10 years or when treated for a contaminated wound if more than 7 years have elapsed since last booster
Tuberculosis	High-risk people; nurses and children in contact with active tubercular cases	Booster doses BCG t needed (contraindicated, as ne, in the U.S. because of l ence in general population`
Typhoid fever	Anyone exposed; travelers	About 80 percent annual booster
Typhus	Anyone exposed	Renew every year d)
Whooping cough	Essential for children by age 3 to 4 months	Highly effective; bo –6 years of age, once
Yellow fever	Anyone exposed; travelers	Highly effective; pro immunity for at least 17 years

Source: adapted from U.S. Public Health Service.

health, periodic health examinations, early detection of disease, and follow-up screening and diagnostic exams.

Good health means many things; in relation to preventing infection with communicable disease it refers to maintaining a good balance of physical exercise, rest, nutrition, and personal hygiene. An individual who is physically fit is less likely to be a susceptible host in the disease cycle.

Chapter 2 was concerned with seeking medical help. We will stress again here the idea that regular physical checkups are important. Many people consult a doctor only when they are sick, but preventive medicine makes more sense. If the doctor is familiar with the patient's history, he can more easily diagnose or predict any problems. The individual who has regular checkups and a good doctor-patient relationship will also be sure to get any booster immunization he may need. Regular checkups become especially important once the male reaches forty or the female reaches thirty-five.

Early diagnosis of any communicable disease is important in controlling the symptoms in the individual and in preventing the spread of the disease in the community.

Follow-up care and treatment are important in the progress of any disease. The patient must be sure, for example, to take all of any drug that has been prescribed; many people stop taking medicine as soon as their symptoms start to disappear. This can be dangerous, for antigens are still present in the body and a relapse may occur. A doctor may also recommend follow-up screening procedures for certain diseases to make sure they have been cured.

COMMON COMMUNICABLE DISEASES

Many of the communicable diseases have been brought under control or have been completely eradicated (smallpox was recently declared to have been eradicated) by immunization. The infectious diseases most commonly occurring in the United States today are the common cold, influenza, streptococcal infections, mononucleosis, hepatitis, and the venereal diseases. Table 15.2 provides information on these diseases and others.

The Common Cold   The common cold is the most widespread contagious disease in the United States today. The average person has four to eight colds a year. The usual mode of transmission is through direct contact with an infected person or by airborne droplets. Colds seem to occur more frequently in crowded conditions and during seasons when people spend more time indoors. A recent study in New York concluded that incidence and prevalence were related to environmental variables, specifically the weather and to a lesser degree environmental pollution. Infants and elderly people face greater risks of contracting colds.

Colds are caused by viruses, predominantly the rhinoviruses, but also enteroviruses and parainfluenza and influenza viruses. There

Table 15.2 Common Communicable Diseases

Disease	Agent	Transmission	Incubation and Communicability	Symptoms	Control
Chickenpox* (Varicella) * (Confers lasting immunity) Shingles—different manifestation of infection by the same virus; characterized by linear eruption along a nerve.	Varicella virus	Contact with previous case; discharges from nose and throat; skin lesions of infected individuals.	a. 13–21 days. b. 1 day before eruption to day 6 after eruption first appeared.	Slight fever; malaise; skin eruption in successive crops; often itching.	No specific treatment other than for relief of itching which prevents children from scratching and causing secondary infection.
Mumps* (Infectious parotitis) * Serious complications in adolescent and adult males; can lead to inflammation of testes which results in sterility.	Virus	Nose and throat discharge of infected person.	a. 14–21 days. b. 7 days before swelling to 9 days thereafter; communicability is greatest at time when swelling begins.	Fever; pain and swelling of salivary gland (paratoid) located in region below and in front of ear.	Mumps vaccine is available; avoid contact with patient having disease.
Measles (Rubeola)	Virus	Nose and mouth discharges of infected patient.	a. 9–12 days. b. 4–5 days before rash appears to 3 days after rash first appears.	Fever followed by head cold symptoms; running nose; sneezing; inflamed and watery eyes; blotchy rash after 3–4 days.	Measles vaccine.
German measles* (Rubella) * Especially dangerous for pregnant woman—during first 3 months of pregnancy often results in stillbirths or deformed babies.	Virus	Contact with previous case; discharges from nose and throat; especially infectious before rash appears.	a. 14–21 days.	Mild illness; head cold symptoms; rash which starts on head and face and spreads to neck and trunk; glands behind ears and in back of neck become swollen.	Gamma globulin is valuable after exposure.

Disease	Cause	How Spread	Incubation Period	Symptoms	Prevention/Control
Whooping cough (Pertussis)	Hemophilus pertussis (affects respiratory tract)	Discharges from mouth and nose of infected person.	a. 5–8 days. b. 7 days after exposure to 3 weeks after onset of spasmodic coughing.	Cough which, in 1–2 weeks, becomes spasmodic with whooping noise and sometimes ends with vomiting.	Isolation of infected person; immunization available.
Diphtheria	Corynebacterium diptheriae (lodges in throat but its toxin is carried via blood to the rest of the body)	Spread by patient, carrier or articles contaminated by bacterium.	a. 2–5 days. b. Communicability period varies.	Headache; fever; sore throat. Complications include heart damage and various paralyses.	Immunization with diphtheria toxoid and boosters in successive years.
Poliomyelitis (infantile paralysis)	Virus	Uncovered cough or sneeze; not washing after bowel movement.	a. 8–10 days.	Sudden fever; dull pain on bending neck forward; headache; vomiting; weakness or paralysis of one or more muscle groups.	Polio vaccine (Sabin-oral).
Tuberculosis	Tubercle bacillus	Contact with patients, indirect contact through contaminated articles, unpasteurized milk; bacillus may be airborne.	4 to 6 weeks.	None (may go undetected for long periods of time).	Proper nutrition, chest X-ray, skin test, BCG vaccine for high-risk individuals.
Tetanus* (lockjaw) *Fatality rate = 35 percent.	Tetanus bacillus (found in soil, intestines, and feces of animals; thrives on dead or devitalized tissue and a lack of oxygen)	When infectious agent enters wound.	a. 4 days–3 weeks.	Characterized by irritability and stiffness of neck, jaw, and limbs; muscle spasms.	Inoculations of tetanus toxoid.
Influenza (flu)	Virus	Sneezing; coughing; contaminated articles.	a. 24–72 hours. b. Up to 3 days after onset of clinical symptoms.	Chills; fever; headache; cough; running nose; sore throat.	Vaccine, valuable if kept up to date.

Table 15.2 *(cont.)*

Disease	Agent	Transmission	Incubation and Communicability	Symptoms	Control
Infectious hepatitis (inflammation of liver)	2 Virus strains (A) and	(A) Transmitted most commonly via food, water or fingers to mouth.	(A) 2–4 weeks.	(A) Lack of appetite; fatigue; abdominal pain; dark urine.	(A) Purification of H_2O supplies; sanitary waste disposal; washing after elimination; fly and roach control; control of fish sources; sterilized needles and syringes.
Serum hepatitis	(B)	(B) Transmitted via blood only.	(B) 2–6 months.	(B) Gradual onset; less likely to have fever; other symptoms are the same.	(B) Sterilized needles and syringes; careful control of persons allowed to give blood transfusions.
Mononucleosis (kissing disease)	Agent is unknown	Close contact.	2–6 weeks.	Fever; sore throat; swollen glands; headache; general poor health. Diagnosis often confirmed by presence of many white blood cells.	Bed rest.

Source: Health Education Package. Massachusetts Department of Public Health, Division of Communicable Diseases.

are as yet no antibiotics to treat and control colds. If a cold lasts more than seven days, a secondary bacterial infection which can be treated by antibiotics is probably involved. Efforts are underway to provide a cold vaccine, especially for the rhinoviruses, which can cause severe illness in children. However, since there are so many viral types involved, control seems unlikely unless a vaccine can combine many antigenic types.

Influenza

Influenza is still a problem because of the probability of widespread epidemics with high morbidity and significant mortality rates. Transmission occurs through direct contact with human reservoirs. Influenza outbreaks have developed into pandemics (worldwide) throughout history. Greatest mortality occurs among infants and older persons.

Influenza is also a viral disease and the viruses involved are subject to changes in their antigenic makeup (a process called *antigenic drift*). In other words, the strain that causes an outbreak one year is likely to be different from that implicated in an epidemic ten years earlier. Thus, development of vaccines is difficult.

The clinical symptoms of influenza are similar to those of a cold: fever, muscle aches, chills, and nasal discharge. However, complications can be severe and illness can last for weeks. Pneumonia is a frequent complication and may be fatal for older people who have a history of chronic respiratory disease.

Prevention measures are basically the same as those for the common cold. The vaccines that have thus far been developed cannot always be successful, but are recommended for high-risk individuals, such as doctors, the elderly, and children with debilitating diseases.

Streptococcal Infections

Most streptococcal bacteria do not cause disease, but one group, the *streptococcus pyrogenes,* is responsible for 95 percent of all acute bacterial upper respiratory infections. Infection can occur through direct or indirect contact; respiratory infections result from direct contact and infection of burns or cuts is attributed to indirect contact. Contamination of milk or food products can often produce outbreaks of throat infections. The rate of transmission is increased in closed areas such as schools or military camps.

Complications from a strep infection include rheumatic fever and heart disease and chronic nephritis (a kidney ailment). Penicillin and erythromycin have been used as control measures.

Mononucleosis   Mononucleosis is thought to be viral in origin, though the viral agent has never been isolated nor successfully reproduced experimentally. Clinical and epidemiological features of the disease strongly suggest that it is communicable. The method of transmission is still unknown; the popular name "kissing disease" suggests direct contact. The population with the highest risk is between the ages of fifteen and thirty. The disease most commonly occurs where large groups of young people are in close contact, such as in college dorms.

The incubation period may last from four days to two months. Symptoms include tiredness or lassitude, sore throat, headache, and fever, with involvement of the lymph nodes. Mononucleosis is almost never fatal, but the liver or spleen may be affected (hepatitis is sometimes a complication), so medical treatment is necessary. Symptoms may last several weeks or even months. One attack of mononucleosis seems to confer a fairly long-lasting immunity.

Hepatitis   Hepatitis is a communicable viral disease that affects the liver. There are two types: infectious hepatitis and serum hepatitis. Infectious hepatitis is believed to be transmitted directly by an infected individual, while serum hepatitis is spread through the use of contaminated blood or plasma. Serum hepatitis has been on the rise in recent years, because of the increasing numbers of drug addicts using nonsterile needles for injections and thereby transmitting the disease.

The incubation period for infectious hepatitis is usually about three or four weeks; for serum hepatitis, it is longer, varying from about seven to twenty-five weeks. In both forms of the disease, the symptoms may be mild or severe and may last from several weeks to several months. The convalescent period is also often months long. Symptoms include fever, loss of appetite and nausea, and exhaustion or general malaise. Jaundice may or may not accompany either form of the disease. Death from infectious hepatitis is rare; the mortality rate for serum hepatitis is somewhat higher.

There is as yet no permanent vaccine against hepatitis. Research has found a vaccine that seems to confer temporary passive immunity against serum hepatitis. Preventive measures include good personal hygiene; it is believed that if everyone washed their hands after using the bathroom and before meals, the incidence of infectious hepatitis would be greatly diminished. Careful checking of blood donors and proper sterilization of medical equipment should reduce the number of cases of serum hepatitis.

The Venereal Diseases   With the discovery of penicillin as an effective treatment against both syphilis and gonorrhea, the incidence of venereal disease

Table 15.3 *Other Sexually Transmitted Diseases*

Name	Causative Agent	Incubation Period	Early Symptoms	Later Developments	Treatment
Chancroid	Haemophilus ducreyi	1–7 days	Small, painful pimples where bacterium entered body become filled with pus and break down to form shallow ulcers.	Infection infiltrates lymph nodes in region causing abscess (bubo). Abscesses erupt, spreading ulcers over skin.	Sulfa drugs, broadspectrum antibiotics except penicillin
Lympho-granuloma Venereum	Chlamydia	1–6 weeks	Tiny pimple where bacterium entered body may be so insignificant as to be unrecognized or ignored.	Infection infiltrates nearest lymph nodes which may fester into abscesses. Abscesses erupt, leaking out blood-stained pus. If chronic, infection may cause gross swelling of penis and scrotum (*elephantiasis*) and may spread from vagina to rectum.	Sulfa drugs, broadspectrum antibiotics except penicillin
Granuloma Inguinale	Donovan body	unknown	Initial painless pimples where bacterium entered body break down into beefy-red, velvety raised masses which bleed and spread over body.	Scar tissue forms over wounds.	Broadspectrum antibiotics
Herpes Simplex 2	Herpes simplex virus	2–20 days	Minor rash or itching in genital area, clusters of painful blisters.	Latency, with possible relapses.	No known cure; treatments to relieve symptoms and shorten duration of outbreak
Trichomoniasis	Trichomonas vaginalis	varies	Vaginal discharge, itching, and burning; possible urethritis in the male.		Antibiotics or vaginal suppositories

rapidly declined in the United States from 1948 to 1958. Since then, however, the number of new venereal disease cases has increased more rapidly with each successive year. Syphilis and gonorrhea are the most common of these diseases. Gonorrhea has reached epidemic proportions in this country. In fact, it is the most common communicable disease in the United States except for the common cold. Well over three million people in the United States will contact one of these diseases in the next year. Herpes simplex, which may not be technically classified as a venereal disease but is related to sexual contact, is also on the rise. Trichomoniasis is another infection becoming more common. There are three other less common venereal diseases: chancroid, lymphogranuloma venereum, and granuloma inguinale. Table 15.3 provides a description of the symptoms and treatments of these diseases.

More than half the reported cases of venereal disease occur in persons under twenty-five years of age. The reported cases may give little indication of the actual proportion of infection; it is estimated that only one out of every nine cases of syphilis and one out of every four cases of gonorrhea are actually reported annually. Infected individuals may not seek treatment because of fear or ignorance; many cases, especially among women, are asymptomatic.

Gonorrhea

Gonorrhea is caused by a bacterium called the *Neisseria gonorrhea*. Transmission is through direct contact with an infected individual, almost always through sexual intercourse. The bacteria that cause both gonorrhea and syphilis are extremely sensitive to dryness and cold and usually can survive only a few seconds outside the human body. The incubation period for gonorrhea may be from three days to three weeks, after which symptoms may or may not appear. Gonorrhea is asymptomatic in at least 80 percent of all infected females and in 5 to 20 percent of infected males.

In the male, the bacteria first attack the urethra. The symptoms of this urethritis are pain or burning upon urination and/or a discharge from the penis. Without treatment, the disease may spread throughout the vas deferens to the epididymis or may attack the prostate gland, seminal vesicles, and/or the bladder. The scar tissue resulting throughout the reproductive system from the infection may result in sterility because of blockage of the sperm.

Only 20 percent (or fewer) women experience any symptoms at all from gonorrhea. Occasionally there is a vaginal discharge. If the infection spreads from the vagina or cervix to the urethra, the woman may also have painful urination. When gonorrhea is left untreated in the female, it can spread throughout the reproductive system. The

Summary of Gonorrhea

Germer: Gonorrhea is caused by a bacterium called *Neisseria Gonorrhea*. It cannot live long in contact with the air, and can enter the body only through the mucous membranes that line body openings.

	MEN	**WOMEN**
Transmission:	Genital, anal, or oral sexual contact	Vaginal, anal, or oral-genital sexual contact
Symptoms:	Three to eight days after contact with an infected partner discharge from the penis and/or burning when urinating. Anal gonorrhea may be recognized through a sensation of wetness or itching around the anus	About 80% of infected women do not have symptoms. Some women have a green or yellow-green vaginal discharge. Symptoms of anal gonorrhea same as male.
Complications:	Sterility if left untreated.	Sterility if left untreated.
Treatment:	Penicillin—if allergic, tetracycline tablets by mouth.	Same as the male.
Considerations:	If you are aware of the fact that you have gonorrhea it is your personal responsibility to inform your partner or partners so they can be treated. Both men and women should have a test for gonorrhea after each ''casual'' sexual encounter.	

fallopian tubes can become scarred, blocking the passage of ova and resulting in sterility.

Both women and men may have anal gonorrhea, and both may develop gonorrhea of the throat from oral-genital sex.

Untreated gonorrhea may cause further complications such as gonococcal arthritis and infection of the valves of the heart. The bacteria can also cause a serious eye infection that may lead to blindness, so infected individuals must be careful not to transfer the germs to their eyes. The bacteria in a woman's system can infect a child during the birth process, so most states now require that an infant's eyes be treated at birth to avoid this possibility.

The tests for the presence of gonorrhea are not always reliable. The most common method of diagnosis relies on the identification of gonococci in ''cultures'' of the male discharge or from the female's cervix. Cultures from the anal canal should also be taken, and throat cultures can detect the presence of the gonococcal bacteria there. A blood test has recently been developed, but so far it has proven less accurate than the cultures.

Treatment of gonorrhea usually involves penicillin; in cases where the individual is allergic to this drug, tetracycline is used. Problems arise from the fact that the strains of gonorrhea now being

> Dr. Ralph H. Henderson said at a meeting of the Society for Adolescent Medicine that the male homosexual, especially within certain communities, is an important vector (transmitter) for syphilis. While national data indicate that about 30% of males with syphilis name contacts of the same sex, there are areas in the U.S. where the total is close to 80%, Dr. Henderson said.
>
> *Source:* "Society's Attitude Major Obstacle To Control of Venereal Disease," *Family Practice News,* March 1, 1974.

found are increasingly resistant to antibiotic treatment, so that much greater dosages are now required for any effect. The resistance of the bacteria means that at least one culture should be taken after treatment to make sure that it was effective. It is also imperative that the infected individual and his sexual partner are treated simultaneously to avoid a "ping-pong" effect of reinfection.

There are some measures that may be helpful in preventing gonorrhea. Washing the genital area with soap and water before and especially after intercourse can be of some use in prevention. Urinating right after sex may also be helpful, especially for the male. A vinegar douche may be effective for the woman (but a woman using a diaphragm and/or spermicides should not douche). If a condom is used carefully and regularly, it may provide some protection.

Syphilis

Syphilis is less rampant in the United States than gonorrhea but it is a far more serious disease with more dangerous complications. While gonorrhea is usually localized in the urogenital tract (or throat or anal canal), syphilis is a blood-borne infection and can be carried throughout the whole body. Syphilis is caused by spiral-shaped bacteria of the spirochete family, known as *Treponema pallidum.* Transmission is always through direct contact with another individual, usually through sexual intercourse. After a person has become infected, there are four stages to the disease; primary, secondary, latent, and tertiary (or late). Syphilis is communicable during the primary and secondary stages and sometimes during the latent period.

The point of entry may be a cut in the skin or any of the mucous membranes of the body. The incubation period for the disease ranges from ten to ninety days. The first symptom of the disease, a chancre —an ulcer-like but painless sore—appears during the primary stage. Chancres are usually found on the penis in males and near the cervix or on the labia in females, but they may also occur on the tongue or

---

Summary of Syphilis

Germp: Syphilis is caused by a spirochete called Treponema Pallidum. It requires both warmth and moisture to survive.

	MEN	**WOMEN**
Transmission:	Genital, anal, or oral-genital sexual contact	Vaginal, anal, or oral-genital sexual contact
Symptoms:	First sign: About 3 to 4 weeks after contact, single painless sore (chancre) on or around genital area, in or around the mouth or anus.	First sign: Sometimes chancre does not appear or is internal and thus overlooked.
	Second sign: Generalized skin rash appears. Possibly low fever, sore throat, sores, falling hair.	Second sign: same as male
Complications:	Destruction of the skin, heart, brain, or other organs. Paralysis, insanity, heart disease, and death.	Same as male, as well as infection of unborn child in women who are pregnant (congenital syphilis).
Treatment:	Syphilis can be cured by a variety of antibiotics.	Same as male
Considerations:	Same as those discussed under gonorrhea.	

---

lips, breasts, fingers, or anal canal. These sores contain massive numbers of infectious agents that can be transmitted through direct contact. In some cases, no chancre will develop. It may also go unnoticed, especially in women, where it may occur within the cervix or be hidden in the folds of the labia. Whether or not treatment is given, the chancre will disappear spontaneously within four to six weeks. However, the bacteria are still increasing and spreading throughout the body.

The signs and symptoms of the secondary stage usually appear within six weeks to six months after infection. This stage lasts from three to six months, but the symptoms may recur for several years thereafter. There are a variety of individual symptoms, but the most common ones are a rash that does not itch, a sore throat or fever and general malaise, loss of patches of hair, infectious raised areas around the genitals and anus, and mucus in the mouth, nose, and cervix. Other symptoms include headaches, weight loss, hoarseness, and aching of the muscles, bones, or joints. Again, these symptoms will eventually disappear without treatment as the disease enters its latent stage.

The latent stage most commonly lasts five to ten years, but it may last for the lifetime of the individual. There are no outward signs

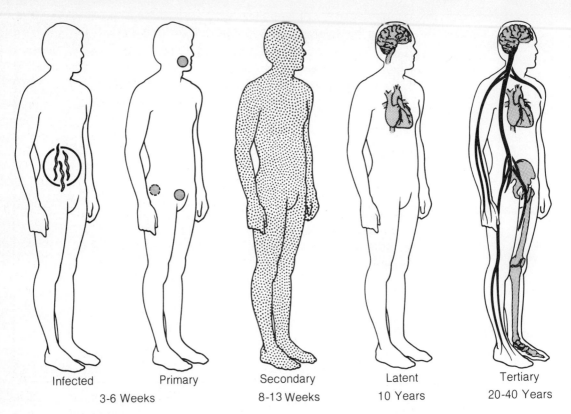

Infected	Primary	Secondary	Latent	Tertiary
3-6 Weeks		8-13 Weeks	10 Years	20-40 Years

FIGURE 15.5 *The Stages of Syphilis. In the early stages, syphilis is easily diagnosed and treated. Unfortunately, in the later stages signs and symptoms are far less obvious and treatment is difficult because the infection has invaded and damaged vital body systems.*

but the bacteria are still present within the body. The disease can be diagnosed during this period only through a blood test. One of the major dangers during this stage is the possibility of transmitting congenital syphilis to a fetus if an infected woman becomes pregnant.

After five or more years, the disease enters the tertiary or late stage, during which the symptoms and complications are most severe. The spirochetes can attack the central nervous and cardiovascular systems, causing various types of heart disease, crippling, insanity, or blindness.

As was mentioned, one of the more dangerous complications of syphilis is the possibility of transmitting the disease to a fetus. Before the eighteenth week of pregnancy the bacteria cannot cross the placenta, so if the mother is treated before this time, the child will not suffer damage. After the eighteenth week the fetus may become infected, but penicillin will also cross the placenta, so treatment of the mother will also cure the fetus.[5] However, if the woman becomes infected late in pregnancy or does not have the disease treated, danger to the fetus is great. Therefore, most states now require blood tests for syphilis before marriage and again at the time pregnancy is confirmed, and congenital syphilis in the United States has almost been eradicated.

The test most commonly used for the diagnosis of syphilis is a blood test that determines the presence of antibodies against the disease. Treatment usually consists of injections of penicillin, but tetracycline or erythromycin are effective if the individual is allergic to penicillin. Any sexual partners should be treated simultaneously to avoid reinfection. Follow-up tests should make sure the disease has been cured.

Again, possible preventive measures include washing the genitalia and douching if possible. A condom is less effective as a preventive measure against syphilis than against gonorrhea because syphilis can enter the body at any point (unlike gonorrhea).

Herpes Simplex

Herpes simplex is a viral disease that is becoming more and more common, especially among young people. There are two types; type 2 is transmitted mainly by sexual intercourse. Herpes simplex 1 usually affects areas above the waist and herpes simplex 2 affects areas below the waist, but each can affect any part of the body (oral-genital sex can cause crossover infection). Herpes appears to be asymptomatic in about 75 percent of infected women; there are no figures for asymptomatic men.

The incubation period for both herpes infections is from two to twenty days. The first symptoms of type 2 may be minor rashes or itching in the genital area. These symptoms are usually followed by the development of a cluster of painful blister-like, fluid-filled lesions or ulcerations. Herpes is believed to be very infectious when the blisters are open. These blisters can be quite painful, especially during intercourse. Symptoms similar to those of the flu may also appear: low-grade fever, aching muscles, and general malaise. Severe cases in the female may cause ulceration of the reproductive organs.

Often the sores heal without treatment in a week to a month, and the disease enters a period of latency. The virus is still in the body and may flare up at various times for several years. These recurrences seem to be related to hormonal changes in women (those

[5] Boston Women's Health Book Collective, *Our Bodies, Ourselves,* New York: Simon and Schuster, 1976, p. 282.

caused by the menstrual cycle, birth control pills and drugs, etc.) or emotional or physical stress (including prolonged intercourse).

Diagnosis is made from the appearance of the sores themselves or through smear or serological tests. When the disease is in a latent period, it becomes very difficult to test for the presence of the virus.

At the present time there is no known cure for herpes. Some treatments can relieve symptom discomfort, and there are other (some of them controversial) medical therapies that may shorten the duration of outbreaks.

Genital herpes has become suspect in the incidence of cervical cancer. Such a correlation would fit in with the theory that certain cancers are caused by viruses. However, this connection is still under debate; Dr. Albert Sabin states that ". . . there is at present no acceptable epidemiological or other evidence that these viruses alone or in conjunction with unknown factors are involved in human cancer."[6]

Trichomoniasis

Trichomoniasis is caused by a one-celled protozoan called *trichomonas vaginalis.* It affects both women and men. Women may have trichomonas in their vaginas without any symptoms and the organism is also found in the male urethra, prostate gland, or seminal vesicles, often (in fact, usually) without symptoms. Trichomoniasis is most often transmitted by intercourse, but it can also be passed on through moist objects such as towels and washcloths or toilet seats.[7]

The symptoms in the female include a thin, foamy, yellowish, often foul-smelling vaginal discharge, itching, and burning. The male is almost always symptomless, but urethritis may occasionally occur.

Treatment is usually with antibiotics or vaginal suppositories. However, early research indicates that the antibiotic most often used (Flagyl) may be linked with gene mutations, birth defects, and/or cancer, so it is recommended that women use vaginal suppositories instead.[8] Both sexual partners should be treated simultaneously to avoid reinfection.

Where to Call for Information or Help

Following is a list of health clinics of Venereal Disease Control Centers in some of the leading cities in the United States.

Atlanta, Ga.
(404) 572-2201

Milwaukee, Wis.
(414) 278-3631

[6] Dr. Albert B. Sabin, "Ethyl Ether Recommended for Use vs. Herpes Simplex Virus Lesions," *Infectious Disease,* January 1976.
[7] Health Collective, *Our Bodies, Ourselves,* p. 138.
[8] Ibid.

Baltimore, Md.
  (301) 494-2713
Berkeley, Calif.
  (415) 845-0197
Birmingham, Ala.
  (205) 324-9571
Boston, Mass.
  (617) 727-2688
Buffalo, N.Y.
  (716) 846-7687
Chicago, Ill.
  (312) 842-0222
Cleveland, Ohio
  (216) 249-4100
Concord, N.H.
  (603) 271-2101
Dallas, Tex.
  (214) 528-4084
Denver, Colo.
  (303) 893-7232
Hartford, Conn.
  (203) 566-6116
Houston, Tex.
  (713) 222-4201
Indianapolis, Ind.
  (317) 630-7192
Kansas City, Kan.
  (913) 321-4803
Los Angeles, Calif.
  (213) 564-6801
Louisville, Ky.
  (502) 584-5281
Memphis, Tenn.
  (901) 522-2987
Miami, Fla.
  (305) 325-2557

Minneapolis, Minn.
  (612) 822-3186
Nashville, Tenn.
  (615) 327-9313
Newark, N.J.
  (201) 733-7584
New Orleans, La.
  (504) 523-6409
New York, N.Y.
  English:
  (212) 269-5300
  Spanish:
  (212) 691-8733
Philadelphia, Pa.
  (215) 546-0141
Phoenix, Ariz.
  (602) 258-6381
Pittsburgh, Pa.
  (412) 355-5781
Richmond, Va.
  (804) 649-4365
San Francisco, Calif.
  (415) 558-3804
Seattle, Wash.
  (206) 583-2590
St. Louis, Mo.
  (314) 453-3523
Syracuse, N.Y.
  (315) 477-7889
  (315) 477-7658
  (4 p.m. to
    8 p.m.)
Washington, D.C.
  (202) 629-7578
Wilmington, Del.
  (302) 571-3400

FURTHER READINGS

Dubos, René. *Mirage of Health.* Garden City, N.Y.: Doubleday & Company, Inc., 1961.

Although more than ten years old, this book remains one of the most readable and comprehensive presentations of the meaning of health as it is related to man's general life and existence.

————. *Man Adapting.* New Haven: Yale University Press, 1965.

The dominant theme of this book, according to the author, "is that the states of health or disease are the expression of the success or failure experienced by the organism in its efforts to respond adaptively to environmental challenges."

Koss, J., Antonovsky, A. and Zola, I. K. (eds.). *Poverty and Health.* Cambridge, Mass.: Harvard University Press, 1969.

The authors contend that present-day health care is a middle-class luxury, but poverty and medical discrimination can be eliminated with the advanced state of American technology.

Maslow, Abraham H. *Toward a Psychology of Being.* New Jersey: D. Van Nostrand Co., Inc., 1962.

The author uses studies of psychologically healthy people and of the healthiest experiences and moments in the lives of average people to demonstrate that human beings can be loving, noble, and creative —that they are capable of pursuing the highest values and aspirations.

Selye, Hans. *The Stress of Life.* New York: McGraw-Hill Book Company, 1956.

This book incorporates the author's well-supported theory on stress as a general factor in the etiology of disease and, in addition, includes his fascinating and logically presented philosophy of life as it relates to health and disease.

Chapter 16

Chronic and Degenerative Diseases

Until recent decades, diseases such as tuberculosis and pneumonia were the leading causes of death in the United States. Today, however, medicine is able to control these diseases more effectively, and the major killers are the chronic and degenerative diseases—specifically cardiovascular disorders and cancer.

CARDIOVASCULAR DISEASE

Cardiovascular diseases include disorders of the heart (*cardio-*) and the blood vessels (*-vascular*). There are three major categories of these conditions: diseases of the heart itself, diseases of the blood vessels, and diseases of the kidneys. Heart and circulatory disorders are the major causes of death in the United States. The major killers are coronary heart disease, degenerative diseases such as rheumatic fever and rheumatic heart disease, arteriosclerosis, hypertension, and stroke.

Causes of Cardiovascular Disease

Research has found that certain factors are implicated in the incidence of the various cardiovascular disorders:

- *age:* the death rate for both sexes climbs with age. The longer a person lives, the more likely it is that extensive arteriosclerosis (hardening of the arteries) will develop
- *sex:* men are more likely than women to suffer from cardiovascular disease. Men contract these diseases an average of twenty years earlier in life than do women, and they are more likely to contract the more severe forms

- *overweight and obesity:* an individual of either sex who is more than 30 percent above his normal weight is twice as likely to develop cardiovascular disease than one who is not overweight. Few studies have shown that moderate overweight itself (without an increase in blood pressure, blood sugar, or cholesterol) does serious harm, but obesity predisposes the individual to high blood pressure, diabetes, increased serum lipids, and high uric acid levels. Consequently, while obesity has not been shown to be an independent risk factor, the usual results of obesity can often lead to heart attacks and other disorders. Furthermore, the Framingham study showed that a subject with an increased blood-cholesterol level who was also overweight faced a greater risk of these diseases than a patient with a high cholesterol level who was of normal weight. Obesity in combination with other dangerous disorders increases the risks.
- *diet:* it is suspected that there is a relationship between high levels of cholesterol in the blood and increased susceptibility to diseases of the arteries and heart. Foods rich in animal fats appear to raise this blood cholesterol level. Some dietary tips related to cholesterol levels and obesity include the following:
  a)   Avoid foods high in cholesterol content.
  b)   Put less emphasis on foods high in unsaturated fats and more emphasis on those high in polyunsaturated fats
  c)   Substitute low-fat or fat-free foods for those high in fats to reduce the total amount of calories received from fats to 25 to 30 percent of the total caloric intake
  d)   Control the total caloric intake to achieve and maintain a desirable weight
- *exercise:* studies have found that heart disease is more prevalent among workers with sedentary jobs than those whose jobs require physical exertion. When one does exercise involving the large back and leg muscles, these muscles act as auxiliary pumps for the circulatory system, taking some of the burden off the heart. Overweight is also more likely to occur when the individual leads a sedentary life. An extensive study in New York showed men who suffered heart attacks but who had always engaged in regular exercise were half as likely to die from the attacks as sedentary men who suffered similar attacks
- *stress:* stress has been shown to produce high blood cholesterol levels. Dr. Meyer Friedman conducted an extensive study in San Francisco and found that individuals could be categorized as either Type A or Type B. Type A individuals are aggressive, competitive, always working against a deadline, and going from one thing to another, never satisfied with what they have accomplished. A Type A individual is far more likely to suffer a heart attack than a Type B, who is relaxed, easygoing, and calm. Exercise can also be helpful in relieving tension, thereby lessening the risk of cardiovascular problems
- *cigarette smoking:* heavy smokers face twice the risk of dying from cardiovascular disease that nonsmokers do. With the increasing number of women who smoke today has come a narrowing of the gap between the number of men and women suffering from these diseases

Are you setting a good example for your kids...

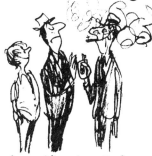

by avoiding cigarettes?

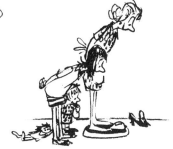

by keeping weight normal?

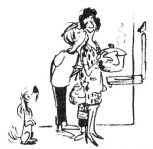

by serving tasty, low-fat foods?

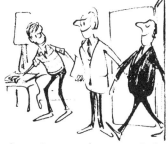

by seeing your doctor regularly?

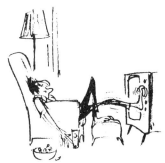

by not being a TV athlete ...

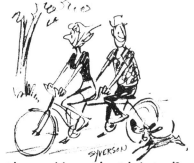

but by exercising moderately instead?

Help your children form good living habits now
to reduce their risk of heart attack later.

GIVE... HEART FUND

FIGURE 16.1

geographic location; it has been found that the mortality rate from coronary heart disease is twice as high in New York City as in the state of New Mexico. Direct causal relationships with various factors have not yet been scientifically established, but tension and atmospheric pollution are possible implications.

Coronary Heart Disease

A coronary heart attack occurs when one of the blood vessels in the heart is blocked, thereby preventing the flow of blood. If a major blood vessel is blocked, death may result. Some of the cells of the heart may die without the blood supply, and the contractions of the heart may cease so that circulation stops. Blockages that affect the smaller vessels are less serious.

Angina pectoris occurs when not enough blood is flowing through the coronary vessels. It causes pain in the chest and shoulders, which may be felt only during exercise or strenuous activity.

Symptoms of a Heart Attack

If people are aware of the symptoms preceding a heart attack, they can be warned and be prepared to deal with it. Among the warning signals are:

- abnormal shortness of breath
- pain in the chest (see Figure 16.2). Many people mistake the warning signals of a heart attack for indigestion
- any unpleasant feelings above the waist that are associated with exercise
- unusual fatigue
- swelling of the feet and ankles (edema), a signal that circulation is poor
- dizziness or fainting spells, caused by lack of oxygen to the brain from poor blood circulation

Any of these symptoms may be caused by other factors than heart disorders, but they can indicate to the individual that he should consult a physician immediately.

Degenerative Cardiovascular Diseases

The degenerative cardiovascular diseases that are the major causes of death in the United States are rheumatic disease, arteriosclerosis, and hypertension.

Rheumatic Fever

Rheumatic fever is an inflammatory disease that occurs most often in children between the ages of five and fifteen. It is caused by strep-

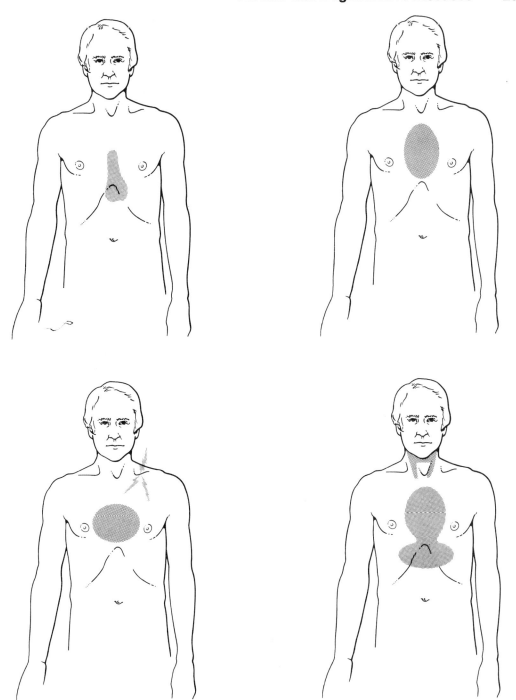

FIGURE 16.2 *The shaded areas in these illustrations indicate pain or pressure patterns involved in heart attacks.*

tococcal infection and commonly follows strep throat or tonsillitis. It can do great damage to the heart valves. After a first attack, one out of every three patients is left with a damaged heart. Rheumatic fever is responsible for about 2 percent of all cardiac deaths.

Prevention of rheumatic fever is therefore an important consideration in reducing heart disease and deaths. Although a strep infection does not automatically mean that a child will contract rheumatic fever, the American Medical Association warns parents to be aware of this possibility with any sore throat or ear infection. A throat culture can determine the presence of streptococcal bacteria; if a child has a positive culture, all the members of the family should also be checked. Penicillin is used to treat such illnesses and has greatly reduced the risk of developing rheumatic fever and heart disease.

Arteriosclerosis and Atherosclerosis

Arteriosclerosis is usually called hardening of the arteries; it involves destructive changes in the walls of these blood vessels. Atherosclerosis is the most common form of arteriosclerosis, affecting the large arteries. The coronary arteries can become narrowed with an accumulation of fatty tissue and other deposits, and damaging blood clots are more likely to occur.

Arteriosclerosis seems to be hereditary. Of the other causative factors, some are more important in the occurrence of vascular disease than others. Long-term anxiety states seem to have an effect on the coronary arteries. Overweight can predispose an individual to conditions resulting in arteriosclerosis. A diet rich in cholesterol increases susceptibility to these diseases. If a person leads a sedentary life, avoiding exercise, excessive amounts of cholesterol and other fatty substances are likely to collect in the artery walls. However, it has been shown that conditioning exercises can help clear the circulatory system of some of these substances. Cigarette smoking is also an important causative factor.

Hypertension

Hypertension means high blood pressure. It can lead to heart or kidney disease, stroke, or other cardiovascular disorders. High blood pressure means the heart must work harder. It also puts excessive pressure on the arteries, damaging them and leading to arteriosclerosis.

Strokes

A stroke occurs when a blood vessel in the brain or neck is ruptured or blocked either partially or completely. When this hap-

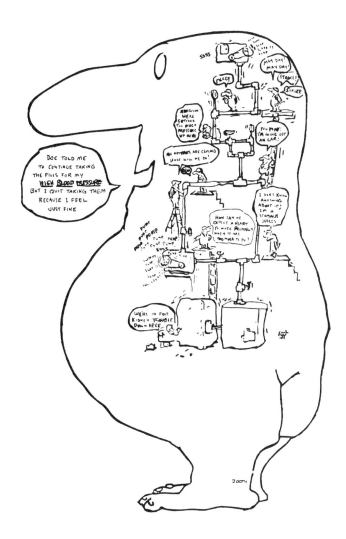

DON'T FOOL AROUND
WITH HIGH BLOOD PRESSURE.
Don't take chances with
a disease you can control.

FIGURE 16.3

pens, brain cells are deprived of blood and are damaged or destroyed. Speech, memory, or vision may be affected, or the part of the body controlled by that part of the brain will be weakened or paralyzed.

A stroke may occur when a blood clot forms in the brain or elsewhere in the body and blocks one of the blood vessels in the brain. Some strokes involve a hemorrhage in the brain, when a weakened blood vessel bursts. Thus, strokes can be related to hypertension, arteriosclerosis, or other of the cardiovascular diseases.

Transient Ischemic Attacks (T.I.A.s)

Some stroke victims may receive a warning signal in the form of a transient ischemic attack, or T.I.A. The symptoms of a T.I.A. are similar to those of a stroke, but they are only temporary, lasting from several minutes to twenty-four hours. Any of the following symptoms may indicate a T.I.A.:

- weakness, clumsiness, or paralysis of one limb or both limbs on the same side
- numbness or tingling in one limb or both limbs on one side
- numbness or tingling of one side, or part of one side, of the face
- sudden alteration of vision
- difficulty in swallowing or speaking
- difficulty in phrasing sentences
- dizziness or fainting
- confusion
- severe unexplained headaches
- a seizure (in a person with no previous history of seizures)

Anyone who experiences these symptoms should immediately consult his doctor. Forty percent of those individuals who experience a T.I.A. will later suffer a stroke.

Prevention and Treatment of Cardiovascular Disease

The prospects for reducing deaths from cardiovascular disease are excellent. Much has been learned through research about causes and prevention, and new developments in medicine have been successfully used for treatment.

The individual can do much to reduce the risk of cardiovascular disease. Lack of exercise, stress, obesity, a high-cholesterol diet, and smoking have all been discovered to be linked to these diseases. If the individual keeps himself in good condition, eats sensibly, and stops or cuts down his smoking, he will be far healthier and less prone to these disorders.

The warning signals of a T.I.A. can be used to cut down on strokes and their debilitating effects. When an individual feels the symptoms of a T.I.A., he can immediately consult a doctor to perform the necessary diagnostic techniques (physical examination, x-rays, brain-wave tracing—an EEG, blood tests). His doctor may find it necessary to consult with a neurologist or neurosurgeon. All these tests should be done as soon as possible after the T.I.A.

Some individuals who experience a T.I.A. may have a correctible condition, so that medical attention can prevent a stroke. Even those whose conditions are not correctible may avoid a stroke. Anticoagulants (drugs that reduce the clotting ability of the blood) can prevent strokes in all but 4 percent of those who have experienced a T.I.A. If a person does suffer a stroke, some of the damaging effects can be lessened with a barbiturate given orally or intravenously immediately after the stroke. Such treatment is only effective for a short time after the stroke—four to six hours afterwards can be too late. Thus, by knowing the signs of a T.I.A. or stroke, an individual can possibly avoid severe aftereffects.

Drug therapy can also help victims of high blood pressure. If this is treated early enough, more severe complications can be avoided. Drugs are useful in treating angina pectoris as well.

Advances in surgery in the last twenty years have helped to save many victims of cardiovascular disease. Until recently, a patient with an aneurysm—a ballooning-out and thinning of the walls of an artery—was almost certain to die within a year from stroke or hemorrhage. Now it is possible to replace the damaged portion with an artificial blood vessel. Open-heart surgery is feasible now because of the development of heart-lung machines that support the patient during surgery. Coronary artery grafts and transplants are now being performed successfully. Congenital or degenerative damage to the valves of the heart can be repaired. Electrical cardiac pacemakers are now implanted to restore a normal beat to a diseased and lethargic heart.

Organ transplants—of the heart, kidneys, lungs, and liver—are becoming more and more successful. Research efforts are even directed toward the development of an artificial heart.

CANCER

Almost 1,300,000 new cases of cancer will be diagnosed in the United States within the coming year. Over 355,000 people will die from cancer within this period.

The term cancer applies to a variety of diseases that are characterized by abnormal cell growth. These cells undergo uncontrolled reproduction and have the ability to spread throughout all parts of

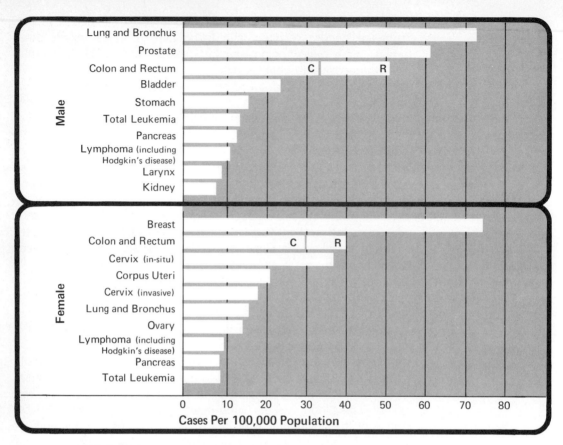

FIGURE 16.4   *Cancer incidence by site and sex, 1969–71 (age-adjusted to 1970 U.S. population). Source: David L. Levin et al.,* Cancer Rates and Risks, *DHEW Pub. No. (NIH)75–691 (2d ed.; Washington, D. C.: Government Printing Office, 1974), Figure 6.*

the body. The difference between the growth of normal cells and cancer cells is that relatively few normal cells multiply continuously; they only reproduce to replace old cells, to maintain a numerical and functional status quo. Cancer cells, in contrast, multiply rapidly, often wildly, and thus begin destroying the normal cells around them. As this process continues, the abnormal cancer cells can invade all parts of the body, in what is called *metastasis.* Once metastasis begins, it is almost impossible to halt the progress of the cancer, and vital organs will be destroyed, resulting in death.

Figure 16.4 shows the major cancer sites in men and women. According to the American Cancer Society, there are over three hundred different forms of cancer; about thirty of these make up 90 percent of all cases. There are three basic types of cancer. *Carcinomas* affect tissue linings, in the breast, prostate, thyroid, lungs, mucous membranes, gastrointestinal tract, etc. *Sarcomas* occur in the connective tissues of the muscles, bones, nerves, and cartilage. *Leukemia* is cancer of the blood.

Not all of these cancers are fatal. The sooner the disease is diagnosed, the better the chances are for survival. For example, 95 percent of all skin cancers can be cured. Lung cancer, on the other hand, is far more likely to result in death. There are about 75,000 cases of lung cancer diagnosed annually in the United States, and this figure is increasing all the time. (This number would be substantially reduced if people stopped smoking.)

Major Forms of Cancer   Progress is definitely being made in treating some types of cancer, while the progress of others is as yet unchecked. According to the American Cancer Society, among the most frequent types of cancer are:

- *lung cancer*—the mortality rate has increased more than fourteen times over the last forty years for men and is steadily rising for women. It now ranks behind only cancer of the colon and rectum and breast cancer as the site of greatest incidence
- *cancer of the colon and rectum*—there has been only a slight change in incidence and mortality rates over the last few years. More of this type of cancer was diagnosed last year than any other type
- *breast cancer*—this is the type of cancer found most frequently among women and causes the most frequent cancer deaths among females. It is the leading cause of all deaths for women forty to forty-four years old and is the second leading cause for several other age groups. Despite all efforts, there has not been any great reduction in the mortality rate over the last thirty-five years; however, when found early, the survival rate from this form can be 85 percent
- *uterine cancer*—deaths from this form are on a steady decline; the rate is one-third what it was thirty-five years ago. The major factors in this decrease are the wide use of the Pap test and better cancer education for women
- *cancer of the pancreas*—this is one of the most frequently fatal forms. For as yet unknown reasons, incidence is up 65 percent in the past generation and 200 percent over the past forty years
- *cancer of the larynx*—very few women are affected by cancer of the larynx. The survival rate for men improved in the 60s but has leveled off since then
- *stomach cancer*—there has been a steady decrease in incidence for both sexes; the death rate is about half what it was twenty years ago. The reasons are as yet unknown
- *cancers of the bladder, kidney, brain, and oral cancer*—the survival rate for all of these improved in the 40s but has plateaued since the 50s
- *prostate and thyroid cancers and Hodgkin's disease*—there has been some decrease in the mortality rate for these three forms

Table 16.1 Reference Chart: Leading Cancer Sites/1974. Source: "Trends in Cancer/1974," American Cancer Society.

Site	Estimated* New Cases 1974	Estimated Deaths 1974	Warning Signal If You Have One, See Your Doctor	Safeguards	Comment
BREAST	90,000	33,000	Lump or thickening in the breast.	Annual checkup. Monthly breast self exam.	Leading cause of cancer death in women.
COLON-RECTUM	99,000	48,000	Change in bowel habits, bleeding.	Checkup including Proctoscopy, especially for those over 40.	Highly curable disease when digital and proctoscopic examinations are included in checkups.
LUNG	83,000	75,000	Persistent cough, or lingering respiratory ailment.	Heed facts about smoking, Annual checkup. Chest X-ray.	Leading cause of cancer death among men. Largely preventable.
ORAL (Including Pharynx)	24,000	8,000	Sore that does not heal. Difficulty in swallowing.	Annual checkup.	Many more lives should be saved because mouth is easily accessible to visual examination.
SKIN	8,000**	5,000	Sore that does not heal, or change in wart or mole.	Checkup, avoidance of overexposure to sun.	Readily detected by observation, and diagnosed by simple biopsy.
UTERUS	46,000***	11,000	Unusual bleeding or discharge.	Checkup, including pelvic exam with Pap test.	With wider application of Pap test, many more lives can be saved from cervical cancer.
KIDNEY AND BLADDER	43,000	16,000	Urinary difficulty or bleeding. Consult doctor at once.	Annual checkup with urinalysis.	Protective measures for workers in high-risk industries help eliminate causes of these cancers.

			Symptoms	Detection	Comments
LARYNX	10,000	3,000	Hoarseness—Difficulty in swallowing.	Checkup, including mirror Laryngoscopy.	Readily curable if caught early.
PROSTATE	54,000	18,000	Urinary difficulty.	Annual checkup, including palpation.	Occurs mainly in men over 60. Can be detected by palpation.
STOMACH	23,000	14,000	Indigestion.	Annual checkup.	A 40% decline in mortality in 20 years, for reasons yet unknown.
LEUKEMIA	21,000	15,000	A cancer of blood-forming tissues characterized by abnormal production of immature white cells. Acute Leukemia strikes mainly children and is treated by drugs which have extended life to as much as ten years. Chronic Leukemia strikes usually after age 25 and progresses less rapidly.		*Drugs or vaccines which might cure or prevent cancers probably would be successful first for Leukemia and Lymphomas.*
LYMPHOMAS	28,000	20,000	These diseases arise in the lymph system and include Hodgkin's and Lymphosarcoma. Some patients with lymphatic cancers can lead normal lives for many years.		

* Based on the *NCI*'s Third National Cancer Survey.
** Estimates vary widely, from 300,000–600,000 or more for superficial skin cancer.
*** If carcinoma-in-situ of the uterine cervix is included, cases total over 86,000.

leukemia—the mortality rate for chronic forms remains unchanged but there is a continuing and dramatic rise in the survival of acute cases

Causes of Cancer

There are many factors that have been implicated in the incidence of cancer, and even more are suspected. Heredity and viruses are suspected to be basic causes and other factors are involved in specific forms of the disease.

Heredity and Cancer

Recent research has shown that some families suffer more cases of cancer than others. This indicates that an individual may inherit a strong predisposition to cancer. The positive aspect of this discovery is that such individuals can be warned of the possibility of cancer and therefore either avoid cancer or have any occurrence diagnosed early enough for treatment. In addition, the existence of a heredity factor can be used in research for prevention and cures.

An inherited predisposition to cancer differs from congenital cancers. With congenital cancers, a special group of tumors can affect the fetus in the womb. Most of these are benign, but some can cause problems in infancy up through young adulthood.

Viruses

Many experts believe at least some forms of cancer are caused by viruses, and evidence to support this theory is increasing. If such viruses exist, theoretically, cancer vaccines can be developed for immunization.

Sunlight

Prolonged exposure to the sun and repeated sunburn has been shown to cause skin cancer. This is most likely to occur in fair-skinned people.

Radiation

There is a greater incidence of cancer among people who work with x-rays and other forms of radiation.

Tobacco Smoking

As was discussed in Chapter 12, tobacco smoking has been linked to both lung cancer and oral cancer. Regular smokers face a far

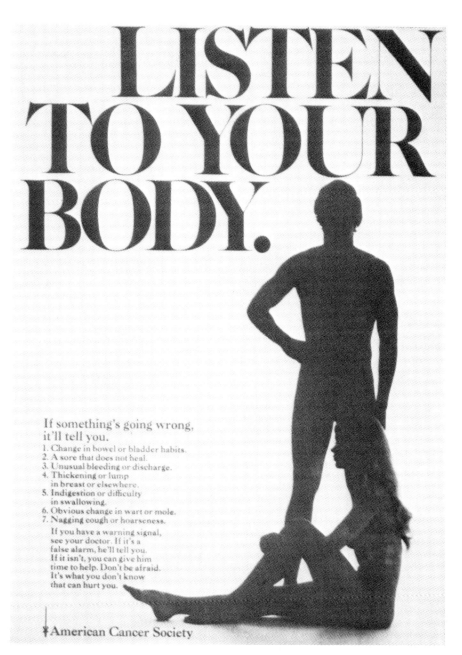

LISTEN
TO YOUR
BODY.

If something's going wrong,
it'll tell you.
1. Change in bowel or bladder habits.
2. A sore that does not heal.
3. Unusual bleeding or discharge.
4. Thickening or lump
   in breast or elsewhere.
5. Indigestion or difficulty
   in swallowing.
6. Obvious change in wart or mole.
7. Nagging cough or hoarseness.

If you have a warning signal,
see your doctor. If it's a
false alarm, he'll tell you.
If it isn't, you can give him
time to help. Don't be afraid.
It's what you don't know
that can hurt you.

American Cancer Society

FIGURE 16.5

greater risk of lung cancer than nonsmokers. Pipe and cigar smokers demonstrate a greater risk of cancer of the lips and tongue.

Hormones and Drugs

Hormone and drug treatments are often used to combat cancers of various types, but recent evidence shows that these treatments can also cause cancer in unaffected individuals. There is suspicion that the hormone programs being used to alleviate the symptoms of menopause may lead to cancer in women. Recently it has been found that many young women are developing vaginal cancer because their mothers were given DES, synthetic estrogen, to prevent miscarriage in pregnancy.

Chemicals and Mycotoxins

There is evidence of a link between chemicals in our food and environment and cancer. Polluted air has been found to contain various carcinogens; certain food additives are now feared to be cancer producing. Many scientists also feel that there is a relationship between mycotoxins (toxic products of fungi) in our food and cancer.

Occupation

Individuals in certain occupations may face a higher risk of certain types of cancer. Workers in certain chemical plants (e.g., those that produce certain plastics or asbestos products) may be breathing in carcinogens all day. Chimney sweeps in England were found to have a higher incidence of cancer because of constant exposure to soot.

Diagnosis of Cancer   During a normal checkup, doctors can detect one-half of all cancers.[1] The earlier a cancer is caught, the more positive the outlook for treatment and cure. An estimated additional ninety thousand lives could be saved if early detection were always possible. Unfortunately, even with regular checkups, early diagnosis is not possible in all cases. Cancers of the larynx, uterus, and bladder are often detected early because of noticeable warning signals, but those of the lung, brain, pancreas, and liver may not be discovered until the later stages.

However, regular checkups and diagnostic procedures can be helpful. Each individual should be aware of the seven warning sig-

[1] *Cancer,* United States Department of Health, Education and Welfare, 1969.

nals for cancer and should know when to consult a doctor. These signals are shown in Figure 16.5.

X-rays are used in the diagnosis of many cancers. Radioisotopes (radioactive atoms of different substances) are also used in both diagnosis and treatment of cancer. Certain radioisotopes injected into the body will be attracted to a tumor if it exists. An x-ray will then show any concentration of the radioisotope in the body.

A rectal examination can be useful for early detection of cancer of the rectum and lower bowel. Since these cancers are among the most prevalent in the United States today, the adult patient should make sure his medical checkup includes a rectal exam.

The mortality rate from uterine cancer has been greatly decreased through cancer education programs and the widespread use of the Pap smear. This form of cancer has a high cure rate if detected early. A change in the pattern of menstrual bleeding or bleeding after menopause may indicate uterine cancer and if these symptoms appear, a doctor should be seen promptly. All women should have a pelvic examination that includes a Pap smear each year. The Pap test, devised by Dr. George N. Papanicolaou, involves scraping some tissue from the cervix and examining the smear in a laboratory. (It is a painless procedure.)

Over 95 percent of all breast cancers are detected first by the patient. Figure 16.6 shows the procedure for detecting a lump in one's breast. Most lumps are not cancerous, but any lump or thickening should be checked by a doctor. He will use palpation in his examination and may then decide upon either of three techniques to screen out the possibility of cancer. *Mammography* is a type of x-ray used especially for detecting breast cancer. *Xeroradiography* is a newer but similar test; it involves less radiation and is more accurate than mammography. These radiation procedures can often identify malignant tumors that otherwise would have gone unnoticed until much later. Figures show that 30 percent of these tumors could not have been otherwise detected at the time of the mammography or xeroradiography. However, recent evidence has suggested a link between use of such radiation techniques and the later appearance of breast cancer. Because of this possible carcinogenic effect, the FDA (as well as the American Cancer Society and the National Cancer Institute) has issued a warning that women under the age of fifty should avoid such tests. In addition, these tests have been shown to be relatively ineffective for younger women.[2] A third method of detection is *thermography,* in which an image is made based on heat variations within the body. Tumorous areas are hotter than healthy areas of the body and will show up lighter.

[2] Boston Women's Health Book Collective, *Our Bodies, Ourselves,* 2d edition, New York: Simon & Schuster, 1976, p. 128.

Did you examine your breasts this month?

If you didn't, you should. If you don't know how, we'll tell you.

Once a month, while you're taking a shower, and your skin is still wet and slippery, begin:

Keep your fingers flat, and touch every part of each breast. Feel gently for a lump or thickening. After the shower, continue with a more thorough check.

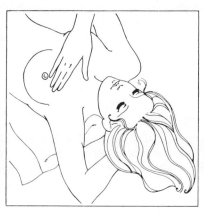

1. Lie down. Put one hand behind your head. With the other hand, fingers flattened, gently feel your breast. Press ever so lightly. Now examine the other breast.

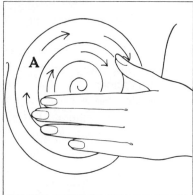

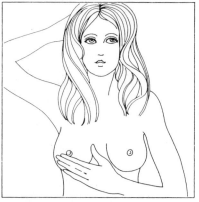

2. This shows you how to check each breast. Begin at the A and follow the arrows, feeling gently for a lump or thickening. Remember to feel all parts of each breast.

3. Now repeat the same procedure sitting up, with the hand still behind your head (right hand if you're checking the right breast, left hand up in checking the left breast).

Don't be afraid. It's what you don't know that can hurt you.

Most women discover breast changes by themselves. If there is a change, the earlier you find it, the better. But some women don't discover it early enough.

You can avoid that mistake by examining your breasts once a month after your menstrual period. Be sure to continue these check-ups after your change of life.

See your doctor as soon as you discover a lump or thickening. In most cases, it turns out to be a perfectly harmless condition. But only the doctor can tell you that for sure. So, for your own peace of mind, see your doctor right away.

Now do your friends a favor: Tell them we'll send free Breast Check booklets to anyone who asks. Just write to your local American Cancer Society Unit; it's in the phone book.

AMERICAN CANCER SOCIETY

FIGURE 16.6

The needle biopsy can be used for detection of breast and some other cancers. A needle is inserted into the lump (often even local anesthesia is unnecessary) and the fluid removed is examined by a pathologist.

Treatment and Cure of Cancer

The major methods of treatment for cancer are surgery, radiation, and chemotherapy (drug therapy). Surgical procedures have accounted for more cures than any other form of treatment, for when the disease is in its early stages it is sometimes possible to remove all of the cancerous cells and prevent any spreading. However, in the later stages, when metastasis has occurred, surgery is less successful. Surgery is often combined with radiation and chemotherapy.

One controversial area now is the treatment of breast cancer. The traditional method has been the radical mastectomy in which the breast, the underlying pectoral muscle, and the lymph nodes of the underarm and chest are removed. Recently, however, many experts have argued that removing only the breast and treating the lymph nodes with radiation therapy is just as successful in preventing the spread of the cancer and causes far less subsequent complications and problems.

Radiation therapy involves the use of x-rays, cobalt treatment, and radioisotopes. Its success is based on the fact that since the cancer cells are rapidly dividing, they are more sensitive to radiation than the normal cells around them.

Radiation has proved effective in controlling cancer of the skin, cervix, esophagus, larynx, pharynx, and sinuses. Hodgkin's disease and certain tumors of the kidney also respond to this treatment.

Over thirty drugs have been found to be successful—often in combination with surgery or radiation therapy—in controlling cancer. There are three main types of drugs used in chemotherapy: hormones, metabolic antagonists, and cell poisons. Hormone injections (and sometimes the removal of hormonal glands) have been successful in restricting, at least temporarily, the spread of cancers of the breast and prostate gland. Metabolic antagonists have been used to slow down or stop the growth of cancer cells. They have often caused remissions of five years or even longer in leukemia patients. Cell poisons can sometimes stop the growth of cancerous cells but they also affect normal cells and are thus quite dangerous.

A new form of chemotherapy has been suggested, involving the specialized use of anticoagulants. It is hoped that this can stop tumor cells from clustering and forming colonies within the blood vessels.

New treatments and drugs are being devised for cancer all the time. Certain drugs have been capable of producing longer and

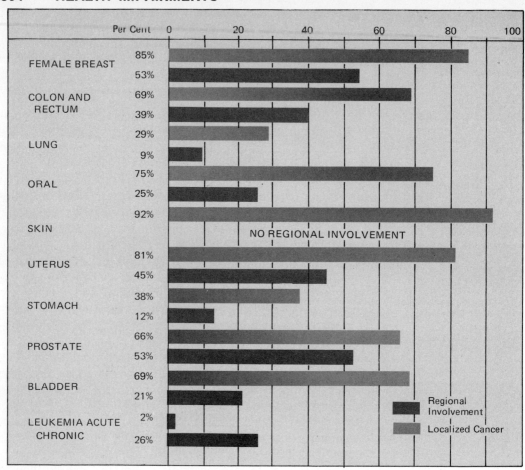

Many patients alive five years after major therapy are classified as cured. This chart shows rates of survival after localized cancer and cancer with regional involvement.

FIGURE 16.7 *Five-year Cancer Survival Rates for Selected Sites (adjusted for normal life expectancy). End Results Group, National Cancer Institute.*

longer remissions for certain cancer patients. Early detection of any type of cancer means that the treatments available will be more effective. Many types of cancer have high cure rates, and as medical technology advances, more and more forms will be easier to eradicate. Realistic hope for cure is important for any cancer victim, and new breakthroughs are occurring.

OTHER CHRONIC AND DEGENERATIVE DISEASES

Other widespread noncommunicable diseases in the United States are diabetes and two respiratory diseases—bronchitis and emphysema. Both chronic bronchitis and pulmonary emphysema are on the rise in this country. Although diabetes has been brought somewhat under control in recent years, it is still a leading cause of death.

Chronic Respiratory Diseases

Chronic bronchitis and pulmonary emphysema, the two most widespread diseases of the respiratory system, were discussed in Chapter 12 as they are often the result of heavy smoking. Air pollution and occupational exposure have been found to be causative factors, but tobacco smoking is the most common factor involved.

Briefly, *chronic bronchitis* is an inflammation that causes destructive changes in the bronchial tubes. It produces persistent coughing and irritation that can damage the alveoli and other lung tissues and lead to emphysema. *Pulmonary emphysema* occurs when the alveoli become damaged to the extent that the individual has great difficulty in exhaling the air from his lungs. This causes wheezing and possible bloating of the chest cavity. It also puts a tremendous strain on the victim's heart.

There are numerous drugs that can be successful in the treatment of these diseases. The most effective treatment is removal of the cause—and usually this means tobacco smoking.

Diabetes

Diabetes is a disease that affects 2 to 4 percent of the population of the United States. Many of these people are ignorant of the symptoms of diabetes and consequently are unaware that they have the disease. Diabetes results from a deficiency or lack of insulin in the body, a hormone produced in the pancreas.

Diabetes is related to heredity; most people who are diabetic have a family history of the disease. Most diabetics are over forty and overweight. Children may have the disease; the childhood form is usually more severe than the type that develops later in life.

The most common symptoms of diabetes are excessive thirst and urination, craving for sweets and starches, slow healing of cuts, and tiredness or weakness. Diabetes can be detected with a urinalysis and a follow-up blood test if indicated.

The treatment of diabetes ranges from controlling diet, to drugs taken orally, to injections of insulin. Childhood diabetes usually requires injections of insulin since the body is probably unable to produce any of this hormone. Drugs are given orally in cases where there is a deficiency but not a total lack of insulin production. Some cases can be controlled merely by following proper diet and exercise routines. An older person with a history of diabetes in the family should avoid being overweight, which may disturb the body's metabolism and bring on the disease.

If diabetes is not properly treated or controlled, the individual may suffer from insulin shock or go into diabetic coma. Insulin shock can result from an overdose of insulin or other imbalance within the system. The individual will experience nervousness and trembling, followed by convulsions and coma. Convulsions and coma may be avoided if the diabetic is aware of what is happening and eats food with sugar in it to restore balance to his system. Diabetic coma can occur when the disease is left untreated; unless medical attention is received immediately, it can be fatal. A diabetic coma may come about more slowly than insulin shock; the symptoms can include nausea, thirst, and deep breathing. There is usually a distinctive breath odor (acetone).

If untreated, diabetes can lead to cardiovascular diseases, kidney infection, or blindness. Since the disease can be treated, it is wise to have a regular urinalysis, especially when a family history exists.

CONCLUSION

The etiological patterns of the various chronic illnesses do not lend themselves to as systematic an analysis as do the communicable diseases. The series of events leading to each type of disease condition tends to be highly specific. There are admittedly certain groups of conditions with much in common, such as the various sequels to atherosclerosis, which include coronary heart disease, stroke, and other vascular disorders. Endocrine diseases, metabolic disorders, and the various cancers constitute other natural groupings, but even within these several categories there are often gross differences in the patterns of causation.

The fact that few steps are absolutely essential in the development of any specific chronic or degenerative disease is another characteristic that makes control difficult. Several factors may contribute to a case of heart disease, but they do not constitute a chain that can be attacked at its weakest link. Many cases of cancer seem to involve a genetic propensity, linked with specific types of irritation to tissues, but it is impossible to identify any one factor as essential.

These characteristics generally have prevented any dramatic technological breakthroughs of the magnitude demonstrated with penicillin or the Salk vaccine in the battle against communicable disease. The synthesizing of insulin and the subsequent control of diabetes is a prominent exception to this generalization, but overall, the most effective preventatives of chronic disease consist of multi-faceted programs designed to combat the numerous causes. Those who seek maximum protection against heart disease, for example, must control their weight and intake of saturated fats, refrain from smoking, maintain a program of regular exercise, and secure treatment for any contributory conditions, such as diabetes or hypertension. A similar level of protection against cancer requires that one learn the recognized danger signals and report them promptly to the physician, endure various types of screening procedures, and avoid known carcinogenic agents, such as cigarette tars, radiation, and known occupational threats.

Many of these measures are inconvenient, time-consuming, and expensive, and they seldom provide a degree of assurance comparable to that guaranteed by a single vaccination against some communicable diseases. Even the most conscientious efforts may merely improve the odds or delay the inevitable. The person who understands the basic principles of disease prevention recognizes most of these measures as being worthwhile in terms of improving his chances of survival, but even informed people disagree as to the proportion of one's time and effort that should be devoted to these activities. Good water treatment generally protects even the most negligent person from typhoid and he will become immunized against the common communicable diseases if public health authorities make it convenient for him, but enticing him to seek medical care in the absence of some painful or advanced condition may be impossible.

These human failings, together with the general lack of simple medical and technological solutions, necessitate a broad front approach to the control of the chronic diseases. This attack must include:

1. Research efforts directed at both the discovery of root causes and improved means of prevention and treatment.
2. The control of all dangerous environmental pollutants, including those affecting air, water, food, and noise levels.
3. Improvement of the health care system to increase the degree to which present medical knowledge can be applied. This requires more doctors and supporting medical personnel, the improvement of methods of financing medical care, and the upgrading and continued development of medical facilities.
4. Improved methods of educating the general public in the individual and community efforts needed to combat these diseases. These efforts must include school programs, public health pro-

grams, and appropriate educational activities by other public service oriented associations.

The multitude of specific measures implied by these four steps will be difficult and expensive to implement fully. However, such a program seems to be at the present time the only way to combat the chronic and degenerative diseases.

FURTHER READINGS

Friedman, Meyer and Rosenman, Ray. *Type A Behavior and Your Heart.* Greenwich, Conn.: Fawcett Publishers, Inc., 1974.

Offers a full discussion of the Type A personality. Excellent reading.

Moore, George E. *The Cancerous Diseases.* Belmont, Calif.: Wadsworth Publishing Company, Inc., 1970.

This book considers the various aspects of the cancerous diseases and provides the reader with some understanding of cancer as a biological phenomenon.

Relax. New York: The Confucian Press, 1976.

A "how to" book on feeling better by reducing tension and stress.

Rosenbaum, Ernest. *Living With Cancer.* New York: Praeger Publishers, Inc., 1976.

A guide for the patient, the family, and friends.

Thommen, George. *Is This Your Day?* New York: Avon Books, 1973.

Drawing on over fifty years of research and experimentation in the field of biorhythm, the author presents the tools you need for a full understanding of your natural biorhythmic cycles.

Chapter 17

Accidents

Accidents are among the major causes of death throughout the world. In the United States, accidents of all types cause more deaths than any illness except cancer and cardiovascular disease. Automobile accidents are a major cause of injury and death, especially for young people. Household accidents affect 180,000 people a year and result in 27,000 fatalities. This chapter is concerned with some of the causes of such accidents as well as the means of preventing them.[1]

FACTORS AFFECTING ACCIDENT RATES

Sex, age, and time of day or year all affect the accident rate. Factors such as emotional stress are also important. Tension and depression can occupy a person so that an accident is more likely to occur. Fatigue and ill health also contribute.

Research on accidents has found the following facts to be significant:

1. The incidence of accidents for people of either sex and any age increases from a low point in February to high points in June and August.
2. Nonindustrial accidents increase in occurrence from a low at 5:00 a.m. to a high at 5:00 p.m.
3. Fifty percent of all accidents involve people under twenty-five; 75 percent involve individuals under thirty-five. Twenty-one is the peak age for accidents.
4. Males have a significantly higher incidence of accidents than females.

[1] The Appendixes contain information on emergency care of the sick and injured and on procedures to be used during natural disasters.

The Accident Prone   Insurance statistics show that only 20 percent of all accidents occur because of mechanical failure or causes. The other 80 percent are related to environmental factors and, in great part, to personality factors. Some people are more likely to be involved in accidents (and are in more accidents) than others—which is accident proneness caused by psychological factors. For such people, an accident has a definite subconscious meaning. It may be a bid for attention, a call for help, compensation, etc. An accident can be viewed as a solution to some sort of unresolvable conflict. The results are usually negative (though positive results include removal from a threatening situation or the attention and sympathy received), but the accident seems easier to deal with than the original problem.

The accident prone person thus may put himself in dangerous or risky situations. Before one of these "self-initiated" accidents occurs, the individual may exhibit increased anxiety and depression in reaction to the conflict he is facing. He may be involved in smaller mishaps, which can serve as a cue to those around him and an unconscious plea for rescue from the situation.

HOUSEHOLD ACCIDENTS

Table 17.1 shows the types of household accidents responsible for the majority of fatalities. Causes of death include falls, fires, suffocation, poisoning, firearms, and other miscellaneous accidents.

Falls   Falls in the home account for 75 percent of all types of fatal falls. The most common causes of such falls are standing on chairs or other unstable objects, skidding on small rugs or slippery surfaces, and tripping over a torn carpet or objects left on the floor or stairs. Improperly lit stairways can contribute to the rate of these accidents.

The possibility of dangerous falls in the home can be reduced by taking some simple precautions. A firm stepladder should be kept handy. (Over 180,000 accidents in the home involve unstable ladders.) Only non-skid rugs and floor waxes should be used. Adequate lighting can be installed. Children should be taught the dangers of climbing on unstable objects. Since approximately 85 percent of the victims of fatal falls are over sixty-five years old, special consideration should be given to accident prevention for the aged. They need handrails as well as good lighting on stairways. Objects left on the floor or stairs are more hazardous to the aged. People are more likely to break bones or suffer other severe consequences from a fall as they get older.

Table 17.1 *How People Were Killed in Home Accidents. Source:* Adapted from *Accident Facts,* 1973 Edition, (Chicago, Ill.: National Safety Council), pp. 80–81.

Type of Injury		Number of People
All Types	All deaths due to accidents in the home or on home premises.	27,000
Falls	Falls on the same level as well as falls from one level to another (down stairs, from roof, from ladder).	9,800
Fires	Burns and deaths associated with fires.	5,700
Suffocation (Ingested)	Deaths from accidental ingestion or inhalation of objects or foods resulting in obstruction of the respiratory passages.	2,600
Suffocation (Mechanical)	Deaths due to smothering by bed clothes, thin plastic materials, cave-ins, mechanical strangulation, or confinement in closed spaces.	800
Poisoning (Solids and Liquids)	Deaths from medicines, and commonly recognized poisons as well as mushroom and shellfish poisoning.	3,100
Firearms	Deaths due to firearms accidents, many of which occur while cleaning or playing with guns.	1,400
Poisoning (Gases and Vapors)	Deaths caused principally by carbon monoxides due to incomplete combustion involving cooking stoves, heating equipment, and standing motor vehicles.	1,100
Others	The accidental deaths making up this group are caused principally by drowning, burns from hot substances, electric current, and blows by falling objects.	2,500

Fires and Burns   Fires account for a large number of household injuries or deaths. One-fifth of all household fatalities result from burns. Severe burns are dangerous not only because of the immediate wound, but also because of the possibility of accompanying shock and toxicity that may affect the kidneys, liver, and blood.

Carelessness is often the cause of household fires and burns. A pack of matches may ignite in a person's hands because he did not close the cover. Cigarettes are not always completely out when thrown into a wastebasket. Many people store oily rags—a fire hazard —and do not follow directions or cautions when using flammable liquids. Grease fires in the kitchen are common—these should be doused with salt, not water, which can splash and spread the flames. Again, special attention should be paid to children and the elderly— 50 percent of those who die from burns are under five years old or over sixty-five.

Suffocation   Mechanical and other types of suffocation are the third major cause of household fatalities. Many people suffocate because food has become lodged in their throat, blocking the air passages. The box

Save a Life: The Cafe Coronary

A few years ago Dr. Heimlich developed a technique for expelling food lodged in an individual's throat. This experience is often referred to as the cafe coronary because the victim may seem to be having a heart attack. He is unable to speak and unable to expire air from the nose or mouth.

In Dr. Heimlich's technique, the person trying to help should grasp the victim around the waist from the back, making a fist with one hand. He should push his fist partly into the victim's abdomen under the rib cage, while holding his own wrist with his other hand. He then "hugs" the person choking, to rapidly and forcibly compress the abdomen. The maneuver forces the diaphragm upward, thereby producing a bellows effect to dislodge the foreign body from the lungs or throat. The maneuver is simple to learn to do properly (although the person should be careful not to grasp the victim too roughly) and it may save a life. (See Figure 17.1.)

If the victim is a small child or an infant, an alternate method can be used. It is occasionally possible to dislodge a piece of food or other foreign body from the larynx of a child by holding him upside down and striking him sharply on the back, so that he will cough hard. Forcible compression of the abdomen in this position sharply elevates the diaphragm in the chest to produce the expulsive expiratory force.

on this page demonstrates emergency procedures to be used if such a situation arises.

Most victims of mechanical suffocation are children under five. Many of these deaths involve suffocation from thin plastic garment bags. Parents should be aware of such potential dangers. Children are also likely to choke on pieces of food or small objects they have picked up; the parent should make sure the child is able to properly chew whatever types of food are given him. (See Figure 17.1 for the technique to use if a child is choking.)

Poisoning   Poisonings of all types account for over 4,000 fatalities yearly. This includes deaths from both medicines and other household products and gases.

Many children die or suffer severe injuries from eating aspirin and other medicines or swallowing household cleansers and other such substances. All of these hazardous products should be kept locked up and out of the reach of children. Child-proof caps are one partial solution to this problem. Adults are also involved in poisoning deaths, often because they pay little attention to proper dosage limits of medicine or to cautions on labels of poisonous substances.

Gas appliances can be dangerous. If ventilation is inadequate, if the flame on a gas stove is accidentally extinguished, or if the appliance is in poor condition, poisoning can result from the fumes. Running a car engine in a closed garage can build up a lethal level of carbon monoxide in the air.

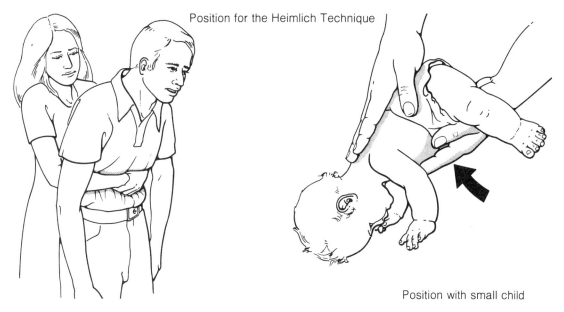

Position for the Heimlich Technique

Position with small child

FIGURE 17.1

Firearms   Firearms are another cause of household deaths and injuries. Many of these accidents involve small children who have found a parent's gun—one that was supposedly well hidden. Adults too are involved in these accidents, when cleaning a gun or using one when they are inexperienced.

Miscellaneous   Electric shocks can often be lethal. Many of these accidents
Causes of   occur in a home workshop. Power tools should only be operated by
Household   a capable adult. These tools should always be properly grounded,
Accidents   and the individual using them should know what he is doing. A person using an electric hair dryer, razor, or other small appliance should keep away from water in the sink or tub. Electrical outlets can be dangerous; household current is strong enough to kill a human being. Therefore, protective covers should be installed on unused outlets when children are around.

Garden tools can be a source of harm. Rakes and hoes should always be left with the teeth pointed downward. Power mowers and hedge clippers should be operated with caution.

Other accidental deaths in the home can be caused by drowning, blows from falling objects, etc. Many of these accidents can be avoided by using common sense and accident prevention tactics.

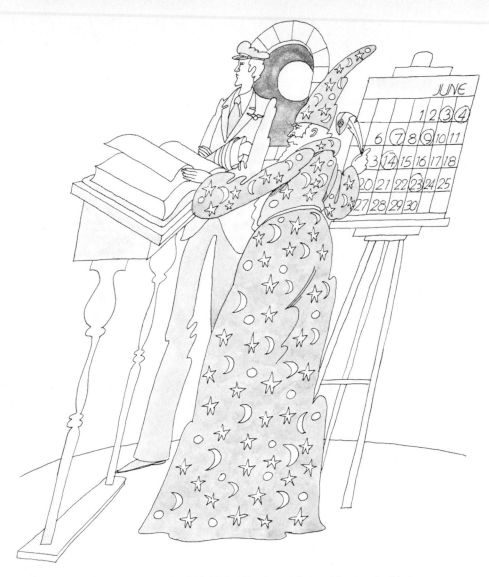

THE FRIENDLY SKIES OF BIORHYTHMS. The theory that accidents and misjudgments can be avoided by observing the "critical" days of a person's physical, emotional and intellectual cycles continues to gain acceptance. United Airlines has recently set aside one of their computers to monitor biorhythms of 28,000 employees. During a 12-month study, the airline found it could cut accidents in half simply by discussing safety with workers during their negative biorhythm periods.

SOURCE: *Practical Psychology for Physicians,*
June 1975, p.3.

FIGURE 17.2

AUTOMOBILE ACCIDENTS

Highway fatalities are the number one accidental killers in the United States. What are some of the causes of these accidents, and how can they be prevented?

Personal Factors Involved in Automobile Accidents

MacFarland and Moore have found four categories of personal factors involved in the "accident process." These categories—characteristics of age, unusual personal susceptibility, personal and social adjustment, and temporary factors influencing behavior—have relevance to most types of accidents but can be particularly applied to a discussion of the causes of automobile accidents.

Age is an especially important factor in automobile accidents. Males under thirty (especially single males from eighteen to twenty-three) are most often involved in auto accidents. This greater frequency of involvement can be attributed in part to immaturity and/or inexperience. Another period of great susceptibility to automobile accidents is age seventy-five and over. Recent research suggests that this increased susceptibility is caused by central nervous system changes that affect the organization of perceptions.

Figure 17.3 shows the percentage of children under age fifteen who were involved in various types of traffic accidents. Injuries suffered as pedestrians or cyclists are the major categories for this age group. Studies have found that children suffer fewer injuries as passengers in automobiles than adults in comparable situations. The types of injuries sustained also differ because of variations in the center of gravity (as well as size).[2]

Accident proneness applies to those involved in auto accidents as well. Typical characteristics of this group such as impatience and a below-average ability to tolerate tension are reflected in both driving and pedestrian behaviors.[3]

An individual's personal and social adjustment is also a factor in automobile accidents. Poor adjustment is often reflected in reckless driving. One study comparing accident-free drivers with individuals involved in many accidents found that 66 percent of the high-accident group was known to local courts or health and service

[2] Ryan, "Children in Traffic Accidents," *Pediatrics*, November 1969, p. 847.
[3] Ross MacFarland and Roland Moore, "The Epidemiology of Accidents," in Maxwell Halsey, ed., *Accident Prevention*, New York: McGraw-Hill Book Co., 1961.

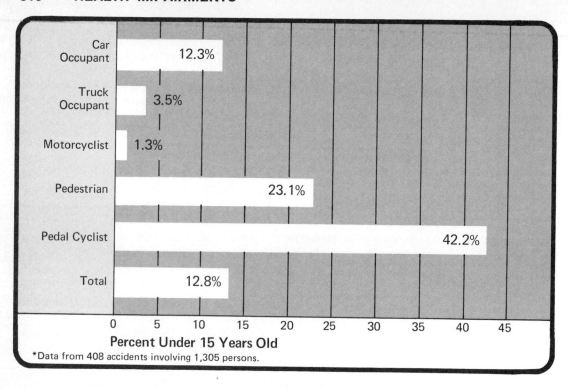

FIGURE 17.3 *Percentage of children injured in various types of traffic accidents.*

agencies for reasons in addition to their accident rate. Only 9 percent of the accident-free group was known to these same agencies.[4]

There is increasing evidence that insecure, neurotic, and psychotic individuals often use the automobile (usually ones with aggressive names such as Charger or Firebird) as a socially acceptable means of drawing attention to themselves and striking back at a society or individual they feel has done them an injustice.[5] An insecure and hostile driver may roar out of intersections and parking lots, screech to a halt at stop signs, or pass with barely enough room to avoid an oncoming car. A paranoid driver may become enraged by a slow driver and attempt to "get back" at him by tailgating or otherwise interfering with his driving. Society (e.g., by referring to automobile *accidents* or drunken *driving*) removes any blame from the driver and places the fault on accidental causes, liquor, or vague

[4] W. A. Tillman and G. E. Hobbs, "The Accident Prone Automobile Driver," in W. Haddon et al. eds., *Accident Research: Methods and Approaches,* New York: Harper and Row, 1964.
[5] Stephen A. Franzmeier, "Driving under the Influence of Emotion," *Today's Health,* October 1969.

qualities such as carelessness. By not condemning the individual driver himself as the direct cause of a fatality or collision, society allows the unstable individual to continue driving unsafely, free of condemnation.

In view of this, it is understandable that young adults between eighteen and twenty are involved in more accidents annually than any other age group. It is during these years that individuals experience a great deal of turmoil and frustration stemming from conflict and societal pressures. The hazard increases when these young people begin to regard their cars as extensions of their personalities, suitable for expressing their own inner tensions.

The relationship between physical defects or disease and accident rates is largely unknown. There is some medical opinion that undiagnosed epilepsy and diabetes may account for many blackouts that have caused accidents, but as yet there is no hard data to support this conclusion. Even so, some states have considered screening for physical problems during license application and renewal. This could be especially important in relation to the elderly, who have been implicated in a large number of traffic accidents.

Temporary factors affecting behavior are also important in automobile accident rates. Although *fatigue* may not be so great as to cause a driver to fall asleep at the wheel, it can have a direct effect on his perceptions and reaction time, making him an unsafe driver. Studies of the effects of fatigue on driving have been limited in so far as this is a difficult state to measure quantitatively.

A person's changing emotional state can be directly related to driving performance. There is increasing statistical support to show that the vast majority of motor vehicle accidents are primarily attributable to the emotional state of the driver.[6] Tension can result in recklessness and inattention.

Alcohol and Drugs

Alcohol is a major cause of automobile accidents. Some of the effects of alcohol on a driver and the related statistics were discussed in Chapter 13. Drunken drivers cause some 800 crashes yearly. Problem drinkers are only a small minority of the population but this minority can be implicated in a majority of all traffic accidents.[7]

Social attitudes still find drinking and driving as acceptable. Yet the drunken driver faces odds of one in five of being involved in an auto accident. (See Figure 17.4.)

[6] Ibid.
[7] U.S., Department of Transportation Research.

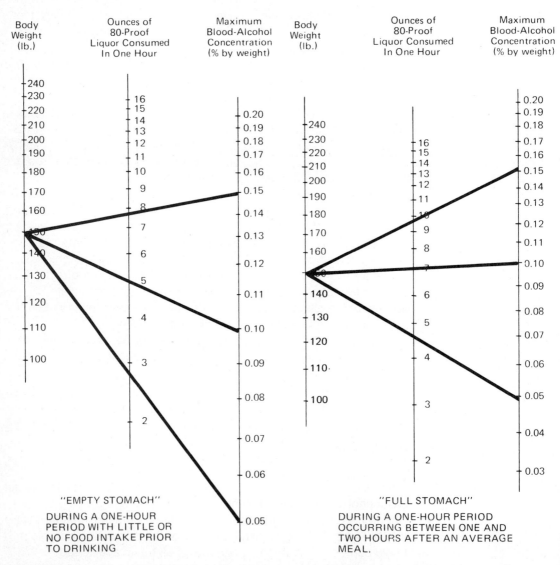

| Body Weight (lb.) | Ounces of 80-Proof Liquor Consumed In One Hour | Maximum Blood-Alcohol Concentration (% by weight) | Body Weight (lb.) | Ounces of 80-Proof Liquor Consumed In One Hour | Maximum Blood-Alcohol Concentration (% by weight) |

"EMPTY STOMACH"
DURING A ONE-HOUR PERIOD WITH LITTLE OR NO FOOD INTAKE PRIOR TO DRINKING

"FULL STOMACH"
DURING A ONE-HOUR PERIOD OCCURRING BETWEEN ONE AND TWO HOURS AFTER AN AVERAGE MEAL.

FIGURE 17.4 *How to Tell What Your Blood Level Is After Drinking. Lay a straightedge across your weight and number of ounces of liquor you've consumed on empty or full stomach. The point where the edge hits in right-hand column is your blood alcohol level. At .05 percent many persons begin to have driving ability affected. At .10 percent, you're at an illegal level in 15 states. In 28 other states, a .15 percent level is considered presumptive guilt of drunken driving. (From* The Safe Driving Handbook, *New York: Grosset & Dunlap Pub., 1970, p. 33.)*

It's official: The caffeine in a couple of cups of coffee will help you stay awake at the wheel and make a better and more alert driver of you. Researchers from Massachusetts General Hospital and the Injury Control Research Laboratory, in the Department of Health, Education, and Welfare, confirmed what many have suspected in tests with a driver simulator at a federal laboratory in Rhode Island. The investigators gave four fast-reaction tests to 24 male drivers, then fed them the equivalent of two cups of coffee and found "significantly enhanced performance." The drivers' reactions were even better after four cups, the report said. However, the researchers did not advise the use of caffeine pills, which they said made users nervous and irritable.

Source: Today's Health, January 1975.

The effects of other forms of drug abuse on driving have not yet been studied in depth, but are sure to be significant.

Preventing Auto Accidents

Preventing automobile accidents depends on the car and even more on the driver himself.

The Car

In 1966 Ralph Nader published a report on the automobile industry, *Unsafe at Any Speed.* He found that most money had been invested in styling, to the detriment of safety research and design. Since the book's publication, federal legislation has made certain safety features mandatory on all cars. Devices such as dual braking systems and collapsible steering wheels are becoming standard. Recent research has involved the air bag as a protective safety device. There is some controversy about its efficiency, but it is expected to become standard equipment. Figure 17.5 shows how the air bag works.

The Driver

Obviously, whether or not a car can be made safer is of little importance if the driver is not concerned with safety. Statistics have shown that seatbelts cut down considerably on automobile injuries and fatalities, yet many people infrequently or never wear them. Some people believe seat belts are only necessary on long, highspeed trips, but actually there are proportionately fewer accidents on major highways than on other roads. The National Safety Council has found

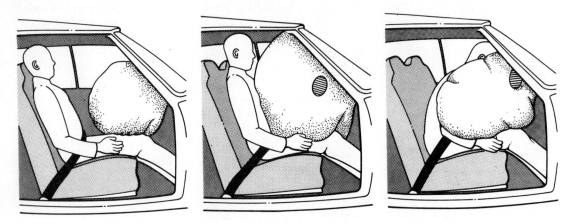

FIGURE 17.5 *The air bag is expected to be offered as optional equipment in all cars. The bag, a large balloon-like device, inflates in 40 thousandths of a second after collision, cushioning the occupants from the impact. The bag is triggered by a sensor behind the front bumper.*

that the majority of traffic deaths occur within twenty-five miles of home and at speeds of 40 miles per hour or less.[8]

The Energy Crisis and Highway Safety

In December 1973, in the height of a fuel crisis, the nationwide speed limit was reduced to 55 miles per hour. One of the side effects of this energy-conserving measure was a dramatic reduction in highway fatalities. Highway deaths dropped almost 25 percent from 1973 to 1974; the percentage of fatalities was the lowest since statistics were first recorded, in 1933. Other factors, such as a reduction of travel in general, were also involved, but the lower speed limit was definitely an important contributor to this drop.

Although the speed limit has remained at 55, more and more people have ignored it in the past few years. Consequently, the fatality rate has increased again. It is unfortunate that people are losing their interest in a measure that can save not only energy but also lives.

[8] National Safety Council, *Seat Belts Save Lives,* Chicago: The National Safety Council, pp. 1–6.

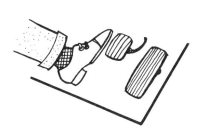

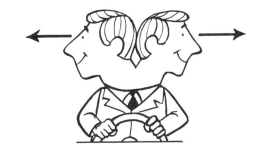

As you approach an intersection, have your foot off accelerator and over brake pedal to give yourself an extra split second of reaction time.

Look first to the left, then to the right, since traffic from the left is closer to you and crosses your path first.

An extremely frequent and costly accident, in terms of liability suits, is collision with the vehicle ahead. Here are four simple steps that will help you avoid being involved in a collision with the car ahead of you:

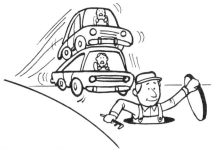

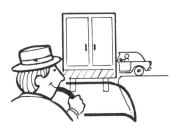

1. Stay alert: Watch for signs from the driver ahead as to what he intends to do. Is his turn signal on? Are his brake lights lit? Is this driver in front of you gradually drifting to the right or left as if to prepare for a turn?

2. Stay ahead of the situation: Look beyond the driver ahead to see situations that may force him to act quickly and become a threat to you. Are there vehicles in the roadway or on shoulder? Are there intersections ahead? Are there parked cars or pedestrians present?

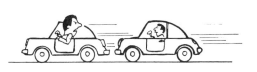

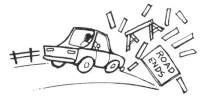

3. Stay back: Allow one car length — using your own car's length as a measure — for every 10 miles of speed. And allow more distance in adverse weather or poor road conditions.

4. Start stopping sooner: Apply brakes the instant you see a hazard developing. Apply them gradually so you don't throw your car into a spin or grind to a stop so quickly that you risk a rear-end collision with the car following.

FIGURE 17.6 *Tips from Defensive Driving Course Workbook.* (Today's Health, *February, 1969.*)

> Traffic deaths for the first half of 1974 have dropped by almost 25 percent compared with the same period in 1973, The National Safety Council announced. The council said that 6,000 fewer fatalities have been reported this year than last, and the death rate per mile has dropped to its lowest since 1933, when statistics were first gathered on highway deaths. Council president Vincent Tofany said the lower speed limit of 55 miles per hour was definitely a "major factor" in the reduced traffic toll.
>
> *Source: Modern Medicine,* September 30, 1974

MOTORCYCLE ACCIDENTS

The use of two-wheeled motor vehicles—motorcycles, motor scooters, and motorized bicycles—for transportation, touring, and sports activities has reached a new peak of popularity in the United States in recent years. With this rise has come a tremendous increase in motorcycle fatalities (an increase of over 80 percent in four years). The death rate for cyclists is five times as great as that for automobile drivers and pedestrians combined.[9] Most of these fatalities involve teenagers or young adults.

Types of Motorcycle Accidents   Accidents in which the motorcycle overturns or leaves the highway account for nearly one-third of all fatalities. Only a small percentage of the deaths can be attributed to collisions with fixed objects. Collisions with other motor vehicles, however, account for about three-fifths of all motorcycle deaths.

A cyclist who is experienced and properly equipped is less likely to be fatally injured, but even when the accident is not fatal, the injuries sustained are unlikely to be minor.[10] The motorcyclist has little protection and is usually thrust forward with his head receiving the major impact. Arms, hands, legs, and feet are also usually injured, but head injuries are by far the most serious (more severe than those suffered in automobile accidents).

Safe Motorcycling   There are no national standards concerning motorcycles; instead, each state makes its own laws, so these may vary greatly.

[9] National Safety Council, Statistics Division, "Motorcycle Facts," Chicago: National Safety Council, August 1969.
[10] Robert Waltz, "Meeting the Motorcycle Menace," *Journal of American Insurance,* March/April 1967, p. 23.

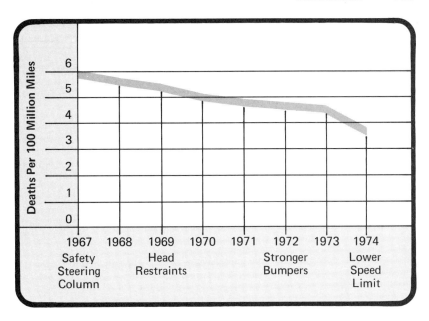

FIGURE 17.7 *Highway death rates, 1967–1974. Source: National Safety Council.*

The National Highway Safety Council has established certain recommended standards:

1. Each operator must pass a special examination for motorcycle operation and must have a special license or a regular license properly endorsed.
2. An approved helmet and eye protection device must be used.
3. Each motorcycle must be equipped with a rear-view mirror.
4. Each passenger must wear an approved helmet and be provided with a seat and foot rest.
5. Each motorcycle must be inspected when originally registered and at least annually thereafter.

A motorcycle operator often directly contributes to his own accidents. He should be familiar with his vehicle and its capabilities and be aware of its operation. He should be aware of accident avoidance techniques and learn to analyze the movements of others in traffic. Studies have shown that over 20 percent of those involved in accidents are riding for the first or second time, often on a rented or borrowed cycle. The individual learning to ride a motorcycle should study the vast amount of educational material available first. Then he should practice on roads that are not heavily traveled, accompanied by an experienced driver.

Mopeds

Mopeds (an acronym from MOtorized PEDal bike) have been popular in resort areas for years and they are now becoming attractive to the American consumer.

One of the positive features of mopeds is that they get excellent gas mileage—from 125 to 150 miles per gallon—and are capable of going up to 30mph. On the negative side is the fact that people are having more and more minor and major accidents while riding them. This may be partially caused by the fact that some states do not require a driver's license, use of helmets, knowledge of rules of the road, etc., for those driving mopeds. Therefore, for those who now own a moped (or are considering the purchase of one), the safety tips offered on motorcycles as well as bike safety should be consulted.

Education for the automobile driver can also help cut down motorcycle accidents. Among the major causes of collisions between cars and motorcycles are surprise or even panic on the part of the automobile driver from the unexpected appearance of a cycle or from its loud noise, improper estimation of the cyclist's speed, and failure to yield the right of way to a cyclist. The cyclist can help the motorist by making sure his motorcycle has mufflers, by driving defensively, and by using his headlights at all times so that other drivers will be more aware of him.

BICYCLE ACCIDENTS

The almost 420,000 people who suffered bicycle-related injuries requiring hospital treatment in a recent year, were injured because of malfunction of the bicycle, unsafe riding, or collisions.

The mechanical difficulties most likely to occur are: brake failure, parting of the steering mechanisms, chain slippage, problems with the pedals or wheels, and hesitation in the shifting mechanism.

A rider is more likely to lose control if his bike is too large, he is riding double, or he is performing stunts. His feet or clothes may become entangled with the bike and cause an accident. Colliding with a fixed obstacle, another bike, or a car are all possibilities.

Bicycle Safety   The U.S. Consumer Product Safety Commission has set up standards that should lead to safer bicycling. These guidelines apply to selection, use, and maintenance.

Selection

1. Buy the right size bike for the user.
2. Buy the type of bike for the type of riding to be done.
3. Use retro-reflective tape to give yourself every chance to be recognized as a bike driver.
4. Always be sure your head and taillights work.
5. Check hand/foot brake for ease of operation and freedom from jams.
6. Avoid plastic pedals, rubber or metal pedals with toe straps are preferable.
7. Look for long protruding bolts or sharp fenders.
8. Avoid a bike with gear controls or any other protruding attachments mounted on the top tube of a man's bike.

Use

1. Observe all traffic laws, just as an automobile.
2. Don't ride double or stunt on a machine not built for these activities.
3. Ride near the curb in the SAME direction as traffic.
4. Select routes for your travel which are not main traffic arteries.
5. Walk your bike through busy intersections and left turn corners.
6. Avoid riding in the rain, brakes are often unresponsive.
7. Strive to make you and your bike visible in the dark.
8. Avoid the use of long or loose clothing when driving your bike.
9. Be aware of large openings in sewer grates near the curb.

Maintenance

1. Routine adjustments and a series of checks is essential for safe riding. An experienced bicycle repair shop should do complicated or technical repairs.

NATIONAL AGENCIES CONCERNED WITH ACCIDENT PREVENTION

Various agencies and organizations have been set up to deal with accident prevention and education. The accident prevention program of the U.S. Public Health Service has developed over two decades. In 1956, the Surgeon General set up the National Advisory Committee on Accident Prevention. In 1961, the Division of Accident Prevention in the Bureau of State Services was established "to strengthen and expand existing programs in accident prevention and to provide more assistance to state and community health departments and other agencies in developing and improving local accident prevention work."[11] The Division performs safety research as well as provides grants for other research programs.

The Consumer Products Safety Commission checks the safety of foods, drugs, cosmetics, and medical devices. It also makes sure that hazardous household products are adequately labeled to warn the user of potential dangers (flammability, poisoning, etc.).

The National Safety Council, organized in 1913, was the first permanent organization with a program devoted entirely to accident prevention. For example, in regard to highway safety, the council has suggested that a national program be effected to (1) judge recklessness and foolhardy driving by the same standards as those applied to murder; (2) emphasize the sense of refraining from driving while emotionally distressed; and (3) suggest means of letting off steam other than driving. The council is made up of a number of sectional organizations that develop its various programs.

There are numerous other organizations promoting safety. Among these are the American Automobile Association (AAA), the National Commission on Safety Education (established in 1944), and the Center for Safety Education at New York University.

FURTHER READING

The Safe Driving Handbook. New York: Grosset & Dunlap. 1970.

This book is based on a multi-media training program developed for the U.S. Air Force to promote good driving techniques which will reduce traffic accidents and fatalities.

[11] U.S., Department of Health, Education and Welfare, *Indicators—Accidents,* Washington, D.C.: U.S. Government Printing Office, December 1964/January 1965, p. 10.

7

ENVIRONMENTAL
HEALTH

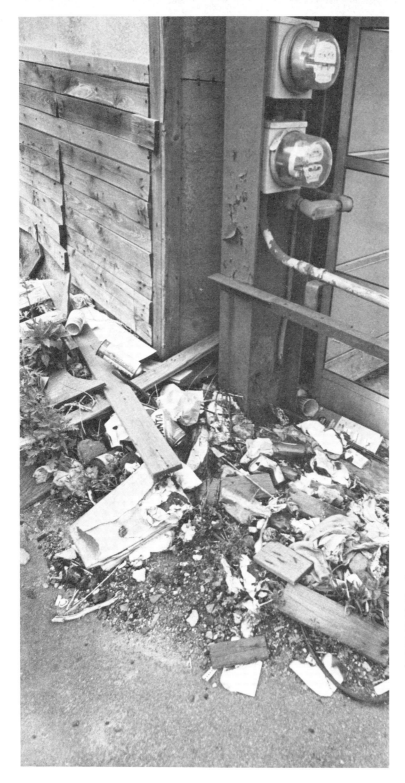

The car has made our cities
uninhabitable. It is also
the best way to escape
them. Hurry and take to the
roadless area, because
it won't be roadless long.
Too much demand.

Jerry and Renny Russell
On the Loose

Chapter 18

Population and Pollution

Once man believed the air and the oceans were boundless, the bounty of nature never ending. Today we have discovered that the world is no more than a fragile sphere of limited resources surrounded by the empty lifelessness of endless space. We know of no other place in the universe that will support us; yet we continue thoughtlessly to destroy our environment in a multitude of ways—careless and wasteful use of precious and irreplaceable resources; pollution of water, air, and silence; destruction of productive farmland in urban and suburban development. This lifestyle can only be called suicidal. We are now beginning to define the limits beyond which we may not progress if we are to continue to live in good health.

WORLD POPULATION

Since 1798, when Thomas Malthus published *An Essay on the Principles of Population,* there have been repeated warnings that man's numbers (which are subject to exponential increase) could—or at some time surely would—overtake food supplies (which Malthus assumed could only increase arithmetically, i.e., a three percent increase in population equals a three percent increase in food demand). Since that book was published, the food problem has been viewed as a food/population problem.

The world growth rate can be quickly seen in a report in *The UNESCO Courier:*

It took at least a million years for human numbers to reach the billion mark. Before the emergence of settled agriculture perhaps 8,000 years ago, the world's entire population may have been from 5 to 10 million. With more elaborate social organization, much larger populations could be sustained, and about 2,000 years ago the world's population had grown to between 200 and 400 million inhabitants.

The billion mark was reached around 1800, and the second billion arrived in about 130 years. But the third billion took only 30 years, and the fourth will have arrived within only 15 years.

World population growth is the result of natural increase—the excess of births over deaths. The fall in the death rate occurred first in the developed regions, but over the last thirty years has been operating spectacularly in Africa, Asia and Latin America. Small families have become the rule in the economically advanced countries but birth rates in the poorer regions have remained high.[1]

In terms of world hunger, the demand for food is determined by the number of people who must be fed and by the level of their consumption.

Though "everybody knows" that there is a population problem, it is not clear what it is, where, and for whom. In the view of the U.S. Government: "population growth is a problem mainly because it retards economic growth, but also because it places an undue burden on food resources; taxes governmental ability to provide schools, housing, etc.; leads to environmental deterioration and resource depletion; and generates social tensions and often political instability."[2]

Most experts do agree on one thing, that world overpopulation is threatening the very survival of the human species. The Population Council in 1974 gave some estimates that are shown in Table 18.1.

This population explosion raises some very basic questions. Already there are people throughout the world dying of starvation. If the food supply is not adequate for the population now, will we be able to upgrade production soon enough to avoid massive famine in the future?

There is obviously not an inexhaustible supply of open land, either for producing food or providing adequate living space. In addition, there is the problem of disposing of solid waste. Each person in the United States, for example, generates about 4.5 pounds of solid waste per day; with population of about 210 million, the daily total for the whole country is almost a billion pounds. There are some alternative measures to our present wasteful use of land (land that could be

[1] "Population Growth or Economic Growth?" *The UNESCO Courier*, May 1974.
[2] Donald P. Warwick, "Ethics and Population Control," *Current History*, November 1974.

used for farming as an example) for open dumps, but these possibilities must be improved and expanded.

POLLUTION

Air pollution, water pollution, and noise pollution are major problems in our technological society. Pesticides are also a matter of concern; although they are essentially part of air and water pollution, they are so dangerous as to warrant separate discussion. The effects of radiation and nuclear power can also be considered a form of pollution, another environmental health hazard.

AIR POLLUTION

The earth's atmosphere extends 600 miles into space, but almost all earthly life exists within a twelve-mile *biosphere,* reaching five miles into space and seven miles into the depths of the ocean. Within the biosphere is a smaller "zone of life" that extends from a depth of 500 feet below sea level to a height of 10,000 feet above sea level. Ninety-five percent of all life exists within this smaller zone. Thus, the air we breathe is really only a narrow layer, far from an inexhaustible supply. A common analogy is that the zone of life is comparable to the skin of an apple (with the apple representing the earth). Mankind is continually pouring vast amounts of pollution into the atmosphere, most of which remains in this thin layer.

The atmosphere of the earth has a remarkable self-cleaning system. It disperses and dissipates the waste products expelled into the air and washes solid particles out with rain and snow. Polluting gases present a different problem, since the atmosphere is a mixture

Table 18.1 *Future Population Estimates. Source:* Bernard Berelson, "World Population: Status Report 1974," *Reports on Population/Family Planning* (New York: The Population Council, January, 1974).

Area	Population 1970 (in billions)	Population size in 2050 if replacement fertility is reached in		
		1980	2000	2040
Developed areas	1.1	1.5	1.6	1.8
Developing areas	2.5	4.7	6.5	11.6
World	3.6	6.2	8.1	13.4

of gases. "Pure" air is composed of about 78 percent nitrogen, 21 percent oxygen, and small proportions of helium, carbon monoxide, and other gases. To maintain this distribution, plants, animals, and bacteria must use and return the gases in the same amounts, through the oxygen and nitrogen cycles. However, pollution can upset this balance so that the levels of oxygen and other atmospheric gases are disturbed. The Air Conservation Commission has stated that the air is termed "polluted" when wastes are produced so rapidly or accumulate in such concentrations that the normal self-cleaning or dispersive propensities of the atmosphere can no longer cope with them.[3]

One problem related to the weather occurs when what is called an *inversion system* exists. An inversion system is created when a cold air mass forms under a warmer air mass. The pollutants contained in the cold air mass are thus trapped in the atmosphere. Inversion systems are usually the cause of the smog over cities such as London and Los Angeles.

Sources of Air Pollution

There are certain chemical substances and gases that are responsible for most air pollution. Carbon monoxide produced in automobile exhaust systems makes up almost half of all the polluting elements in the air. Sulfur dioxide is another dangerous pollutant. It comes mainly from coal and oil heating systems and is an increasing problem as fuel with high sulfur content is used more frequently. Particulates—minute solid or liquid particles—come largely from burning coal. Nitrogen oxides come from automobile exhaust systems and chemical factory processes. Ozone is a foul-smelling poison produced through the effect of the sun's rays on nitrogen oxides. Hydrocarbons are another major element of air pollution, produced usually by automobile exhaust systems and refineries.

Health Problems Caused by Air Pollution

Figure 18.1 shows the effects of air pollution on various parts of the body. The primary effect of air pollution is an aggravation of the symptoms of people with respiratory and cardiovascular disorders, with a consequent increase in mortality from these diseases. Those affected may have only mild or asymptomatic forms of chronic bronchitis, emphysema, asthma, pneumonia, and other such illnesses. Recent evidence suggests that air pollution can actually cause these diseases in otherwise healthy individuals.

Air pollution has also been linked with lung and bronchial cancer. Hydrocarbons are suspected carcinogens, as are some of the

[3] Lloyd E. Burton and Hugh H. Smith, *Public Health and Community Medicine,* Baltimore: Williams & Wilkins, 1970, p. 438.

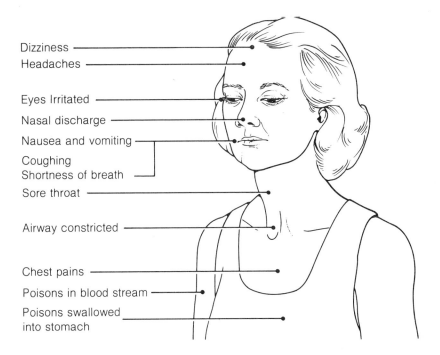

Dizziness
Headaches

Eyes Irritated
Nasal discharge
Nausea and vomiting
Coughing
Shortness of breath
Sore throat

Airway constricted

Chest pains
Poisons in blood stream
Poisons swallowed
into stomach

FIGURE 18.1 *Effects of Air Pollution on the Human Body. Air pollution can be a contributing factor to chronic bronchitis, emphysema, and lung cancer; it can also increase the discomfort of those suffering from allergies, the common cold, pneumonia, and bronchial asthma.*

particulates, such as arsenic (produced in smelting operations and found in certain pesticides) and asbestos. This link is substantiated by the higher death rates from lung cancer in urban areas than in rural areas.[4]

Carbon monoxide, the most prevalent air pollutant, can produce moderate to severe symptoms and death. Carbon monoxide affects the oxygen-carrying capacity of the blood. Concentrations of 100 ppm (parts per million), a level that has been found in city traffic, can produce dizziness, headache, and lassitude.[5] Greater amounts can inhibit complex responses. Carbon monoxide poisoning can sometimes be mistaken for drunkenness, as the affected individual may have difficulty in talking or walking and his eyes may fail to track.[6] Severe carbon monoxide poisoning can result in death. It is likely that a number of auto accidents have been caused by drivers in various stages of carbon monoxide poisoning.

[4] Ibid., p. 440.
[5] Ibid., p. 439.
[6] Donald E. Carr, *The Breath of Life,* New York: W. W. Norton, 1965, p. 56.

Air Pollution and Disease

Scientists are convinced that air pollution is a very real contributing factor to the three major types of disease that cause sickness and death in our society—heart disease, lung disease, and cancer.

The six major pollutants and their effects are:

- *Sulfur oxides*—acrid, corrosive, poisonous gases, produced mainly by fossil fuel-burning electric power plants and industrial plants. Coal burning produces about sixty percent of all sulfur oxide emissions. Sulfur oxide pollution aggravates lung and heart disease, and asthma.
- *Hydrocarbons*—produced by motor vehicles, refineries, petroleum processing and storage facilities, and the use of organic solvents in dry cleaning, painting, etc. Hydrocarbons affect human beings indirectly by contributing to photochemical oxidants, which cause irritation of the eyes and respiratory system.
- *Nitrogen oxides*—produced by high temperature fuel combustion in furnaces and transportation vehicles, and by chemical plants. Occupational exposure to nitrogen oxides has had severe health effects, and tests on laboratory animals indicate a lower resistance to influenza and an effect on lung tissue. Nitrogen oxides react with hydrocarbons to form photochemical smog.
- *Photochemical oxidants*—produced when automobile exhaust, hydrocarbons, and nitrogen oxides are exposed to sunlight, producing ozone, peroxyacyl nitrate, formaldehyde, acrolein, nitrogen peroxide, and organic peroxides. Health effects include worsening of asthma, respiratory and eye irritation, lung problems, and impaired athletic performance.

Lead poisoning can also be related to pollution; the major contributor is the combustion of leaded gasoline in automobiles. Lead poisoning can cause blood disorders, cardiovascular and renal injury, and damage to the central nervous system. It is especially dangerous to pregnant women and children, because it can cause mental retardation in young children.

There are other destructive results of air pollution. Many urban dwellers experience mild symptoms daily, such as watery eyes and headaches. Arsenic has been implicated in outbreaks of dermatitis (skin irritation). Asbestos has been linked to a form of pulmonary fibrosis. Sulfur trioxide (from inexpensive fuels used in heating and power generation) combines with water to form sulfuric acid, a highly caustic and corrosive substance. Air pollution can damage buildings, destroy crops and plants—as well as injure human beings and animals.

(*Continued*)

- *Carbon monoxide*—produced mostly by automobiles and other vehicles, it interferes with the blood's ability to carry a normal supply of oxygen. It also weakens heart function. Carbon monoxide is particularly dangerous for people with heart problems, but also affects those with anemia and lung and cerebral-vascular diseases. It also affects mental function, visual perception, and alertness.
- *Particulates* include all particles in the air, including soot, mists, and sprays, caused by a wide variety of factors. Major health effects are on the respiratory system, and some chemicals can cause cancer when inhaled.

How do we stand on cleaning up these six pollutants? Environmental Protection Agency Administrator Russell E. Train says, "The nation has made significant progress in cleaning up the air, but there is still a long way to go. If citizens, industries, and officials at all levels of government work hard together, we can and will attain the health protection goals established in the Clean Air Act. I am confident that we have both the will and the means to do so."

Source: Environment News, U.S. Environmental Protection Agency, September 1976, p. 9.

Controlling Air Pollution

The need for massive controls to prevent air pollution is obvious. Air pollution is not a new problem, but it has only recently become a major public concern. Laws were enacted several decades ago to fight air pollution, but most of these have been ineffective in that most regulation or prevention of pollution has been left to the discretion of individuals or communities. Therefore, pollution has been increasing, rather than decreasing.

In 1955, the Air Pollution Control Act delegated to the states primary responsibility for controlling air pollution. Federal authority was limited to research and technical assistance although the Surgeon General was authorized (upon request by a state or local government) to conduct investigations of specific local pollution problems. The next major legislation, the Clean Air Act of 1963, extended federal government authority to situations involving interstate pollution. It also made grants available to more communities, extending local and regional programs from 85 in 1961 to 130 in 1966. The Clean Air Act also gave increasing recognition to the automobile as a principal source of air pollution. In 1965, Congress enacted the Motor Vehicle Air Pollution Control Act, which was aimed at emission control. However, the emission standards were based on "technological feasibility and economic cost" and the changes made were minimal.

The Aerosol Controversy

In recent years, increasing quantities of fluorocarbon compounds have been used as aerosol propellants in a wide variety of consumer products, such as cosmetics, perfumes, deodorants, insect sprays, and automotive products. Evidence now indicates that worldwide release of these compounds may endanger the ozone layer, a natural gaseous barrier in the upper atmosphere that shields life on earth from biologically harmful radiation from the sun. Experts estimate that if the present production trends of these fluorocarbon compounds continue, there will be a 16 percent reduction of the ozone layer within twenty-five years.

The most important consequence in terms of human health is that the loss of ozone would allow greater amounts of ultraviolet radiation to reach the earth's surface. This increase could result in greater incidence of skin cancer.

Many manufacturers have stopped manufacturing aerosol sprays propelled by fluorocarbons and legislation is pending on a ban of such sprays. The Environmental Protection Agency (EPA) has already banned the distribution and sale of pesticide aerosols that use vinyl chloride as a propellant. This gas has been linked to a form of liver cancer.

Established in 1963, the National Environmental Policy Act is the only statute designed to function as an environmental mandate to all federal agencies. NEPA does not explicitly establish pollution control programs. Rather, it states a broad policy that federal agencies must consider environmental factors as an integral part of their decision-making process. In 1970, the Clean Air Act required an arbitrary 90 percent reduction by 1975–76 from the 1970–71 levels of the three main auto pollutants: hydrocarbons, carbon monoxide, and oxides of nitrogen.

The solution to the problem of the automobile as a major source of air pollution may be found in efficient mass transit systems within and between cities. However, present patterns suggest that use of mass transit by the majority of the population would have to be enforced by legislation—perhaps a limit would be imposed on the number of cars one family can own.

We know that there is indeed a limit to the available fresh air and that the balance nature has provided in the past is seriously threatened by mankind. There is no longer any real excuse for air pollution; we know where our faults lie and we must work now to eliminate them. Our alternatives are limited—we must deal with air pollution today if we want air to breathe tomorrow.

Is This Trip Really Necessary?

· If you *must* have a car, buy a small one that gets high mileage per gallon and has a long life expectancy.

· Take good care of your car. Use lead-free gas. Keep the engine well tuned—one dead spark plug can increase pollution 10 times! A misfiring spark plug can triple pollution. Install anti-pollution devices and have them checked when your car is serviced. But don't have too much faith in the "clean air car" as a panacea.

· Make the most efficient use of your car—join car pools. At the very least, *plan* your errands so that one trip includes the grocery, the cleaners, etc., instead of going out several times.

· Turn off the engine whenever you're going to be stopped more than a minute. It uses more gas in 60 seconds than is needed to start it again.

· Use public transportation as much as possible. You may think buses are bad polluters, but one bus with 45 passengers is much less guilty than 30 cars with 1½ passengers each.

· Better still, get a bicycle.

· Best of all, *walk*. Bicycles are pollution free but require resources and power for their production and eventually become solid waste.

· *Don't* have a snowmobile, ATV (all-terrain vehicle), or dune buggy. These noisy, unnecessary resource users have the potential of upsetting the fragile eco-systems they intrude on.

WATER POLLUTION

Water pollution is viewed by many people as one of the most serious problems we now face. Senator Frank Moss of Utah says:

> For the next generation of Americans, I believe it is not an exaggeration to say that water—its competing uses and the conflicts that arise out of these uses—may be the most critical national problem.[7]

In 1900, the daily national water demand was less than 50 billion gallons and the supply just under 100 billion gallons per day, but by 1980 the demand may be 600 billion gallons per day while

[7] Frank E. Moss, *The Water Crisis,* New York: Frederick A. Praeger, 1967, p. ix.

the estimated supply will be only 540 billion gallons.[8] Our requirements may soon outstrip our demands unless we can control water pollution. Since water is a fixed commodity and even technology cannot increase the available supply beyond a certain limit, we must depend on conservation and re-use.

Sources of Water Pollution

Industry uses the vast majority of our water supply, far more than half. Consequently, factories and industries are the greatest polluters of our water; they dump various pollutants into waterways or otherwise contaminate the supply. Water processing facilities are not adequate to supply the water needed by industry or for the amounts used by municipalities. Agriculture also uses and pollutes much of our water supply. Commercial and recreational ships and boats are another source of water pollution; recent oil spill disasters have publicized this aspect of the problem.

All of these sources release various types of chemical pollutants into our water, while making tremendous demands on the supply. The dangers of nitrates and phosphates, which are found in municipal and industrial sewage, have only recently been made known. Detergents have been a major cause of this type of pollution, and many brands now contain lower levels of these harmful chemicals. Other polluting chemicals enter the water supply through industrial and agricultural processes. Power plants often use the waterways for their cooling processes, thereby heating up the waterways with destructive results.

Effects of Water Pollution

Nearly undrinkable water, resulting either from inadequate treatment processes or from the addition of numerous chemicals necessary to overcome the pollutants, may be the first aspect of water pollution noticed by many people. Increasing pollution also makes health hazards out of recreational water sources and kills wildlife. As various pollutants infiltrate our waterways, the growth of algae and other plant life is stimulated. Eventually, in a process called *eutrophication,* the oxygen content of the body of water decreases, so that the fish die off. The plant life clogs the water, and it becomes a site of pollution—and little else.

Controlling Water Pollution

There are no swift and simple solutions to the problems of water pollution or shortages, but there is a need for some sort of imme-

[8] U.S., Department of Health, Education and Welfare, Public Health Service, *Clean Water,* Washington, D.C.: Surgeon General's National Conference on Water Pollution, 1960.

diate action. Former Secretary of the Interior Stewart L. Udall has stated:

> To speak of use and abuse, of grace and disgrace is to tell the story of water in the fewest possible words. . . . Unprecedented and continuing population and economic growth, increasing urbanization, and technological changes, all are major contributors toward a water problem which can no longer be ignored.[9]

Unless more effective methods of controlling water pollution are used, we may soon be facing severe shortages.

The two major ways of dealing with the problem are the development of more and better water treatment facilities and the prevention of various forms of pollution at the source. It is—at least at the present time—impossible to recycle severely polluted water. Laws relating to pollution control and water quality have been in effect since the 1940s, but harsher legislation is needed. Senate committees and Congressional hearings have dealt with various facets of the problem; the U.S. Public Health Service has conducted comprehensive water quality investigations of all the river basins in the country. Legislation in 1970 was directed against pollution-causing industrial practices and authorized fines or jail sentences for those responsible for the use of such practices. Other laws have included appropriations for research and development of improved sewage treatment and recycling plants. Efforts at solving pollution and shortage problems have involved a viable desalination process to use the oceans' waters, weather modification and rain-making techniques, specific solutions to certain types of pollution, and research on a multitude of new and old approaches to water conservation.

PESTICIDES

In 1962 Rachel Carson published *The Silent Spring,* a frightening but scientific documentation of the hazards of the numerous pesticides in our environment. Pesticides are used in agriculture and for disease prevention, but they can be harmful and even fatal.

Pesticides have been implicated in massive killings of fish, birds, and other animals. They affect the reproductive abilities of various forms of wildlife. They upset the balance of nature by killing

[9] Jim Wright, Jr., *The Coming Water Famine,* New York: Coward-McCann, 1966, p. 10.

Policy on Preventive Pesticide Use Issued by EPA

Using a pesticide to prevent an insect or other pest outbreak where none is actively occurring has been a common practice in the home, on the farm, and in commercial buildings. But until recently, the legality of this practice has been in doubt. The problem arises from language in the 1972 federal pesticides law that makes it unlawful for "any person to use any registered pesticide in a manner inconsistent with its labeling." As a result, professional pest control operators, farmers, and occasional users have been unsure as to whether they could use a product in a preventive manner without running the risk of a fine for misuse. Typical preventive treatments include wood impregnation to discourage insect damage, rat and mouse control, plant protection from diseases, and the use of herbicides to discourage weeds. Few pesticide labels state affirmatively that preventive uses are allowable.

EPA, responsible for pesticide regulation, has taken action to clarify this area of pesticide use. A policy statement defining when preventive treatments are permissible was issued recently by EPA. It is one of several statements on controversial pesticide enforcement questions published by the Agency during the past fifteen months.

According to the preventive use statement, it is acceptable to use a pesticide to thwart an anticipated pest problem if [1] the label of the pesticide which is used does not affirmatively prohibit preventive treatments; [2] the target pest is reasonably expected to infest the treated area; and [3] the pesticide is normally safe and effective against the target pest when used in a preventive manner.

Source: Environment News, U.S. Environmental Protection Agency, September 1976.

---

off certain pests that are the natural enemies of other insects or animals. Pesticides have been responsible for the poisoning and deaths of human beings. Individuals may be affected either through the presence of pesticides in their immediate environment or through eating contaminated fish, meat, or other agricultural products. Certain pesticides are now suspected of being carcinogenic.

Many people are returning to the use of safer, organic pesticides rather than synthetic chemicals. Indiscriminate pesticide use can have widespread damaging effects; pesticide use is another form of environmental pollution that must be controlled. Certain governmental and private or public consumer agencies are working towards safe and controlled use of pesticides, but more research and stronger preventive legislation is necessary.

NOISE POLLUTION

In recent years the volume of noise surrounding us has changed from a simple annoyance to a damaging health hazard. Noise is measured in decibels. One decibel (db) represents the smallest difference in sound intensity a human being can detect.[10] A level of sound under 85 db is considered safe, but many sources of noise produce much louder sounds than this. Research has shown that the age of technology has raised the average noise level in the United States by one decibel a year over the last twenty-five years.

Sources of Noise Pollution   One of the major sources of noise pollution is motor vehicle traffic. The Federal Council for Science and Technology has found that ". . . traffic noise radiating from the freeways and expressways and from midtown shopping and apartment districts of our large cities probably disturbs more people than any other source of outdoor noise." According to General Motors, "The biggest single source from passenger cars is usually exhaust noise." (A car without a muffler may generate up to 160 decibels of noise through the exhaust system alone.) "After exhaust noises are reduced, tires become the main noise source, particularly at freeway speeds."

Jet aircraft are another source of serious noise pollution. A comprehensive study by the Environmental Protection Agency has found that aircraft noise adversely affects some 16 million residents near the nation's airports.

Industrial and other occupations may expose employees to dangerous levels of noise. Many states recognize partial deafness as an occupational hazard for some forms of employment.

Rock music, with electronic amplification, can reach dangerous decibel levels. A sound level of over 120 decibels is commonly recorded at rock concerts so that frequent concert attendance can result in some permanent hearing loss.

Other sources of noise pollution are subway systems, police and fire engine sirens, construction work, and various household appliances. The modern city dweller may be continuously exposed to excessive and dangerous levels of noise in his everyday life.

Effects of Noise Pollution   Noise can cause hearing damage, ranging from slight temporary hearing loss to permanent deafness. Daily exposure to high decibel levels can result in permanent hearing loss in varying degrees. Extremely loud noise, as from an explosion, can rupture the eardrum or damage some of the sensitive inner organs of the ear.

Researchers have discovered that noise pollution can raise blood pressure levels and increase the heart rate. Thus, excessive noise can eventually cause cardiovascular disease. Noise pollution can also interfere with relaxation and sleep, causing general fatigue.

[10] The decibel scale is logarithmic rather than linear, which means that an increase of ten decibels signifies ten times as much loudness.

Decibel Scale		
Eardrum Ruptures	140	Jet taking off
Painful to Ear	120	Siren Jet revving its motors for takeoff Maximum allowable for hearing Roar of a two-engine prop plane
Deafening	100	Thunder Car horn at 3 feet Loud motorcycle Loud power lawn mower
Very Loud	80	Portable sander Have to shout to be heard Food blender Continued daily exposure brings about loss of hearing Noisy cocktail party Impossible to use telephone
Loud	60	City playground Vacuum cleaner Noisy office Average traffic Point at which use of the telephone becomes difficult
Moderate	40	Suburban playground All right for a restaurant Average living room
Faint	20	Quiet enough for courtroom or classroom Private office A whisper at 5 feet
Threshold of Audibility	0	Rustling leaves Breathing

It can set off the alarm reaction described by Selye (see Chapter 5), so that production of adrenalin is stimulated, with accompanying effects. Stress and nervousness are common reactions to noise pollution—symptoms of tension such as irritability and insomnia may appear. Extremely high decibel levels (such as the 175 db of a rocket blast) can actually impede breathing to the extent that convulsions and death may occur.

Controlling Noise Pollution　　Noise pollution is the form of pollution that we can most easily control. Industrial and environmental noise pollution can be decreased through our present technology and through effective legislation.

Various protective devices can be used by those working with aircraft and in other jobs that expose them to dangerous decibel levels. Selective attenuators protect against sudden explosive noises and are used on firing ranges. Protective booths can provide a shield against noise for others in industrial jobs.

The individual can do much to cut down on the noise level in his environment. He can make sure his car has a proper muffler, which will cut the sound level down from 160 db to 85. Rugs, curtains, and acoustical tiles can also cut down noise levels; even furniture choice and arrangement can affect the amount of sound in a house. Weather stripping and well-fitting doors and windows can help block sound.

The technology for controlling noise pollution exists; adequate legislation is necessary to make sure this technology is used. The American Academy of Ophthalmology and Otolaryngology has recommended that if any industrial workers are exposed to more than five continuous hours daily of sound at 85 db or more they should be supplied with protective devices. Yet only four states (New York, California, Wisconsin, and Missouri) have enacted such safety recommendations, and they allow workers to be exposed to noise levels up to 95 db before protection is required.

The U.S. Congress enacted a Noise Control Act in 1972. Many states are now beginning to establish noise control standards for machinery, appliances, and other equipment. Hawaii, Illinois, and Colorado have adopted major laws and regulatory structures concerning noise pollution. Industrial noise is not the only target—many states (including Vermont, Maine, Washington, and California) now regulate noise caused by "leisure-time" vehicles and products. Anti-noise ordinances can be effective in many communities. Major cities such as Chicago, New York, and San Francisco have enacted comprehensive noise ordinances, and others are sure to follow. Such controls are necessary to protect our health against one more form of pollution.

RADIATION

The effect of radiation on health is becoming an increasingly important question. Mankind has always been exposed to some amount of radiation in his environment, through what is called *natural background radiation.* However, man-made radiation pollution is now a problem as nuclear energy is used more and more frequently by the field of medicine and by utilities and industry.

Sources of Radiation

The positive effects of radiation must be carefully weighed against the negative effects. *Radioiodine* has been found effective in treating certain thyroid disorders and some thyroid cancers. Radioisotopes are used in research and industry as well as in medical diagnosis and treatment. Radiation therapy can help stop the progress of certain cancers. (See Chapter 16.) *Radiography* is used in industry to detect flaws in certain products. X-rays are commonly used in dentistry and in other medical diagnoses.

With the explosion of the first atomic bomb in the mid-1940s, we were faced with the problem of fallout. Radioactive material that is sent up into the earth's atmosphere by such explosions eventually returns to earth in the form of radioactive fallout. It can contaminate all parts of the environment.

The use of nuclear power as a solution to the problems of the energy crisis is becoming an extremely controversial issue today. The major problem with such use is the disposal of the radioactive wastes created. Much radioactive material takes years to completely deteriorate. The effect of leakage of such wastes into our environment would be disastrous.

Effects of Radiation

The biological effects of radiation are both *somatic* (affecting the cells and tissues of an organism) and *genetic* (affecting the germ cells of the organism in such a way that effects are carried to future generations). Exposure to large amounts of radiation (e.g., through radiation therapy or industrial accidents) can produce such somatic effects as radiation burns and radiation sickness, with symptoms of nausea, vomiting, and diarrhea. The central nervous system and blood cell formation can also be involved. Death may result from a massive exposure to radiation. Long-term effects that may appear after prolonged exposure to smaller amounts of radiation are leukemia and bone and other cancers, cataracts, and shortened life span. Genetic effects in offspring may appear as nonspecific health ailments, which may be minor or may result in serious illness or death. Leukemia is one such genetic effect, and birth defects are also a possibility.

Controlling Radiation Pollution　　　Certain steps are now being taken to cut down the amount of radiation in our environment but the major questions at present seem to be to a great extent political. Medical x-rays are used less casually and greater protection is provided for the patient. The benefits of such radiation must be carefully considered against the negative possibilities. Reduced nuclear testing will reduce the amounts of radioactive fallout, but the fallout that has already been released into our environment will remain there for decades. The use of nuclear power involves the most serious debate. Nuclear wastes pile up from nuclear power plants, but the extent of possible destruction from leakage or other industrial accidents is only now beginning to be known. Many experts believe that the use of nuclear power should be shelved until better safeguards—if any exist—can be found.

FURTHER READINGS

Bender, Tom. *Environmental Design Primer.* New York: Schocken Books, 1973.

Tom Bender's book recalls the traditional wisdom concerning nature and the earth.

Carr, Donald, *The Breath of Life.* New York: Berkley Medallion Book, 1970.

The full report on a subject of deadly fascination: our poisoned air.

Caudill, Harry. *My Land Is Dying.* New York: E. P. Dutton & Co., Inc., 1973.

The author warns of the coming devastation of the continent—the creation of an "American Carthage, plowed and salted."

Dubos, René. *A God Within.* New York: Charles Scribner's Sons, 1972.

A positive philosophy for a more complete fulfillment of human potentials.

Ehrlich, Paul. *Population Bomb.* New York: Ballantine Books, 1968.

The potential for the loss of rights in the years to come.

Fallows, James. *The Water Lords.* New York: Bantam Books, 1971.

Ralph Nader's study group report on industry and environmental crisis in Savannah, Georgia.

Goldman, Marshall. *Controlling Pollution.* Englewood Cliffs, N.J.: Prentice-Hall, Inc., 1967.

Documents the shocking conditions of pollution in our "affluent society."

Graham, Frank. *Since Silent Spring.* Greenwich, Conn.: Fawcett Pub., Inc., 1970.

The author describes the background of Rachel Carson, her book, and the furor it caused.

Hall, Gus. *The Energy Rip-Off*. New York: International Pub., 1974.

Discussion of the problem, structure, and victims of the so-called energy crisis.

Rall, David P. "Tracking Down the Chemical Culprits That Endanger Man." *Prism*. April 1974.

The Crisis of Survival. New York: Morrow Paperbacks, 1970.

This book covers such areas as the famine of resources, nuclear war, overpopulation, and pollution.

The Grass Roots Primer. San Francisco: Sierra Club Books, 1975.

A book about the grassroots environmental movement by the people who are making it happen.

8

THE FINAL CHAPTER

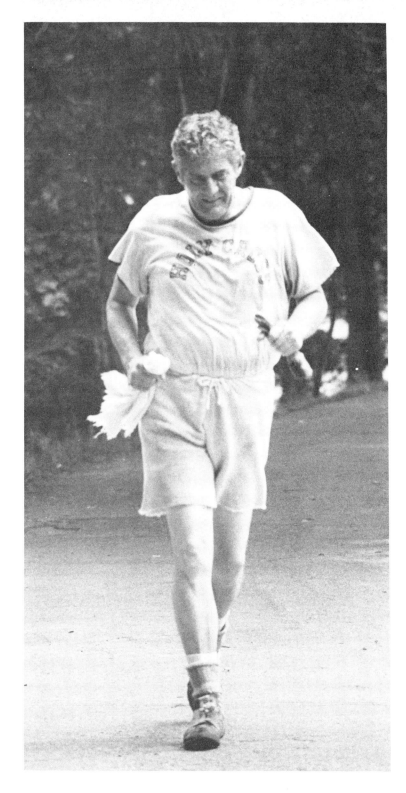

It takes some little time to accept and realize the fact that while you have been growing old, your friends have not been standing still.

Mark Twain

Chapter 19

Aging
and Death

Eternal youth and immortality are among the most persistent fantasies in American society. Ours is a youth-oriented culture. The elderly are, in effect, ignored, and old age is surrounded by myths and stereotyped ideas. The idea of death, whether as the natural result of the aging process or because of a terminal illness, is a taboo subject.

Yet facing the inevitable prospects of aging and death is important to a healthy life. Many other cultures have open and positive attitudes towards these processes, and a few "brave pioneers" are beginning a re-evaluation (and re-formation) of the attitudes of our society.

AGING

Although we have been able to eradicate or control many debilitating diseases, it is unlikely that we will be able to halt the process of aging. But aging need not remain the depressing spectre many people fear. Dr. Nathan W. Shock, one of the world's leading gerontologists, says that instead of concentrating on an extension of the life span itself (and there will occur through our technology a gradual "continuing drift upward in the average age at death"), "the ultimate goal of all research on aging should be to improve the performance and well-being of older people." We can "improve the quality of life in the later years by reducing the incidence of the disabilities."

Dr. Alex Comfort is one authority who believes the quality of life for older people can be changed drastically. A dramatic improvement can be achieved just through a re-evaluation of the whole aging

> In our long and obsessive passion for youth, we have—more than any other modern society—avoided direct approach to age and to dying by denying them in word, in fact, and—above all—in worth. Like sex, until the last three decades, death has been unmentionable in what was known as "polite society." We "pass away," not die. We do not tell our children about dying.
>
> —Marya Mannes, *Last Rights*

process. His book *A Good Age* destroys many of the myths that surround the quality of life in the later years and provides a positive discussion of old age.

Aging will have no effect upon you as a person. When you are "old" you will feel no different and be no different from what you are now or were when you were young, except that you will have had more experiences. Your appearance will change and you may have more physical problems—they will affect you only as physical problems affect a person of any age. An "aged" person is simply a person who has been there longer than a young person. Aging is not a radical change, but by the time you reach it, you will have been thoroughly indoctrinated by society to think it is.[1]

DEATH AND DYING

Even if our technology were to become so effective that disease were eradicated, it is unlikely that the life span would be extended radically or indefinitely. Diploid cells in tissue cultures have been shown to have finite life spans; they reach the end of the period of existence that is programmed in their chromosomes and they die. It is likely that our own cells wear out in a similar manner, regardless of disease.

Adjusting to Death   Facing death at a relatively young age (e.g., because of a chronic illness) requires a different type of psychological preparation than accepting death after a "good" old age as the natural culmination of a long and productive life. Elisabeth Kübler-Ross deals with various aspects of this subject in *On Death and Dying*. She recognizes four stages of coping mechanisms used by terminally ill individuals in the process of adapting to approaching death.

[1] Alex Comfort, *A Good Age,* New York: Crown Publishers, 1976.

She sees the first response to news of imminent death as one of *denial,* followed by a period of isolation. The first statement of such an individual may be, "No! Not me! It can't be true!" The reaction of flat denial is usually temporary and is replaced by partial acceptance during a time of isolation and withdrawal from others. This first response is exhibited by people without regard to their religious convictions or beliefs.

The second stage is one of *anger.* The individual may feel cheated by fate, picked out unjustly. He may feel that his friends have less valuable or virtuous existences but are granted perfect health and long life. The question is "Why me?"

Kübler-Ross defines the third stage as a *bargaining* period. The dying hope for a miracle. Perhaps they feel that they will be rewarded for good behavior and granted life in exchange for special services.

The final stage is one of *acceptance.* This final adjustment may involve peace, bitterness, or continued fear, depending on the circumstances and the patient's philosophical resources. Throughout all four stages, even acceptance, a feeling of hope persists—"hope of a miracle cure, of getting 'better,' etc."[2]

Some authorities disagree with the theories of Kübler-Ross. Dr. Melvin Krant, for example, feels that the four-stage cycle is applicable only to specific individuals rather than to all patients suffering from terminal illnesses. He rejects "the notion that most people . . . regress to denial or fantasy stages." He believes that a substantial number can simply achieve a feeling of resignation or acceptance. The difference between the individual who denies and represses the fact of his dying and the one who accepts the inevitable is in great part related to basic personality traits, but the availability of support in dealing honestly with death is also important.[3]

Looking at Life   Sometimes an escape from death or an acceptance of dying may enhance one's appreciation and understanding of life. After recovering from a near-fatal illness, Abraham Maslow felt:

> . . . everything gets doubly precious, gets piercingly important. You get stabbed by things, by flowers, and by babies and by beautiful things—just the very act of living, of walking and breathing and eating and having friends and chatting. Everything seems to look more beautiful

[2] Elisabeth Kübler-Ross, *On Death and Dying,* New York: Macmillan, 1969.
[3] Melvin Krant, "Dying," *Medical Insight,* January 1973, p. 28.

rather than less, and one gets the much intensified sense of miracles.[4]

Those individuals who grow wise as well as old often experience such feelings. Such a love of life is one positive aspect of a realistic acceptance of eventual death.

The Right To Die   Many people are now concerned that our medical technology is being used to prolong the pain and suffering of terminally ill patients. Dr. Krant states, "An important philosophical final question we must ask ourselves is whether, in our modern technological culture, we have not arranged our medical thinking and education so as to deprive us of the ultimate understanding of suffering and death."[5]

California enacted legislation in early 1977 allowing the terminally ill a voice in their own deaths. Any adult can draft a "living will" (in the presence of two witnesses who are neither relatives nor involved in the individual's medical treatment). If two doctors determine that the patient is suffering from a terminal illness, under the authorization of such a will, life-sustaining machinery can be shut off without any legal repercussions for the physicians or the surviving family members.

Professor Richards has . . . written about death—which does not depress him. "Seems to me the most interesting set of undetermined possibilities, so I'm rather curious," he said. "I watch the leaves falling off the tree outside my window. I know there couldn't be a healthy tree next year unless the leaves fall off. The life of the thing that matters—a tree or forest—depends on their departure. And the leaves seem to delight in the purge: they put on a great show."

But he is upset about life. "I'm afraid I'm going to live to 100," he explained. "That's a serious thing, and I'm rather in favor of euthanasia."

Why is he afraid? "May be gaga quite soon," he replied. "I wouldn't like to go on living after I'd forgotten the things that really matter."

—From a New York *Times* interview with I.A. Richards, eighty, by Israel Shenker.

---

[4] Abraham Maslow, in an editorial in *Psychology Today,* 4, no. 3, August 1970, p. 16.
[5] Krant, "Dying," p. 28.

Is There a Life After?

I had a heart attack, and I found myself in a black void, and I knew I was dying. . . . I could see a gray mist, and I was rushing toward it. . . . Beyond the mist I could see people. . . . The whole thing was permeated with the most gorgeous light—a living, golden-yellow glow, a pale color, not like the harsh gold color we knew on earth. As I approached more closely, I felt certain that I was going through that mist. It was such a wonderful, joyous feeling; there are just no words in human language to describe it. Yet it wasn't my time to go through the mist, because instantly from the other side appeared my Uncle Carl, who had died many years earlier. He blocked my path, saying: "Go back. Your work on earth has not been completed. Go back now." I didn't want to go back, but I had no choice, and immediately I was back in my body. I felt that horrible pain in my chest, and I heard my little boy crying, "God, bring my mommy back to me."

This experience, related by a woman who nearly died, is one of many from *Life After Life,* a book written by Dr. Raymond Moody, a physician from Augusta, Georgia. This is just one of the true experiences of a person declared clinically "dead," that means Dr. Moody cannot "dismiss out of hand the notion that there could be other realms of existence."

In his book, Moody states that "At the present time, I know of approximately 150 cases of this phenomenon (of a near-death experience). The experiences which he has studied fall into three distinct categories.

1. The experiences of persons who were resuscitated after having been thought, adjudged, or pronounced clinically dead by their doctors.
2. The experiences of persons who, in the course of accidents or severe injury or illness, came very close to physical death.
3. The experiences of persons who, as they died, told them to other people who were present. Later, these other people reported the content of the death experience to me.*

Moody says that nearly every survivor says ordinary language is inadequate to describe this extraordinary experience. Often the survivors have heard themselves pronounced dead by doctors or spectators at the scene of an accident. This, many say, is followed by a great sense of release, peace, even euphoria.

* Raymond A. Moody, *Life After Life.* New York: Bantam Book, 1975, p. 16.

FURTHER READINGS

Becker, Ernest. *The Denial of Death.* New Jersey: The Free Press, 1973.

Becker's book, with its penetrating critiques of the key insights of Freud, Jung, and others, discusses the limitations of psychoanalysis and of reason itself in helping man transcend his conflicting fears of both death and life.

Halsell, Grace. *Los Viejos.* Emmaus, Pa.: Rodale Press, Inc., 1976.

The author examines the physical aspects of health and longevity: genetics, exercise, environment, diet, and other life habits of the Viejos; the longest-living people in the Western Hemisphere.

Keleman, Stanley. *Living Your Dying.* New York: Random House, 1974.

This book is about dying, not about death. For those who are curious about what dying is for them.

Koenig, Ronald. "Dying vs. Well-Being," *Omega.* Fall 1973, pp. 181–194.

Koenig says that the terminally ill are less fearful of death itself than of pain, abandonment, loss of function and control, and burdening their families.

Kübler-Ross, Elisabeth. *On Death and Dying.* New York: The Macmillan Publishing Co., 1969.

This book discusses, nontechnically, the final stages of life with all its anxieties, fears, and hopes. Most important, it focuses on the dying person as a human being.

Mack, Arien, ed. *Death in the American Experience.* New York: Schocken Books, 1973.

This book, which reprints the papers from the Fall, 1972 issue of *Social Research,* includes "The Sacral Power of Death," by William May; "Being and Becoming Dead," by Eric Cassell; and "The 'Gift of Life' and Its Reciprocation," by Parsons, Fox, and Lidz.

Mannes, Marya. *Last Rights: The Case for the Good Death.* New York: William Morrow & Co., 1974.

This is a highly personal and somewhat emotional statement of the tragic "vegetable-like" last days of the terminally ill.

Weisman, Avery D. *On Dying and Denying: A Psychiatric Study of Terminality.* New Jersey: Behavioral Science Books, 1973.

The most complete and thorough study of the psychological mechanisms of approaching death and ways clinicians can confront them.

APPENDICES

Appendix A   Food Values*

The following abbreviations are used: Cal. for calory; Gm. for gram; Mg. for milligram; I.U. for International Unit; Tr. for trace; tbs. for tablespoon.

Food and Approximate Measure	Food Energy (Cal.)	Protein (Gm.)	Fat (Gm.)	MINERALS Calcium (Mg.)	Iron (Mg.)	VITAMINS Vitamin A Value (I.U.)	Thiamine B_1 (Mg.)	Riboflavin B_2 (Mg.)	Niacin Value (Mg.)	Ascorbic Acid (Mg.)
Apple, raw, 1 medium 2½″ in diam.	76	.4	.5	8	.4	120	.05	.04	.2	6
Apple juice, fresh or canned, 1 cup	124	.2	—	15	1.2	90	.05	.07	Tr.	2
Applesauce, canned unsweetened, 1 cup	100	.5	.5	10	1.0	70	.05	.02	.1	3
Bacon, crisp, 2 slices	97	4.0	8.8	4	.5	—	.08	.05	.8	—
Bananas, raw, 1 large, 8 × 1½″	119	1.6	.3	11	.8	570	.06	.06	1.0	13
Beans:										
Red kidney, canned or cooked, 1 cup	230	14.6	1.0	102	4.9	—	.12	.12	2.0	—
Baked—pork and molasses, 1 cup	325	15.1	7.8	146	5.5	90	.13	.09	1.2	7
Beef cuts, cooked:										
Chuck, 3 ounces without bone	265	22.0	19.0	9	2.6	—	.04	.17	3.5	—
Flank, 3 ounces without bone	270	21.0	20.0	9	2.6	—	.04	.17	3.5	—
Hamburger, 3 ounces	316	19.0	26.0	8	2.4	—	.07	.16	4.1	—
Porterhouse, 3 ounces without bone	293	20.0	23.0	9	2.6	—	.05	.15	4.0	—
Rib roast, 3 ounces without bone	266	20.0	20.0	9	2.6	—	.05	.15	3.6	—
Round, 3 ounces without bone	197	23.0	11.0	9	2.9	—	.06	.19	4.7	—
Sirloin, 3 ounces without bone	257	20.0	19.0	9	2.5	—	.06	.16	4.1	—
Beef and vegetable stew, 1 cup	252	12.9	19.3	31	2.6	2,520	.12	.15	3.4	15
Breads:										
Cracked-wheat, unenriched, 1 sl. ½″ thick	60	2.0	.5	19	2.2	—	.03	.02	.3	—
Italian, unenriched, 1 pound	1,195	39.5	3.6	59	3.2	—	.23	.30	4.5	—

Item										
Raisin, unenriched, 1 slice ½" thick	65	1.6	.7	18	.3	Tr.	.02	.02	.2	—
Rye, American, 1 slice ½" thick	57	2.1	.3	17	.4	—	.04	.02	.4	—
White, unenriched, 4 percent nonfat milk solids, 1 slice ½" thick	63	2.0	.7	18	.1	—	.01	.02	.2	—
Toasted, 1 slice ½" thick	63	2.0	.7	18	.1	—	.01	.02	.2	—
Whole wheat, 1 slice ½" thick	55	2.1	.6	22	.5	—	.07	.03	.7	—
Butter, 1 tbs.	100	.1	11.3	3	—	460	Tr.	Tr.	Tr.	—
Cakes:										
Cupcake, 1 2¾" in diam.	131	2.6	3.3	62	.2	50	.01	.03	.1	—
Pound, 1 sl. 2¾ × 3 × ⅝"	130	2.1	7.0	16	.5	100	.04	.05	.3	—
Sponge, 2" sector	117	3.2	2.0	11	.6	210	.02	.06	.1	—
Candy:										
Butterscotch, 1 ounce	116	—	2.5	6	.5	—	—	Tr.	Tr.	Tr.
Caramels, 1 ounce	118	.8	3.3	36	.7	50	.01	.04	Tr.	Tr.
Chocolate, sweetened milk, 1 ounce	143	2.0	9.5	61	.6	40	.03	.11	.2	—
Peanut brittle, 1 ounce	125	2.4	4.4	11	.6	10	.03	.01	1.4	—
Carrots, raw, 1, 5½ × 1"	21	.6	.2	20	.4	6,000	.03	.03	.3	3
Catsup, tomato, 1 tbs.	17	.3	.1	2	.1	320	.02	.01	.4	2
Cheese:										
Cheddar, 1 ounce (1" cube)	113	7.1	9.1	206	.3	400	.01	.12	Tr.	—
Cottage from skim milk, 1 cup	215	43.9	1.1	216	.7	50	.04	.69	.2	—
Cream cheese, 1 ounce	106	2.6	10.5	19	.1	410	Tr.	.06	Tr.	—
Swiss, 1 ounce	105	7.8	7.9	262	.3	410	Tr.	.11	Tr.	—
Chicken, raw, broiler, ½ bird (8 oz. bone out)	332	44.4	15.8	31	3.3	—	.18	.36	22.4	—
Roasters, 4 oz. bone out	227	22.9	14.3	16	1.7	—	.09	.18	9.1	—
Hens, stewing, 4 oz. bone out	342	20.4	28.3	16	1.7	—	.09	.18	9.1	—
Fryers, 1 breast, 8 oz. bone out	210	47.0	1.0	28	2.2	—	.13	.18	21.1	—
1 leg, 5 oz. bone out	159	29.1	3.8	21	2.6	—	.14	.34	8.0	—
Canned, boned, 3 oz.	169	25.3	6.8	12	1.5	—	.03	.14	5.4	—

*This section was adapted from *Handbook No. 8*, U.S. Department of Agriculture by the Research Department of the New York Times and presented in *The New York Times Encyclopedic Almanac* (New York: The New York Times, 1972), pp. 484, 485.

Food Values (continued)

Food and Approximate Measure	Food Energy (Cal.)	Protein (Gm.)	Fat (Gm.)	Calcium (Mg.)	Iron (Mg.)	Vitamin A Value (I.U.)	Thiamine B_1 (Mg.)	Riboflavin B_2 (Mg.)	Niacin Value (Mg.)	Ascorbic Acid (Mg.)
		MINERALS					**VITAMINS**			
Chocolate syrup, 1 tbs.	42	.2	.2	3	.3	—	—	—	—	—
Clams, raw, meat only, 4 ounces	92	14.5	1.6	109	7.9	120	.11	.20	1.8	—
Cocoa, breakfast, plain dry powder, 1 tbs.	21	.6	1.7	9	.8	Tr.	.01	.03	.2	—
Cola beverage, carbonated, 1 cup	107	—	—	—	—	—	—	—	—	—
Coffee, black, 1 cup	—	—	—	—	—	—	—	—	—	—
Coleslaw, 1 cup	102	1.6	7.3	47	.5	80	.06	.05	.3	50
Corn, 1 ear, 5″ long	84	2.7	.7	5	.6	390	.11	.10	1.4	8
Corn flakes, 1 cup	96	2.0	.1	3	.3	—	.01	.02	.4	—
Corn flour, 1 cup sifted	406	8.6	2.9	7	2.0	370	.22	.06	1.6	—
Cream, light, table, 1 tbs.	30	.4	3.0	15	—	120	Tr.	.02	Tr.	Tr.
Heavy or whipping, 1 tbs.	49	.3	5.2	12	—	220	Tr.	.02	Tr.	Tr.
Doughnuts, cake type, 1	136	2.1	6.7	23	.2	40	.05	.04	.4	—
Eggs, boiled, poached, 1	77	6.1	5.5	26	1.3	550	.05	.14	Tr.	—
Omelet, 1 egg	106	6.8	7.9	50	1.3	640	.05	.17	Tr.	—
Scrambled, 1 egg	106	6.8	7.9	50	1.3	640	.05	.17	Tr.	—
Fats, cooking (vegetable), 1 tbs.	110	—	12.5	—	—	—	—	—	—	—
Flounder, 4 oz. (raw) edible portion	78	16.9	.6	69	.9	—	.07	.06	1.9	—
Frankfurters, 1	124	7.0	10.0	3	.6	—	.08	.09	1.3	—
Fruit cocktail, canned, 1 cup (solids & liquid)	179	1.0	.5	23	1.0	410	.03	.03	.9	5
Grapefruit, raw, 1 cup sections	77	1.0	.4	43	.4	20	.07	.04	.4	78
Canned in syrup, 1 cup solids & liquid	181	1.5	.5	32	.7	20	.07	.05	.5	74
Juice, fresh, 1 cup	87	1.2	.2	20	.7	20	.09	.05	.5	99
Haddock, cooked, 1 fillet 4 × 3 × ½″	158	19.0	5.5	18	.6	—	.04	.09	2.6	—
Halibut, broiled, 1 steak 4 × 3 × ½″	228	33.0	9.8	18	1.0	—	.08	.09	13.9	—
Honeydew melon, 1 wedge 2 × 7″	49	.8	—	26	.6	60	.07	.04	.3	34
Ice cream, plain, ⅐ of quart brick	167	3.2	10.1	100	.1	420	.03	.15	.1	1

Jellies, 1 tbs.	50	—	—	2	.1	Tr.	Tr.	Tr.	Tr.	1
Lamb:										
Rib chop, cooked, 3 ounces without bone	356	20.0	30.0	9	2.6	—	.12	.22	4.8	—
Shoulder roast, 3 ounces without bone	293	18.0	24.0	8	2.2	—	.10	.19	3.9	—
Leg roast, 3 ounces without bone	230	20.0	16.0	9	2.6	—	.12	.21	4.4	—
Liver, beef, 2 ounces cooked	118	13.4	4.4	5	4.4	30,330	.15	2.25	8.4	18
Calf, 3 ounces raw	120	16.2	4.2	5	9.0	19,130	.18	2.65	13.7	30
Chicken, 3 ounces raw	120	18.8	3.4	14	6.3	27,370	.17	2.10	10.0	17
Lobster, canned, 3 ounces	78	15.6	1.1	55	.7	—	.03	.06	1.9	—
Luncheon meat: Boiled ham, 2 ounces	172	12.9	12.9	5	1.5	—	.57	.15	2.9	—
Canned, spiced, 2 ounces	164	8.4	13.8	5	1.2	—	.18	.12	1.6	—
Macaroni & cheese, baked, 1 cup	464	17.8	24.2	420	1.1	990	.07	.35	.9	Tr.
Margarine, 1 tbs.	101	.1	11.3	3	—	460	—	—	—	—
Mayonnaise, 1 tbs.	92	.2	10.1	2	.1	30	Tr.	Tr.	—	—
Milk, cow: fluid, whole, 1 cup	166	8.5	9.5	288	.2	390	.09	.42	.3	3
Fluid, nonfat (skim), 1 cup	87	8.6	.2	303	.2	10	.09	.44	.3	3
Canned, evaporated (unsweetened), 1 cup	346	17.6	19.9	612	.4	1,010	.12	.91	.5	3
Malted beverage, 1 cup	281	12.4	11.9	364	.8	680	.18	.56	—	3
Mushrooms, canned, 1 cup solids & liquid	28	3.4	.5	17	2.0	—	.04	.60	4.8	—
Nuts:										
Almonds, shelled, 1 cup	848	26.4	76.8	361	6.2	—	.35	.95	6.5	Tr.
Peanuts, roasted, 1 cup medium halves	805	38.7	63.6	107	2.7	—	.42	.19	23.3	—
Oatmeal or rolled oats, 1 cup dry	312	11.4	5.9	42	3.6	—	.48	.11	.8	—
Cooked, 1 cup	148	5.4	2.8	21	1.7	—	.22	.05	.4	—
Oils, salad or cooking, 1 tbs.	124	—	14.0	—	—	—	—	—	—	—
Oranges, 1 medium, 3" diam.	70	1.4	.3	51	.6	290	.12	.04	.4	77
Orange juice, fresh, 1 cup	108	2.0	.5	47	.5	460	.19	.06	.6	122
Oysters, meat only, raw, 1 cup (13–19 med.)	200	23.5	5.0	226	13.4	770	.35	.48	2.8	—
Stew, 1 cup (6–8 oysters)	244	16.6	13.2	262	7.0	820	.21	.46	1.6	—
Pancakes (griddlecakes):										
Wheat, 1 cake, 4" diam.	59	1.8	2.5	43	.2	50	.02	.03	.1	Tr.
Buckwheat, 1 cake, 4" diam.	47	1.6	2.3	67	.3	30	.04	.04	.2	Tr.
Peaches, raw, 1 medium	46	.5	.1	8	.6	880	.02	.05	.9	8
Peanut butter, 1 tbs.	92	4.2	7.6	12	.3	—	.02	.02	2.6	—

Food Values (continued)

Food and Approximate Measure	Food Energy (Cal.)	Protein (Gm.)	Fat (Gm.)	Calcium (Mg.)	Iron (Mg.)	Vitamin A Value (I.U.)	Thiamine B₁ (Mg.)	Riboflavin B₂ (Mg.)	Niacin Value (Mg.)	Ascorbic Acid (Mg.)
Pies: Apple, 4″ sector	331	2.8	12.8	9	.5	220	.04	.02	.3	1
Blueberry, 4″ sector	291	2.8	9.3	14	.7	160	.02	.04	.3	5
Cherry, 4″ sector	340	3.2	13.2	14	.5	530	.04	.02	.3	2
Pineapple, raw, 1 cup diced	74	.6	.3	22	.4	180	.12	.04	.3	33
Pork, cured:										
Ham, smoked, cooked, 3 ounces without bone	339	20.0	28.0	9	2.5	—	.46	.18	3.5	—
Potatoes, baked, 1 medium, 2½″ diam.	97	2.4	.1	13	.8	20	.11	.05	1.4	17
Peeled and boiled, 1 medium, 2½″ diam.	105	2.5	.1	14	.9	20	.12	.04	1.3	17
French fried, 8 pieces 2 × ½ × ½″	157	2.2	7.6	12	.8	20	.07	.04	1.3	11
Hash-browned, 1 cup	470	6.4	22.8	35	2.3	60	.15	.11	3.3	14
Mashed, milk added, 1 cup	159	4.3	1.4	53	1.2	80	.16	.10	1.7	14
Prune juice, canned, 1 cup	170	1.0	—	60	4.3	—	.07	.19	1.0	2
Puffed rice, 1 cup	55	.8	.1	3	.3	—	.06	.01	.8	—
Rice, brown, raw, 1 cup	784	15.6	3.5	81	4.2	—	.66	.10	9.6	—
Cooked, 1 cup	204	4.2	.2	14	.5	—	.10	.02	1.9	—
White, cooked, 1 cup	201	4.2	.2	13	.5	—	.02	.01	.7	—
Rolls, 1 plain, pan rolls unenriched (12 per pound)	118	3.4	2.1	21	.3	—	.02	.04	.4	—
Salad dressing:										
Commercial, plain (mayonnaise type), 1 tbs.	58	.2	5.5	1	.1	20	Tr.	Tr.		—
French, 1 tbs.	59	.1	5.3	—	—	—	—	—	—	—
Mayonnaise, 1 tbs.	92	.2	10.1	2	.1	30	Tr.	Tr.	—	—
Salad oil, 1 tbs.	124	—	14.0	—	—	—	—	—	—	—
Salmon, broiled, baked, 1 steak 4 × 3 × ½″	204	33.6	6.7	—	1.4	—	.12	.33	9.8	—
Shredded wheat, 1 large biscuit, plain	102	2.9	.7	13	1.0	—	.06	.03	1.3	—

Shrimp, canned, 3 ounces drained solids	110	23.0	1.2	98	2.6	50	.01	.03	1.9	—
Soups, canned:										
Bouillon, broth, and consommé, ready-to-serve, 1 cup	9	2.0	—	2	1.0	—	—	.05	.6	—
Chicken, ready-to-serve, 1 cup	75	3.5	2.5	20	.5	—	.02	.12	1.5	—
Clam chowder, ready-to-serve, 1 cup	86	4.6	2.3	36	3.6	—	—	—	.7	10
Tomato, ready-to-serve, 1 cup	90	2.2	2.2	24	1.0	1,230	.02	.10	.7	8
Vegetable, ready-to-serve, 1 cup	82	4.2	1.8	32	.8	—	.05	.08	1.0	—
Spaghetti, dry, unenriched, 1 cup 2″ pieces	354	12.0	1.3	21	1.4	—	.09	.06	1.9	—
Cooked, 1 cup	218	7.4	.9	13	.9	—	.03	.02	.7	—
Spinach, raw, 4 ounces edible portion	22	2.6	.3	92	3.4	10,680	.13	.23	.7	67
Cooked, 1 cup	46	5.6	1.1	223	3.6	21,200	.14	.36	1.1	54
Sugars:										
1 teaspoon	16	—	—	—	—	—	—	—	—	—
1 lump 1⅛ × ⅝ × ⅛″	27	—	—	—	—	—	—	—	—	—
Swordfish, broiled, 1 steak 3 × 3 × ½″	223	34.2	8.5	25	1.4	2,880	.06	.07	12.9	—
Tongue, beef, medium fat, raw, 4 ounces	235	18.6	17.0	10	3.2	—	.14	.33	5.7	—
Tuna fish, canned, 3 oz. drained solids	169	24.7	7.0	7	1.2	70	.04	.10	10.9	—
Turkey, medium fat, raw, 4 oz. edible portion	304	22.8	22.9	26	4.3	Tr.	.10	.16	9.1	—
Veal, cooked, cutlet, 3 ounces without bone	184	24.0	9.0	10	3.0	—	.07	.24	5.2	—
Shoulder roast, 3 ounces without bone	193	24.0	10.0	10	3.1	—	.11	.27	6.7	—
Stew meat, 3 ounces without bone	252	21.0	18.0	9	2.6	—	.04	.20	3.9	—
Watermelon, ½ slice ¾ × 10′	45	.8	.3	11	.3	950	.08	.08	.3	10
Wheat germ, 1 cup stirred	246	17.1	6.8	57	5.5	—	1.39	.54	3.1	—
Yeast, dried, brewer's, 1 tbs.	22	3.0	.1	8	1.5	—	.78	.44	2.9	—
Yogurt, commercial made with whole milk, 1 cup	170	11.0	8.0	560	.2	380	.10	.45	—	3

Appendix B

Emergency Care of The Sick and Injured

The material in this section is taken from the booklet *In Time of Emergency* published by the Office of Civil Defense.* Although this booklet was designed primarily as a guide to the management of emergencies which might result from such widespread disasters as nuclear warfare, floods, earthquakes, and so forth, it has obvious applications to the more common emergencies experienced by individuals and small groups. During these infrequent but often serious situations those involved may have little more on which to rely than their own knowledge of first aid and emergency medical care.

Both adults and teenagers can acquire these valuable skills now by taking free courses that are offered in many communities, such as the Medical Self-Help course or a First Aid course.

The following information is no substitute for one of these courses. This basic guidance may save lives during a nuclear emergency, however, by helping untrained persons take care of the sick and injured when professional medical assistance may not be immediately available.

GENERAL RULES FOR ANY MEDICAL EMERGENCY

1. **First of all, do no harm.** Often, well-meaning but untrained persons worsen the injury or illness in their attempts to help. Get competent medical assistance, if possible. Do not assume responsibility for a patient if you can get the help of a doctor, nurse, or experienced first-aid worker. But if no one better qualified is available, take charge yourself.

*Office of Civil Defense (Department of Defense), *In Time of Emergency: A Citizen's Handbook on Nuclear Attack, Natural Disasters* (H–14), Washington, D.C., 1968.

2. **Look for stoppage of breathing, and for serious bleeding.** These are the two most life-threatening conditions you can do something about. They demand *immediate* treatment. . . .

3. **Prevent shock, or treat it.** Shock, a serious condition of acute circulatory failure, usually accompanies a severe or painful injury, a serious loss of blood, or a severe emotional upset. If you *expect* shock, and take prompt action, you can prevent it or lessen its severity. This may save the patient's life. . . .

4. **Don't move the patient immediately.** Unless there is real danger of the patient receiving further injury where he is, he should not be moved until breathing is restored, bleeding is stopped, and suspected broken bones are splinted.

5. **Keep calm, and reassure the patient.** Keep him lying down and comfortably warm, but do not apply heat to his body, or make him sweat.

6. **Never attempt to give liquids to an unconscious person.** If he is not able to swallow, he may choke to death or drown. Also, don't give him any liquids to drink if he has an abdominal injury.

IF THE PATIENT HAS STOPPED BREATHING

Quick action is required. You must get air into his lungs again immediately or he may die. The best and simplest way of doing this is to use mouth-to-mouth artificial respiration. Here is how to do it:

1. Place the patient on his back. Loosen his collar (Figure F-1).

FIGURE F-1

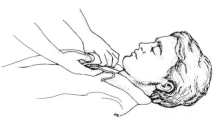

2. Open his mouth and use your fingers to remove any food or foreign matter. If he has false teeth or removable dental bridges, take them out.

3. Tilt the patient's head back so that his chin points upward. Lift his lower jaw from beneath and behind so that it juts out (Figure F-2). This will move his tongue away from the back of his throat, so it does not block the air passage to his lungs. Placing a pillow or something else

FIGURE F-2

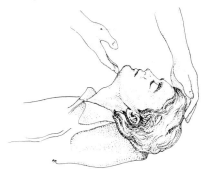

under his shoulders will help get his head into the right position. Some patients will start breathing as soon as you take these steps, and no further help is necessary.

4. Open your mouth as wide as possible, and place it tightly over the patient's mouth, so his mouth is completely covered by yours. With one hand, pinch his nostrils shut. With your other hand, hold his lower jaw in a thrust-forward position and keep his head tilted back (Figure F-3). With a baby or small child, place your mouth over both his nose and mouth, making a tight seal.

FIGURE F-3

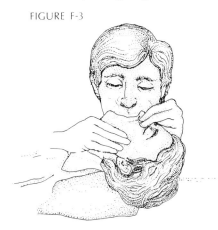

5. Blow a good lungful of air into an adult patient's mouth, continuing to keep his head tilted back and his jaw jutting out so that the air passage is kept open (Figure F-4). (Air can be blown through an unconscious person's teeth, even though they may be clenched tightly together.) Watch his chest as you blow.

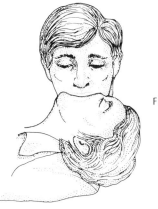

FIGURE F-4

When you see his chest rise, you will know that you are getting air into his lungs.

6. Remove your mouth from the patient's mouth, and listen for him to breathe out the air you breathed into him. You also may feel his breath on your cheek and see his chest sink as he exhales.

7. Continue your breathing for the patient. If he is an adult, blow a good breath into his mouth every 5 seconds, or 12 times a minute, and listen for him to breathe it back out again. *Caution:* If the patient is an infant or small child, blow *small puffs* of air into him about 20 times a minute. You may rupture his lung if you blow in too much air at one time. Watch his chest rise to make sure you are giving him the right amount of air with each puff (Figure F-5).

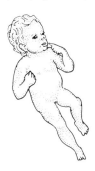

FIGURE F-5

8. If you are *not* getting air into the patient's lungs, or if he is not breathing out the air you blow into him, first make sure that his head is tilted back and his jaw is jutting out in the proper position. Then use your fingers to make sure nothing in his mouth or throat is obstructing the air passage to his lungs. If this does not help, turn him on his side and strike him sharply with the palm of your hand several times between his shoulder blades (Figure F-6). This

FIGURE F-6

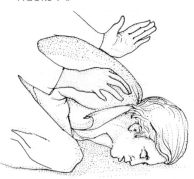

should dislodge any obstruction in the air passage. Then place him again on his back, with his head tilted back and his jaw jutting out, and resume blowing air into his mouth. If this doesn't work, try closing his mouth and blowing air through his nose into his lungs.

9. If you wish to avoid placing your mouth directly on the patient's face, you may hold a cloth (handkerchief, gauze or other porous material) over his mouth and breathe through the cloth (Figure F-7). But don't waste precious time looking for a cloth if you don't have one.

FIGURE F-7

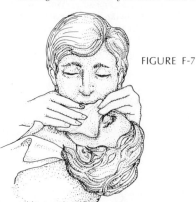

10. *Important:* Even if the patient does not respond, continue your efforts for 1 hour or longer, or until you are completely sure he is dead. If possible, have this confirmed by at least one other person.

TO STOP SERIOUS BLEEDING

1. Apply firm, even pressure to the wound with a dressing, clean cloth, or sanitary napkin (Figure F-8). If you don't have

FIGURE F-8

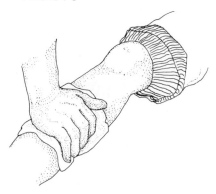

any of these, use your bare hand until you can get something better. Remember, you must keep blood from running out of the patient's body. Loss of 1 or 2 quarts will seriously endanger his life.

2. Hold the dressing in place with your hand until you can bandage the dressing in place. In case of an arm or leg wound, make sure the bandage is not so tight as to cut off circulation; and raise the arm or leg above the level of the patient's heart (Figure F-9). (But if the arm or leg appears broken, be sure to splint it first.)

FIGURE F-9

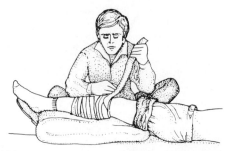

3. Treat the patient for shock. . . .
4. If blood soaks through the dressing, do *not* remove the dressing. Apply more dressings.
5. SPECIAL ADVICE ON TOURNIQUETS: Never use a tourniquet unless you cannot stop excessive, life-threatening bleeding by any other method. Using a tourniquet increases the chances that the arm or leg will have to be amputated later (see Figure F-10). If

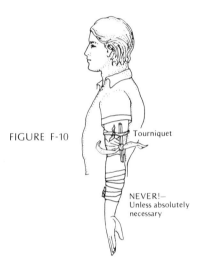

FIGURE F-10 — Tourniquet

NEVER!—
Unless absolutely
necessary

you are *forced* to use a tourniquet to keep the patient from bleeding to death (for example, when a hand or foot has been accidentally cut off), follow these instructions carefully:

☐ Place the tourniquet *as close to the wound as possible,* between the wound and the patient's heart.
☐ After the tourniquet has been applied, do not permit it to be loosened (even temporarily, or even though the bleeding has stopped) by anyone except a physician, who can control the bleeding by other methods and replace the blood that the patient has lost.
☐ Get a physician to treat the patient as soon as possible.

[*Note:* When tourniquets are not applied tightly enough they may encourage bleeding by preventing the normal return of the blood through the veins.—Au.]

PREVENTING AND TREATING SHOCK

Being "in shock" means that a person's circulatory system is not working properly, and not enough blood is getting to the vital centers of his brain and spinal cord.

These are the symptoms of shock: The patient's pulse is weak or rapid, or he may have no pulse that you can find. His skin may be pale or blue, cold, or moist. His breathing may be shallow or irregular. He may have chills. He may be thirsty. He may get sick at his stomach and vomit.

A person can be "in shock" whether he is conscious or unconscious.

Important: All seriously injured persons should be treated for shock, even though they appear normal and alert. Shock may cause death if not treated promptly, even though the injuries which brought on shock might not be serious enough to cause death. In fact, persons may go into shock without having any physical injuries.

Here is how to treat any person who may be in shock:

1. Keep him lying down and keep him from chilling, but do *not* apply a hot water bottle or other heat to his body. Also, loosen his clothing.
2. Keep his head a little lower than his legs and hips. But if he has a head or chest injury, or has difficulty in breathing, keep his head and shoulders slightly higher than the rest of his body.
3. Encourage him to drink fluids if he is conscious and not nauseated, and if he does not have abdominal injuries. Every 15 minutes give him a half-glass of this solution until he no longer wants it: One teaspoonful of salt and a half-teaspoonful of baking soda to one quart of water.
4. Do *not* give him alcohol.

FRACTURES

Any break in a bone is called a fracture. If you think a person may have a fracture, treat it as though it were one. Otherwise, you may cause further injury. For example, if an arm or leg is injured and bleeding, splint it as well as bandage it.

With any fracture, first look for bleeding and control it. Keep the patient comfortably warm and quiet, preferably lying down. If you have an ice bag, apply it to the fracture to ease the pain. Do not move the patient (unless his life is in danger where he is) without first applying a splint or otherwise immobilizing the bone that may be fractured. Treat the patient for shock.

A fractured arm or leg should be straightened out as much as possible, preferably by having 2 persons gently stretch it into a normal position. Then it should be "splinted"—that is, fastened to a board or something else to prevent motion and keep the ends of the broken bone together. As a splint, use a board, a trimmed branch from a tree, a broomstick, an umbrella, a roll of newspapers, or anything else rigid enough to keep the arm or leg straight (Figure F–11). Fasten the arm or leg to the splint with

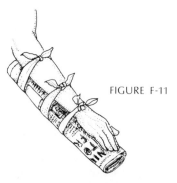

FIGURE F-11

bandages, strips of cloth, handkerchiefs, neckties, or belts. After splinting, keep the injured arm or leg a little higher than the rest of the patient's body (Figure F–12). From time to time, make sure that the splint

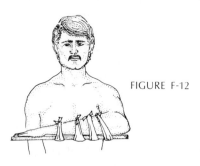

FIGURE F-12

is not too tight, since the arm or leg may swell, and the blood circulation might be shut off. If the broken bone is sticking out through the skin but the exposed part of it is clean, allow it to slip back naturally under the skin (but don't push it in) when the limb is being straightened. However, if the exposed part of the bone is dirty, cover it

with a clean cloth and bandage the wound to stop the bleeding. Then splint the arm or leg without trying to straighten it out, and try to find a doctor or nurse to treat the patient.

A fractured collarbone should also be prevented from moving, until the patient can get professional medical attention. It can be immobilized by placing the arm on that side in a sling and then binding the arm close to the body (Figure F–13).

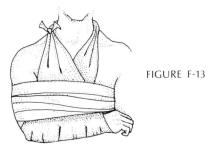

FIGURE F-13

A fractured rib should be suspected if the patient has received a chest injury or if he has pain when he moves his chest, breathes, or coughs. Strap the injured side of his chest with 2-inch adhesive tape if available, or with a cloth bandage or towel wrapped around and around his entire chest. (See Figure F–14.)

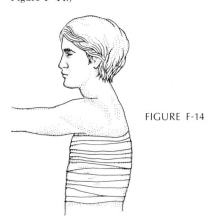

FIGURE F-14

Fractured bones in the **neck or back** are very serious, because they may injure the patient's spinal cord and paralyze him or even kill him. He should not be moved until a doctor comes (or a person trained in first aid), unless it is absolutely necessary to move him to prevent further injury. If a person with a back injury has to be moved, he should be placed gently on his back on a

FIGURE F-16

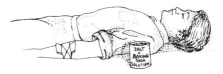

stiff board, door or stretcher. His head, back, and legs should be kept in a straight line at all times (Figure F–15).

A person with a neck injury should be moved gently with his head, neck, and shoulders kept in the same position they were when he was found. His neck should not be allowed to bend when he is being moved.

from the burn (Figure F-17). The dressing will help prevent surface washings from getting into the burned area.

FIGURE F-17

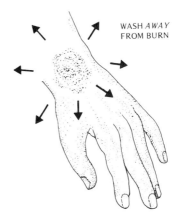

WASH *AWAY* FROM BURN

BURNS

Non-serious or superficial (first degree) burns should not be covered—in fact, nothing need be done for them. However, if a first degree burn covers a large area of the body, the patient should be given fluids to drink as mentioned in item 2 following.

The most important things to do about serious (second or third degree) burns are: (a) Treat the patient for shock, (b) Prevent infection, and (c) Relieve pain. These specific actions should be taken:

1. Keep the patient lying down, with his head a little lower than his legs and hips unless he has a head or chest wound, or has difficulty in breathing.
2. Have him drink a half-glass every 15 minutes of a salt-and-soda solution (one teaspoonful of salt and a half-teaspoonful of baking soda to a quart of water, Figure F-16). Give him additional plain water to drink if he wants it.
3. Cover the burned area with a *dry,* sterile gauze dressing. If gauze is not available, use a clean cloth, towel, or pad.
4. With soap and water, wash the area *around* the burn (not the burn itself) for a distance of several inches, wiping *away*

5. Use a bandage to hold the dry dressing firmly in place against the burned area. This will keep moving air from reaching the burn, and will lessen the pain. Leave dressings and bandage in place as long as possible.
6. If adjoining surfaces of skin are burned, separate them with gauze or cloth to keep them from sticking together (such as between toes or fingers, ears and head, arms and chest) (Figure F–18).
7. If the burn was caused by a chemical—or by fallout particles sticking to the skin or hair—wash the chemical or the fallout

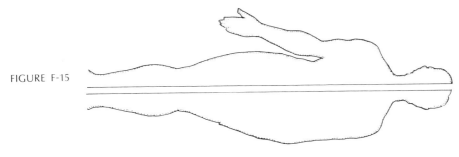

FIGURE F-15

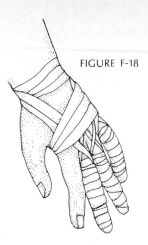

FIGURE F-18

particles away with generous amounts of plain water, then treat the burn as described above.

What NOT to do about burns:

☐ Don't pull clothing over the burned area (cut it away, if necessary, Figure F–19).

FIGURE F-19

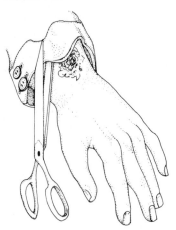

☐ Don't try to remove any pieces of cloth, or bits of dirt or debris, that may be sticking to the burn.
☐ Don't try to clean the burn; don't use iodine or other antiseptics on it; and don't open any blisters that may form on it.
☐ Don't use grease, butter, ointment, salve, petroleum jelly, or any type of medication on severe burns. Keeping them dry is best.
☐ Don't breathe on a burn, and don't touch it with anything except a sterile or clean dressing.

☐ Don't change the dressings that were initially applied to the burn, until absolutely necessary. Dressings may be left in place for a week, if necessary.

RADIATION SICKNESS

Radiation sickness is caused by the invisible rays given off by particles of radioactive fallout. If a person has received a large dose of radiation in a short period of time—generally, less than a week—he will become seriously ill and probably will die. But if he has received only a small or medium dose, his body will repair itself and he will get well. No special clothing can protect a person from gamma radiation, and no special medicines can protect him or cure him of radiation sickness.

Symptoms of radiation sickness may not be noticed for several days. The early symptoms are lack of appetite, nausea, vomiting, fatigue, weakness, and headache. Later, the patient may have sore mouth, loss of hair, bleeding gums, bleeding under the skin, and diarrhea. But these same symptoms can be caused by other diseases, and not everyone who has radiation sickness shows all these symptoms, or shows them all at once.

If the patient has headache or general discomfort, give him one or two aspirin tablets every 3 or 4 hours (half a tablet, for a child under 12). If he is nauseous, give him "motion sickness tablets," if available. If his mouth is sore or his gums are bleeding, have him use a mouth wash made up of a half-teaspoonful of salt to 1 quart of water. If there is vomiting or diarrhea, he should drink slowly several glasses each day of a salt-and-soda solution (one teaspoonful of salt and one-half teaspoonful of baking soda to 1 quart of cool water), plus bouillon or fruit juices. If available, a mixture of kaolin and pectin should be given for diarrhea. Whatever his symptoms, the patient should be kept lying down, comfortably warm, and resting.

Remember that radiation sickness is *not* contagious or infectious and one person cannot "catch it" from another person.

Appendix C

*Major Natural Disasters**

GENERAL GUIDANCE

There are certain things you can learn and do that will help you get ready for, and cope with, almost any type of natural disaster.

Perhaps the most basic thing to remember is to *keep calm*. This may mean the difference between life and death. In many disasters, people have been killed or injured needlessly because they took thoughtless actions when they should have done something else—or done nothing at all just then.

In a time of emergency, taking proper action may save your life. *Take time to think,* and then take the considered action that the situation calls for. Usually, this will be the action you have planned in advance, or the action you are instructed to take by responsible authorities.

Here is other guidance that applies to most types of natural disasters.

Warning

LEARN YOUR COMMUNITY'S WARNING SIGNALS. In most communities having outdoor warning systems, the Attack Warning Signal is a wavering sound on the sirens, or a series of short blasts on whistles, horns, or other devices. This signal will be used only to warn of an attack against the United States.

Many communities also are using an *Attention or Alert Signal,* usually a 3- to 5-minute *steady blast* to get the attention of

*This section is reprinted from the Office of Civil Defense (Department of Defense), *In Time of Emergency: A Citizen's Handbook on Nuclear Attack, Natural Disasters* (H-14), Washington, D.C., 1968.

their people in a time of threatened or impending peacetime emergency. In most places, the Attention or Alert Signal means that people should turn on their radio or television sets to hear important emergency information being broadcast.

You should find out now, before any emergency occurs, what warning signals are being used in your community, what they sound like, what they mean, and what actions you should take when you hear them.

Also, whenever a major storm or other peacetime disaster threatens, keep your radio or television set turned on to hear Weather Bureau reports and forecasts (issued by the Environmental Science Services Administration of the U.S. Department of Commerce), as well as other information and advice thay may be broadcast by your local government.

When you are warned of an emergency, get your information on the radio or television. Use your telephone only to *report* important events (such as fires, flash floods, or tornado sightings) to the local authorities. If you tie up the telephone lines simply to get information, you may prevent emergency calls from being completed.

Emergency Supplies

A major disaster of almost any kind may interfere with your normal supplies of water, food, heat, and other day-to-day necessities. You should keep on hand, in or around your home, a stock of emergency supplies sufficient to meet your needs for a few days or preferably for a week.

If you stayed at home during the disaster, these supplies would help you live through the period of emergency without hardship. If you had to evacuate your home and move temporarily to another location, your emergency supplies could be taken with you and used en route or after you arrived at the new location (where regular supplies might not be available). Even if you only had to move to an emergency shelter station set up by a local agency, these supplies might be helpful to you, or make your stay easier.

The most important items to keep on hand are water (preferably in plastic jugs or other stoppered containers); canned or sealed-package foods that do not require refrigeration or heat for cooking; medicines needed by family members, and a first aid kit; blankets or sleeping bags; flashlights or lanterns; a battery-powered radio; and perhaps a covered container to use as an emergency toilet. In addition, an automobile in good operating condition with an ample supply of gasoline may be necessary in case you have to leave your home.

In those parts of the country subject to hurricanes or floods, it is also wise to keep on hand certain emergency materials you may need to protect your home from wind and water—such as plywood sheeting or lumber to board up your windows and doors, and plastic sheeting or tarpaulins to protect furniture and appliances.

Fire Protection and Fire Fighting

Fires are a special hazard in a time of disaster. They may start more readily, and the help of the fire department may not be available quickly. Therefore, it is essential that you

1. Follow . . . fire prevention rules . . . and be especially careful not to start fires.
2. Know how to put out small fires yourself. . . .
3. Have on hand simple tools and equipment needed for fire fighting. . . .

After a Natural Disaster

Use extreme caution in entering or working in buildings that may have been damaged or weakened by the disaster, as they may collapse without warning. Also, there may be gas leaks or electrical short circuits.

Don't bring lanterns, torches, or lighted cigarettes into buildings that have been flooded or otherwise damaged by a natural disaster, since there may be leaking gas lines or flammable material present.

Stay away from fallen or damaged electric wires, which may still be dangerous.

Check for leaking gas pipes in your home. Do this by *smell only*—don't use matches or candles. If you smell gas, do this: (1) Open all windows and doors. (2) Turn off the main gas valve at the meter. (3) Leave the house immediately. (4) Notify the gas company or the police or fire department. (5) Don't reenter the house until you are told it is safe to do so.

If any of your electrical appliances are wet, first turn off the main power switch in your house, then unplug the wet appliance, dry it out, reconnect it, and finally, turn on the main power switch. (Caution: Don't do any of these things while *you* are wet or standing in water.) If fuses blow when the electric power is restored, turn off the main power

switch again and then inspect for short circuits in your home wiring, appliances, and equipment.

Check your food and water supplies before using them. Foods that require refrigeration may be spoiled if electric power has been off for some time. Also, don't eat food that has come in contact with flood waters. Be sure to follow the instructions of local authorities concerning the use of food and water supplies.

If needed, get food, clothing, medical care or shelter at Red Cross stations or from local government authorities.

Stay away from disaster areas. Sightseeing could interfere with first aid or rescue work, and may be dangerous as well.

Don't drive unless necessary, and drive with caution. Watch for hazards to yourself and others, and report them to local authorities.

Write, telegraph, or telephone your relatives, after the emergency is over, so they will know you are safe. Otherwise local authorities may waste time locating you—or if you have evacuated to a safer location, they may not be able to find you. (However, do not tie up the phone lines if they are still needed for official emergency calls.)

Do not pass on rumors or exaggerated reports of damage.

Follow the advice and instructions of your local government on ways to help yourself and your community recover from the emergency.

FLOODS AND HURRICANES

In addition to the general guidance at the beginning of this section, there are certain emergency actions particularly associated with major floods, hurricanes, and storm tides or surges. These types of disasters usually are preceded by extended periods of warning. People living in areas likely to be most severely affected often are warned to move to safer locations.

Evacuation

If you are warned to evacuate your home and move to another location temporarily, there are certain things to remember and do. Here are the most important ones:

Follow the instructions and advice of your local government. If you are told to evacuate, do so promptly. If you are instructed to move to a certain location, go there—don't go anywhere else. If certain travel routes are specified or recommended, use those routes rather than trying to find short cuts of your own. (It will help if you have previously become familiar with the routes likely to be used.) If you are told to shut off your water, gas, or electric service before leaving home, do so. Also find out on the radio where emergency housing and mass feeding stations are located, in case you need to use them.

Secure your home before leaving. If you have time, and if you have not received other instructions from your local government, you should take the following actions before leaving your home:

☐ Bring outside possessions inside the house, or tie them down securely. This includes outdoor furniture, garbage cans, garden tools, signs, and other movable objects that might be blown or washed away.

☐ Board up your windows so they won't be broken by high winds, water, flying objects, or debris.

☐ If flooding is likely, move furniture and other movable objects to the upper floor of your house. Disconnect any electrical appliances or equipment that cannot be moved—but don't touch them if you are wet or are standing in water.

☐ Do *not* stack sandbags around the outside walls of your house to keep flood waters out of your basement. Water seeping downward through the earth (either beyond the sandbags or over them) may collect around the basement walls and under the floor, creating pressure that could damage the walls or else raise the entire basement and cause it to "float" out of the ground. In most cases it is better to permit the flood waters to flow freely into the basement (or flood the basement yourself with clean water, if you feel sure it will be flooded anyway). This will equalize the water pressure on the inside and outside of the basement walls and floor, and thus avoid structural damage to the foundation and the house.

☐ Lock house doors and windows. Park your car in the garage or driveway, close the windows, and lock it (unless you are driving to your new temporary location).

Travel with care. If your local government is arranging transportation for you, precautions will be taken for your safety. But if you are walking or driving your own car to another location, keep in mind these things:

☐ Leave early enough so as not to be marooned by flooded roads, fallen trees, and wires.

☐ Make sure you have enough gasoline in your car.

☐ Follow recommended routes.

☐ As you travel, keep listening to the radio for additional information and instructions from your local government.

☐ Watch for washed-out or undermined roadways, earth slides, broken sewer or water mains, loose or downed electric wires, and falling or fallen objects.

☐ Watch out for areas where rivers or streams may flood suddenly.

☐ Don't try to cross a stream or a pool of water unless you are certain that the water will not be above your knees (or above the middle of your car's wheels) *all the way across.* Sometimes the water will hide a bridge or a part of the road that has been washed out. If you decide it is safe to drive across it, put your car in low gear and drive very slowly, to avoid splashing water into your engine and causing it to stop. Also, remember that your brakes may not work well after the wheels of your car have been in deep water. Try them out a few times when you reach the other side.

During a Hurricane

☐ If your house is on high ground and you haven't been instructed to evacuate, stay indoors. Don't try to travel, since you will be in danger from flying debris, flooded roads, and downed wires.

☐ Keep listening to your radio or television set for further information and advice. If the center or "eye" of the hurricane passes directly over you, there will be a temporary lull in the wind, lasting from a few minutes to perhaps a half-hour or more. *Stay in a safe place during this lull.* The wind will return—perhaps with even greater force—from the *opposite* direction.

Special Advice on Flash Floods

In many areas, unusually heavy rains may cause quick or "flash" floods. Small creeks, gullies, dry streambeds, ravines, culverts or even low-lying grounds frequently flood very quickly and endanger people, sometimes before any warning can be given.

In a period of heavy rains, be aware of this hazard and be prepared to protect yourself against it. If you see any possibility of a flash flood occurring where you are, move immediately to a safer location (don't wait for instructions to move), and then notify your local authorities of the danger, so other people can be warned.

TORNADOES

When a tornado watch (forecast) is announced, this means that tornadoes are expected in or near your area. Keep your radio or television set tuned to a local station for information and advice from your local government or the Weather Bureau. Also, keep watching the sky, especially to the south and southwest. (When a tornado watch is announced during the approach of a hurricane, however, keep watching the sky to the east.) If you see any revolving, funnel-shaped clouds, report them by telephone immediately to your local police department, sheriff's office or Weather Bureau office. But do not use the phone to get information and advice—depend on radio or TV.

When a tornado warning is issued, take shelter immediately. The warning means that a tornado has actually been sighted, and this (or other tornadoes) may strike in your vicinity. You must take action to protect yourself from being blown away, struck by falling objects, or injured by flying debris. Your best protection is an underground shelter or cave, or a substantial steel-framed or reinforced-concrete building. But if none of these is available, there are other places where you can take refuge:

☐ If you are *at home,* go to your underground storm cellar or your basement fallout shelter, if you have one. If not, go to a corner of your home basement and take cover under a sturdy workbench or table (but not underneath heavy appliances on the floor above). If your home has no basement, take cover under heavy furniture on the ground floor in the center part of the house, or in a small room on the ground floor that is away from outside walls and windows. (As a last resort, go outside to a nearby ditch, excavation, culvert or ravine.) Doors and windows on the sides of your house *away from* the tornado may be left open to help reduce damage to the building, but stay away from them to avoid flying debris. Do not remain in a trailer or mobile home if a tornado is approaching; take cover elsewhere.

☐ If you are *at work* in an office building, go to the basement or to an inner hallway on a lower floor. In a factory, go to a shelter area, or to the basement if there is one.

☐ If you are *outside in open country,* drive away from the tornado's path, at a right angle to it. If there isn't time to do this—or if you are walking—take cover and lie flat in the nearest depression, such as a ditch, culvert, excavation, or ravine.

WINTER STORMS

Here is advice that will help you protect yourself and your family against the hazards of winter storms—blizzards, heavy snows, ice storms, freezing rain, or sleet.

Keep posted on weather conditions. Use your radio, television and newspapers to keep informed of current weather conditions and forecasts in your area. Even a few hours' warning of a storm may enable you to avoid being caught outside in it, or at least be better prepared to cope with it. You should also understand the terms commonly used in weather forecasts:

☐ A *blizzard* is the most dangerous of all winter storms. It combines cold air, heavy snow, and strong winds that blow the snow about and may reduce visibility to only a few yards. A *blizzard warning* is issued when the Weather Bureau expects considerable snow, winds of 35 miles an hour or more, and temperatures of 20 degrees Fahrenheit or lower. A *severe blizzard warning* means that a very heavy snowfall is expected, with winds of at least 45 miles an hour and temperatures of 10 degrees or lower.

☐ A *heavy snow warning* usually means an expected snowfall of 4 inches or more in a 12-hour period, or 6 inches or more in a 24-hour period. Warnings of *snow flurries, snow squalls,* or *blowing and drifting snow* are important mainly because visibility may be reduced and roads may become slippery or blocked.

☐ *Freezing rain or freezing drizzle* is forecast when expected rain is likely to freeze as soon as it strikes the ground, putting a coating of ice or glaze on roads and everything else that is exposed. If a substantial layer of ice is expected to accumulate from the freezing rain, an *ice storm* is forecast.

□ *Sleet* is small particles of ice, usually mixed with rain. If enough sleet accumulates on the ground, it will make the roads slippery.

Be prepared for isolation at home. If you live in a rural area, make sure you could survive at home for a week or two in case a storm isolated you and made it impossible for you to leave. You should:

□ Keep an adequate supply of heating fuel on hand and use it sparingly, as your regular supplies may be curtailed by storm conditions. If necessary, conserve fuel by keeping the house cooler than usual, or by "closing off" some rooms temporarily. Also, have available some kind of *emergency* heating equipment and fuel so you could keep at least one room of your house warm enough to be livable. This could be a camp stove with fuel, or a supply of wood or coal if you have a fireplace. If your furnace is controlled by a thermostat and your electricity is cut off by a storm, the furnace probably would not operate and you would need emergency heat.

□ Stock an emergency supply of food and water, as well as emergency cooking equipment such as a camp stove. Some of this food should be of the type that does not require refrigeration or cooking.

□ Make sure you have a battery-powered radio and extra batteries on hand so that if your electric power is cut off you could still hear weather forecasts, information, and advice broadcast by local authorities. Also, flashlights or lanterns would be needed.

□ See previous section on "General Guidance" for other supplies and equipment that you may need if isolated at home. Be sure to keep on hand the simple tools and equipment needed to fight a fire. Also, be certain that all family members know how to take precautions that would prevent fire at such a time, when the help of the fire department may not be available.

Travel only if necessary. Avoid all unnecessary trips. If you must travel, use public transportation if possible. However, if you are forced to use your automobile for a

trip of any distance, take these precautions:

□ Make sure your car is in good operating condition, properly serviced, and equipped with chains or snow tires.

□ Take another person with you if possible.

□ Make sure someone knows where you are going, your approximate schedule, and your estimated time of arrival at your destination.

□ Have emergency "winter storm supplies" in the car, such as a container of sand, shovel, windshield scraper, tow chain or rope, extra gasoline, and a flashlight. It also is good to have with you heavy gloves or mittens, overshoes, extra woolen socks, and winter headgear to cover your head and face.

□ Travel by daylight and use major highways if you can. Keep the car radio turned on for weather information and advice.

□ Drive with all possible caution. Don't try to save time by travelling faster than road and weather conditions permit.

□ Don't be daring or foolhardy. Stop, turn back, or seek help if conditions threaten that may test your ability or endurance, rather than risk being stalled, lost, or isolated. If you are caught in a *blizzard,* seek refuge immediately.

Keep calm if you get in trouble. If your car breaks down during a storm, or if you become stalled or lost, don't panic. Think the problem through, decide what's the safest and best thing to do, and then do it slowly and carefully. If you are on a well-traveled road, show a trouble signal. Set your directional lights to flashing, raise the hood of your car, or hang a cloth from the radio aerial or car window. Then stay in your car and wait for help to arrive. If you run the engine to keep warm, remember to open a window enough to provide ventilation and protect you from carbon monoxide poisoning.

Wherever you are, if there is no house or other source of help in sight, do not leave your car to search for assistance, as you may become confused and get lost.

Avoid overexertion. Every winter many unnecessary deaths occur because people—especially older persons, but younger ones as well—engage in more strenuous physical activity than their bodies can stand. Cold weather itself, *without* any physical exertion, puts an extra strain on your heart. If you add to this physical exercise, especially exercise that you are not accustomed to—such as shovelling snow, pushing an automobile, or even walking fast or far—you are risking a heart attack, a stroke, or other damage to your body. In winter weather, and especially in winter storms, be aware of this danger, and avoid overexertion.

[*Note:* Although it is true that overexertion can be dangerous as a result of undiagnosed heart disease, particularly prevalent in older persons, it should be noted that there is little evidence that a healthy heart can be damaged by excessive exercise. Moreover, those who exercise appropriately on a regular basis are less likely to experience overexertion while coping with occasional emergencies.—Au.]

EARTHQUAKES

If your area is one of the places in the United States where earthquakes occur, keep these points in mind:

□ When an earthquake happens, *keep calm.* Don't run or panic. If you take the proper precautions, the chances are you will not be hurt.

□ REMAIN WHERE YOU ARE. If you are outdoors, stay outdoors; if indoors, stay indoors. In earthquakes, most injuries occur as people are entering or leaving buildings (from falling walls, electric wires, etc.).

□ If you are indoors, sit or stand against an inside wall (preferably in the basement), or in an inside doorway; or else take cover under a desk, table or bench (in case the wall or ceiling should fall). Stay away from windows and outside doors.

□ If you are outdoors, stay away from overhead electric wires, poles or anything else that might shake loose and fall (such as the cornices of tall buildings).

□ If you are *driving an automobile,* pull off the road and stop (as soon as possible, and with caution). Remain in the car until the disturbance subsides. When you drive on, watch for hazards created by the earthquake, such as fallen or falling objects, downed electric wires, and broken or undermined roadways.

After an Earthquake

For your own safety and that of others, you should follow carefully the advice given in the section, "After a Natural Disaster"

REFERENCES

Chapter 1   Health: What Does It Mean?

Apple, D. "How Laymen Define Illness," *Journal of Human Behavior,* 1960.

Dunn, H. L. "Points of Attack for Raising The Level of Wellness," *Journal of the National Medical Association,* 1957.

Feinstein, A. R., and E. N. Brandt. "New Concepts in Diagnostic Decision-Making," *Continuing Education for the Family Physician.* 1974.

Robbins, L. C., and J. H. Hall. *How to Practice Prospective Medicine.* Indianapolis, Ind.: Methodist Hospital of Indiana, 1970.

Roemer, M. I. "A Program of Preventive Medicine for the Individual," *Milbank Memorial Fund Quarterly,* 1945.

Sehnert, K. W., and M. Osterweis. "A Concept for Health Education," *Continuing Education,* October 1974.

Chapter 2   Making Wise Health Decisions

Brownfeld, Allan C. "The Manufactured Health Care 'Crisis' and the Demand That Wasn't There," *Private Practice,* December 1973.

"Cheaper Drugs?" *The National Observer,* January 12, 1974.

McMahon, John A. "How Much Care Can We Afford?" *Prism,* October 1974.

The Consumer Union Report on Life Insurance, Orangeburg, N.Y.: Consumer Union, 1972.

Chaper 4   Concepts of Positive Mental Health

"Anxiety and Coping Behavior," *Medical Tribune,* March 13, 1974.

Berne, Eric. *What Do You Say After You Say Hello?* New York: Bantam Books, 1973.

Chesler, Phyllis. *Women & Madness.* Garden City, N.Y.: Doubleday & Co., Inc., 1972.

"Competent Coping," *Medical Tribune,* February 13, 1974.

Fast, Julius. *Body Language.* New York: J. B. Lippincott Co., 1970.

Fisher, Seymour. *Body Consciousness.* Englewood Cliffs, N.J.: Prentice-Hall, Inc., 1973.

Fisher, Seymour and Sidney Cleveland. *Body Image and Personality.* New York: Dover Publications, Inc., 1968.

Chapter 5   Coping With Stress and Anxiety

"Anxiety and Coping Behavior," *Medical Tribune.* March 13, 1974.

Chesler. *Women and Madness.* Garden City, New York: Doubleday & Co., Inc., 1972.

"Competent Coping," *Medical Tribune,* February 13, 1974.

Jourard, Sidney M. *Disclosing Man to Himself.* Princeton, N.J.: D. Van Nostrand Co., Inc., 1968.

Menninger, Karl. *The Vital Balance.* New York: The Viking Press, 1963.

Selye, Hans. *The Stress of Life.* New York: McGraw-Hill Book Co., 1956.

Fletcher, Joseph. "New Definitions of Death," *Prism,* January 1974.

Frankl, Viktor E. *Man's Search For Meaning.* New York: Washington Square Press, Inc., 1968.

Hendin, Herbert. *Black Suicide.* New York: Harper Colophon Books, 1969.

Kübler-Ross, Elisabeth. *On Death and Dying.* New York: The MacMillan Co., 1969.

Meerloo, Joost A. M. *Suicide and Mass Suicide.* New York: E. P. Dutton & Co., Inc., 1968.

Shneidman, Edwin S. and Norman Farberow. *Clues to Suicide.* New York: McGraw-Hill Book Co., Inc., 1957.

Chapter 6   Maintaining Physical Well-Being

Cooper, Kenneth H. *Aerobics.* New York: Bantam Books, 1968.

Cooper, Kenneth H. *The New Aerobics.* New York: Bantam Books, 1970.

"Exercise: How to Conduct In Office Tests," *Patient Care,* March 15, 1974.

McGlynn, George H. *Issues in Physical Education and Sports.* Palo Alto, Calif.: National Press Books, 1974.

Chapter 7   Nutrition and Health

Bruch, Hilde. "Psychological Aspects of Obesity," *Medical Insights,* July-August 1973.

Engel, Mary, and Mae Rudolph. "Let's Talk About Good Foods," *Family Health,* July 1970.

"Good Food for Good Health," *Family Health,* June 1971.

Harris, T. George. "Affluence, the Fifth Horseman of the Apocalypse: A Conversation with Jean Mayer," *Psychology Today,* January 1970.

Hegsted, D. Mark. "The Recommended Dietary Allowances for Iron," *American Journal of Public Health,* April 1970.

Lee, D. "Food and Human Existence," *Nutritional News,* June 1962.

Setizer, Carl C., and Jean Mayer. "An Effective Weight Control Program in a Public School System," *American Journal of Public Health,* April 1970.

Seltzer, Carl C., and Frederick J. Stare.

"Obesity: How It Is Measured—What Causes It—How To Treat It," *Medical Insights,* July-August 1973.

White, Philip S. *Let's Talk About Food.* Chicago: American Medical Association, 1968.

White, Philip S., and Edward Rynearson. "The Dangers in Diet Advice," *Medical Insights,* July-August 1973.

Chapter 8   Healthy Sex and Sexuality

Otto, Herbert A. (Ed.). *The New Sexuality.* Palo Alto, Calif.: Science and Behavior Books, Inc., 1971.

Reich, Wilhelm. *The Sexual Revolution.* New York: Farrar, Straus and Giroux, 1970.

Chapter 9   Female Sexuality

Amir, Menachem. "Forcible Rape," *Sexual Behavior,* November 1971.

Boston Women's Health Book Collective, *Our Bodies Ourselves.* New York: Simon and Schuster, 1973.

"Does A Woman's Attractiveness Influence Men's Nonsexual Reactions?" *Medical Aspects of Human Sexuality,* November 1971.

Henley, Arthur. "The Mind of the Victim," *Physician's World,* August 1973.

Lee, Betty. "Precautions Against Rape," *Sexual Behavior,* January 1972.

Llewellyn-Jones, Derek. *Everywoman And Her Body.* New York: Lancer Books, 1971.

Miller, Jean Baker. *Psychoanalysis and Women.* New York: Penguin Books, 1973.

Montague, Ashley. *The Natural Superiority of Women.* New York: Collier Books, 1968.

Pengelley, Eric T. *Sex and Human Life.* Reading, Mass.: Addison-Wesley Pub., Co., 1974.

Pierson, Elaine. *Sex Is Never An Emergency.* New York: J. B. Lippincott Co., 1970.

Pierson, Elaine and William V. D'Antonio. *Female and Male.* New York: New York: J. B. Lippincott Co., 1974.

Time, "Special Issue: The American Women," March 20, 1972.

The Sensuous Woman by "J". New York: Dell Publishing Co., Inc., 1969.

"Women and Rape," *Medical Aspects of Human Sexuality,* May 1974.

Chapter 10   Male Sexuality

Belliveau, Fred and Lin Richter. *Understanding Human Sexual Inadequacy.* New York: Bantam Books, 1970.

Bowers, Faubion. "The Sexes: Getting It All Together," *Saturday Review,* January 9, 1971.

Katchadourian, Herant A., and Donald T. Lunde. *Fundamentals of Human Sexuality.* New York: Holt, Rinehart & Winston, 1972.

Masters, William H., and Virginia E. Johnson. *Human Sexual Inadequacy.* Boston: Little Brown, 1970.

Pengelley, Eric T. *Sex and Human Life.* Reading, Mass.: Addison-Wesley Pub., Co., 1974.

Chapter 11   Human Reproduction

Altchek, Albert. "The Art of Abortion," *Emergency Medicine,* September 1973.

Edwards, R. G., and Ruth E. Fowler. "Human Embryos in the Laboratory," *Scientific American,* December 1970.

Eggerz, S. "Childbirth Through The Ages," *Private Practice,* October 1973.

Friedman, Theodore. "Prenatal Diagnosis of Genetic Disease," *Scientific American,* November 1971.

Greenblatt, Robert B. "Risks of Oral Contraceptives," *Continuing Education,* August 1973.

Guild, Warren R., and Robert E. Fuisz et al. *The Science of Health.* Englewood Cliffs, N.J.: Prentice-Hall, Inc., 1969.

Hon, Edward H. "New Help for High Risk Pregnancies," *Modern Medicine,* September 3, 1973.

"IUDs: The Progress and the Problems," *Medical World News,* September 13, 1974.

Karmel, Marjorie. *Thank You, Dr. Lamaze.* Garden City, N.J.: Dolphin Books, 1959, 1965.

Netter, Frank H. *Reproductive System,* The CIBA Collection of Medical Illustrations. Summit, N.J.: The CIBA Pharmaceutical Co., 1965.

Rugh, Roberts, and Landrum B. Shettles. *From Conception to Birth—The Drama of Life's Beginnings.* New York: Harper & Row, 1971.

"Sterilization: The Patient's Final Choice," *Patient Care,* April 1, 1974.

"Vasectomy: Best Permanent Option?" *Patient Care,* April 1, 1974.

Chapter 12   Tobacco and Health

Chester, Eustace. *When and How to Quit Smoking.* New York: Emerson Books, 1964.

Cohen, Jacob, and R. K. Heimann. "Heavy Smokers with Low Mortality," *Industrial Medicine and Surgery,* March 1962.

Diehl, Harold. *Tobacco and Your Health.* New York: McGraw-Hill, 1969.

National Clearing House for Drug Abuse Information, *Resource Book for Drug Abuse Education, Second Edition.* Washington, D.C.: U.S. Government Printing Office, 1971.

Smoking and Health: Report of the Advisory Committee to the Surgeon General of the U. S. Public Health Service. Washington, D. C.: U. S. Government Printing Office, 1964.

Smoking and Health: A Report of the Royal College of Physicians. New York: Pitman Publishing, 1962.

U. S. Public Health Service, *The Health Consequences of Smoking.* Washington, D. C.: U. S. Government Printing Office, 1967.

Chapter 13   Alcohol Use and Abuse

"Alcohol and Health Notes," Rockville, Md.: Department of HEW, (ongoing series).

"Alcoholism—A Call for Early Detection, Aggressive Management," *Medical World News,* October 13, 1972.

"Alcoholism: Is It A Treatable Disease?" *Modern Medicine,* October 1, 1973.

"Alcoholism: New Victims, New Treatments," *Time,* April 22, 1974.

"Distinction Needed Between Alcoholism as Disease and 'Problem,'" *Family Practice News,* January 15, 1974.

Dunn, Robert B., and Allan G. Hedlberg. "Treating The Two Faces of Alcoholism," *Modern Medicine,* June 10, 1974.

"For The Alcoholic, Drinking Is More Than A Pleasant Interlude—It Is A Way of Life," *Physician's World,* August 1973.

"Good Food Won't Help Alcoholics," *Medical World News,* October 19, 1973.

Jones, Ben Morgan and Oscar A. Parsons. "Alcohol and Consciousness: Getting High, Coming Down," *Psychology Today,* January 1975.

"Sudden Death From an Older Drug," *Emergency Medicine,* December 1971.

Willner, William F. "Drinking in America—And How It Grew," *Medical Times,* August 1974.

Chapter 14   The Mood Modifiers

"Are We Winning the War Against Drug Addiction," (Special Drug Abuse Issue), *Medical Times,* September 1974.

Amiel, H. F. "Dream Drugs," *MD,* October 1973.

Gay, George et al. "The New Junkie," *Emergency Medicine,* February 1974.

Grinspoon, L., and P. Hedblom. "Amphetamine Abuse," *Drug Therapy,* January 1972.

"More on Marijuana," *American Family Physician,* October 1972.

Murphee, Henry B. "The Continuing Problem of Barbiturate Poisoning," *American Family Physician,* August 1973.

Nahas, Gabriel G. "Marijuana: Toxicity, Tolerance, and Therapeutic Efficacy," *Drug Therapy,* January 1974.

"Search and Destroy—The War on Drugs," *Time,* September 4, 1972.

"The Deadly Downer," *Time,* March 5, 1973.

"The Jigsaw Puzzle of Drugs," *Courier,* May 1973.

Chapter 15   The Communicable Diseases

Asper, Ronald, and Andrew Schwartz. "The Newer Penicillins," *American Family Physician,* January 1975.

Chang, Te-Wen. "Genital Herpes—Another VD on the Rise," *Medical Times,* January 1975.

"Countering the Complications of This Year's Flu," *Drug Therapy,* January 1975.

"First Human Ca Virus: Enter a New Candidate," *Medical World News,* January 13, 1975.

"Urinary Tract Infection," *Consultant,* January 1975.

Chapter 16   Chronic and Degenerative Diseases

"Controlling Type A Behavior," *Practical Psychology,* July-August, 1974.

"Coping With Cancer," *Medical Tribune,* April 10, 1974.

"Coping With Cardiovascular Disease," *Medical Tribune,* June 12, 1974.

"Hypertension: Conquering the Quiet Killer," *Time,* January 13, 1975.

Smith, A. et al. "The Staging of Hodgkin's Disease," *JAMA,* May 14, 1973.

"Stroke: It Has An 'Early' Warning System," *Marion Laboratories,* May 1973.

Wolfe, John N. "Xeroradiography of the Breast," *Geriatrics,* April 1974.

Chapter 17   Accidents

Nader, Ralph. *Unsafe at Any Speed.* New York: Pocket Books, 1966.

The Safe Driving Handbook. New York: Grosset & Dunlap, 1970.

Chaper 18   Population and Pollution

Air Pollution. New Haven, Conn.: Department of United Illuminating, n.d.

Dubos, René. "The Hidden Menace of Pollution," *Prism,* April 1974.

"Eco-Logic," Published under a Title I Grant, Higher Education Act of 1965, 1972.

"Help! Air Pollution . . . ," *Medical Tribune,* February 20, 1974.

Rall, David P. "Tracking Down the Chemical Culprits That Endanger Man," *Prism,* April 1974.

Train, Russell E. "Noise: The Government's View," *Medical Times,* March 1974.

Watson, John E. "Noise Pollution: Just How Bad Is It?" *Medical Times,* March 1974.

Watson, John E. "Noise Pollution: Just How Bad Is It?" *Medical Times,* March 1974.

"Why We're Disturbed About Noise," *Medical Times,* March 1974.

Chapter 19   Aging and Death

Allport, Gordon W. *Becoming.* New Haven, Conn.: Yale University Press, 1955.

Alvarez, A. *The Savage God.* New York: Bantam Books, 1971.

INDEX